GENERALIZED ANXIETY DISORDER

Generalized Anxiety Disorder

ADVANCES IN RESEARCH AND PRACTICE

Edited by
Richard G. Heimberg
Cynthia L. Turk
Douglas S. Mennin

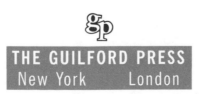

THE GUILFORD PRESS
New York   London

Last digit is print number: 9 8 7 6 5 4 3 2 1

Library of Congress Cataloging-in-Publication Data

Generalized anxiety disorder : advances in research and practice /
edited by Richard G. Heimberg, Cynthia L. Turk, Douglas S. Mennin.
   p. cm.
Includes bibliographical references and index.
 ISBN 1-57230-972-5
 1. Anxiety. I. Heimberg, Richard G. II. Turk, Cynthia L. III. Mennin,
Douglas S.
 RC531.G465 2004
 616.85′22—dc22

                                                               2003015738

About the Editors

Richard G. Heimberg, PhD, is Professor of Psychology, Director of Clinical Training, and Director of the Adult Anxiety Clinic at Temple University. He is well known for his efforts in developing and evaluating cognitive-behavioral treatments, especially for social anxiety. Dr. Heimberg has published more than 225 articles and chapters on anxiety disorders and related topics. He is coeditor or coauthor of several books, including *Social Phobia: Diagnosis, Assessment, and Treatment* (1995, Guilford Press) and *Cognitive-Behavioral Group Therapy for Social Phobia: Basic Mechanisms and Clinical Strategies* (2002, Guilford Press). Dr. Heimberg is past president of the Association for Advancement of Behavior Therapy. He was recently named one of the four most influential psychological researchers in anxiety in a survey of members of the Anxiety Disorders Association of America, and he serves on the Scientific Advisory Board of that association. Dr. Heimberg is a founding fellow of the Academy of Cognitive Therapy and was the inaugural recipient of the Academy's A. T. Beck Award for Significant and Enduring Contribution to Cognitive Therapy.

Cynthia L. Turk, PhD, joined the psychology faculty at La Salle University in 2002 and is currently the Director of the La Salle Anxiety Disorders Treatment and Research Program. She received her doctoral degree from Oklahoma State University in 1996. Prior to her current position, Dr. Turk was Associate Director of the Adult Anxiety Clinic at Temple University and Director of its Generalized Anxiety Program. Her main interests are in the assessment and treatment of anxiety disorders, particularly generalized anxiety disorder and social phobia.

Douglas S. Mennin, PhD, is currently Assistant Professor in the Department of Psychology at Yale University and Director of Yale Anxiety and Mood Services. He received his doctoral degree from Temple University in 2001, and with Drs. Heimberg and Turk, helped to establish the Generalized Anxiety Program at the Adult Anxiety Clinic at Temple University. Dr. Mennin's primary interests are generalized anxiety disorder, the role of difficulties in emotion regulation in generalized anxiety disorder and other mental disorders, and the integration of cognitive-behavioral and emotion-focused therapies.

Contributors

Anne Marie Albano, PhD, Child Study Center, New York University School of Medicine, New York, New York

Oscar M. Alcaine, MA, Department of Psychology, Pennsylvania State University, University Park, Pennsylvania

Patricia M. Averill, PhD, University of Texas–Houston Harris County Psychiatric Center, Houston, Texas

J. Gayle Beck, PhD, Department of Psychology, University at Buffalo, State University of New York, Buffalo, New York

Evelyn Behar, MS, Department of Psychology, Pennsylvania State University, University Park, Pennsylvania

Thomas D. Borkovec, PhD, Department of Psychology, Pennsylvania State University, University Park, Pennsylvania

Kristin Buhr, MA, Department of Psychology, Concordia University, Montreal, Quebec, Canada

Louis G. Castonguay, PhD, Department of Psychology, Pennsylvania State University, University Park, Pennsylvania

Katherine Crits-Christoph, PhD, Center for Psychotherapy Research, Department of Psychiatry, University of Pennsylvania, Philadelphia, Pennsylvania

Paul Crits-Christoph, PhD, Center for Psychotherapy Research, Department of Psychiatry, University of Pennsylvania, Philadelphia, Pennsylvania

Michel J. Dugas, PhD, Department of Psychology, Concordia University, Montreal, Quebec, Canada

Mary Beth Connolly Gibbons, PhD, Center for Psychotherapy Research, Department of Psychiatry, University of Pennsylvania, Philadelphia, Pennsylvania

Robert A. Gould, PhD, (deceased) Department of Psychiatry, Massachusetts General Hospital and Harvard Medical School, Boston, Massachusetts

Jack M. Gorman, MD, Department of Psychiatry, Mt. Sinai Medical School, New York, New York

Sabine Hack, MD, Child Study Center, New York University School of Medicine, New York, New York

Richard G. Heimberg, PhD, Adult Anxiety Clinic, Department of Psychology, Temple University, Philadelphia, Pennsylvania

Jennifer L. Hudson, PhD, Department of Psychology, Macquarie University, Sydney, Australia

Ronald C. Kessler, PhD, Department of Health Care Policy, Harvard Medical School, Boston, Massachusetts

Robert Ladouceur, PhD, Ecole de Psychologie, Université Laval, Ste-Foy, Quebec, Canada

Robert L. Leahy, PhD, American Institute for Cognitive Therapy, New York, New York

R. Bruce Lydiard, MD, Department of Neuropsychiatry and Behavioral Science, University of South Carolina School of Medicine, Columbia, South Carolina, and Southeast Health Consultants, Charleston, South Carolina

Colin MacLeod, PhD, Department of Psychology, University of Western Australia, Nedlands, Perth, Australia

Douglas S. Mennin, PhD, Department of Psychology, Yale University, New Haven, Connecticut

Jan Mohlman, PhD, Department of Psychology, Syracuse University, Syracuse, New York

Christine Molnar, PhD, Brain Stimulation Laboratory, Medical University of South Carolina, Charleston, South Carolina

Jeannine Monnier, PhD, Department of Psychiatry and Behavioral Sciences, Medical University of South Carolina, Charleston, South Carolina

Michelle G. Newman, PhD, Department of Psychology, Pennsylvania State University, University Park, Pennsylvania

Michael W. Otto, PhD, Department of Psychiatry, Massachusetts General Hospital and Harvard Medical School, Boston, Massachusetts

Ronald M. Rapee, PhD, Department of Psychology, Macquarie University, Sydney, Australia

Elizabeth Rutherford, PhD, Department of Psychology, University of Western Australia, Nedlands, Perth, Australia

Steven A. Safren, PhD, Department of Psychiatry, Massachusetts General Hospital and Harvard Medical School, Boston, Massachusetts

Smit S. Sinha, MD, Department of Psychiatry, Columbia University, New York, New York

Cynthia L. Turk, PhD, Department of Psychology, La Salle University, Philadelphia, Pennsylvania

Ellen E. Walters, MS, Department of Health Care Policy, Harvard Medical School, Boston, Maasachusetts

David O'Neill Washington, PhD, Department of Psychiatry, Massachusetts General Hospital and Harvard Medical School, Boston, Massachusetts

Adrian Wells, MSc, PhD, Department of Clinical Psychology, University of Manchester, Manchester, United Kingdom

Hans-Ulrich Wittchen, PhD, Institute of Clinical Psychology and Psychotherapy, Technical University of Dresden, Dresden, Germany, and Max Planck Institute of Psychiatry, Clinical Psychology and Epidemiology, Munich, Germany

Preface

One might say that we are living in an "age of anxiety" (Twenge, 2000, p. 1007). Given an unstable economy, war, terrorist threats, shooting sprees, and the renewed spread of deadly disease, it may seem that our sense of security has diminished. Indeed, it appears that anxiety may be a more prominent reaction in modern times: Anxiety levels have increased steadily in birth cohorts over the past 50 years (Twenge, 2000). With this rise in anxiety has come an increase in our understanding of its adaptive and maladaptive aspects. Most notably, the study of the pathological forms of anxiety—anxiety disorders—has increased tremendously over the past 20 years (Cox, Wessel, Norton, Swinson, & Direnfeld, 1995; Norton, Cox, Asmundson, & Maser, 1995).

Anxiety disorders have been shown to be associated with functional disability, poor quality of life, and increased health care costs, and are experienced in some form by over 20% of the population (Kessler et al., 1994). These findings suggest a significant public health care concern. In response to the clinical importance of anxiety, theories about pathological mechanisms have been generated and have demonstrated considerable empirical support (e.g., Barlow, 2002; Clark, 1986; Rapee & Heimberg, 1997). Novel treatments also have been developed that specifically address these difficulties and have been shown to be quite effective in treating anxiety disorders and ameliorating the suffering of those afflicted with them (Barlow, Gorman, Shear, & Woods, 2000).

One notable exception to this growth is the study and treatment of generalized anxiety disorder (GAD). Unlike panic disorder (e.g., McNally, 1994), social phobia (e.g., Heimberg & Becker, 2002; Heimberg, Liebowitz, Hope, & Schneier, 1995), or obsessive–compulsive disorder (Swinson, Antony, Rachman, & Richter, 1998), in which considerable advances are clearly evident, GAD remains an understudied (Dugas,

2000), misunderstood (Persons, Mennin, & Tucker, 2001), and treatment-resistant (Borkovec & Ruscio, 2001) disorder. Much of the confusion surrounding the disorder comes from its checkered past as a residual diagnosis in the third edition of the *Diagnostic and Statistical Manual of Mental Disorders* (DSM-III; American Psychiatric Association, 1980). This early form of the diagnosis resulted in poor reliability and led many to question its validity. In recent years, the reliability of GAD has improved considerably (Brown, DiNardo, Lehman, & Campbell, 2001; Starcevic & Bogojevic, 1999). With this improvement and better definition of the key features of GAD, research into its nature and treatment has begun to catch up to research on the other anxiety disorders. As will be demonstrated throughout this book, GAD is now recognized as a widely prevalent disorder associated with substantial functional impairment and reduced life satisfaction. Thus it is appropriate that the field has turned its attention to this important problem.

We are excited to have the opportunity to present this volume, one of the first of its kind to focus on GAD. We have brought together many of the world's leading authorities to address the phenomenology, etiology, pathological mechanisms, and treatment of GAD. These investigators and clinicians shed light on this important but neglected syndrome and help provide direction for future inquiry. In the book's chapters, the contributors present state-of-the-art reviews and analyses of almost every aspect of GAD. We believe that this work will prove useful to both novices and experts and to both researchers and clinicians interested in GAD.

The book is organized into four sections. In Part I ("Generalized Anxiety Disorder in the Clinic and in the Community"), the three of us examine the history of the diagnosis of GAD and its essential feature, excessive and uncontrollable worry. Kessler, Walters, and Wittchen provide an in-depth analysis of the epidemiology of the disorder. Hudson and Rapee examine the role of temperament and environment in the development of GAD.

In Part II ("Theoretical and Empirical Approaches"), five chapters examine diverse perspectives on the understanding of GAD. Borkovec, Alcaine, and Behar present the most comprehensive review to date on the role of worry in GAD. MacLeod and Rutherford provide a similarly detailed analysis of the information-processing problems that are evident in persons with GAD. Dugas, Buhr, and Ladouceur examine the role of intolerance of uncertainty in the etiology and maintenance of GAD, and Wells gives us a comprehensive account of his cognitive model of GAD. From a very different, and equally important, perspective, Sinha, Mohlman, and Gorman provide an up-to-the-minute examination of the rapidly developing study of the neurobiology of GAD.

Part III ("Assessment and Treatment") begins with a detailed presentation of the assessment of worry and GAD, again by the three of us.

Gould and colleagues present a meta-analytic review of various forms of cognitive-behavioral treatment (CBT) for GAD, and Leahy provides a valuable perspective on the application of one form of CBT to patients with GAD in clinical practice. Crits-Christoph and colleagues describe their supportive–expressive psychodynamic therapy for GAD and present some new data on its efficacy. Newman and colleagues provide a detailed description of their integrative approach to treatment of GAD. Lydiard and Monnier do the same for pharmacotherapy of GAD.

Part IV is devoted to "Special Populations." Albano and Hack give us a complete and thorough look at the assessment and treatment of GAD in children and adolescents. Beck and Averill do the same for GAD in older adults. These are areas that call for our greatest attention.

Generalized Anxiety Disorder: Advances in Research and Practice is a comprehensive guide to the understanding and treatment of GAD. However, there is still much to learn, so research continues. We hope that this volume will stimulate you to think about GAD in new ways, and lead to new and productive directions in treatment and research on this important disorder.

Many people have played an important part in the development of this book, and we can never adequately express our gratitude to all of them. Thanks to the chapter contributors. Thanks to Barbara Watkins of The Guilford Press, who helped us in many ways from the first thought to the final product. Thanks to David M. Fresco for his many contributions to our thinking about GAD. Thanks to Ismael Alvarez, administrative assistant to Richard G. Heimberg at the Adult Anxiety Clinic of Temple University, for his many contributions to this book. Most of all, thanks to the patients with GAD who have let us learn from them as we have attempted to help them.

RICHARD G. HEIMBERG
CYNTHIA L. TURK
DOUGLAS S. MENNIN

REFERENCES

American Psychiatric Association. (1980). *Diagnostic and statistical manual of mental disorders* (3rd ed.). Washington, DC: Author.

Barlow, D. H. (2002). *Anxiety and its disorders* (2nd ed.). New York: Guilford Press.

Barlow, D. H., Gorman, J. M., Shear, K. M., & Woods, S. W. (2000). Cognitive-behavioral therapy, imipramine, or their combination for panic disorder: A randomized controlled trial. *Journal of the American Medical Association, 283*, 2529–2536.

Borkovec, T. D., & Ruscio, A. M. (2001). Psychotherapy for generalized anxiety disorder. *Journal of Clinical Psychiatry, 62*, 37–42.

Brown, T. A., DiNardo, P. A., Lehman, C. L., & Campbell, L. A. (2001). Reliability of

DSM-IV anxiety and mood disorders: Implications for the classification of emotional disorders. *Journal of Abnormal Psychology, 110,* 49–58.

Clark, D. M. (1986). A cognitive approach to panic. *Behaviour Reserach and Therapy, 24,* 461–470.

Cox, B. J., Wessel, I., Norton, G. R., Swinson, R. P., & Direnfeld, D. M. (1995). Publication trends in anxiety disorders research: 1990–1992. *Journal of Anxiety Disorders, 9,* 531–538.

Dugas, M. J. (2000). Generalized anxiety disorder publications: So where do we stand? *Journal of Anxiety Disorders, 14,* 31–40.

Heimberg, R. G., & Becker, R. E. (2002). *Cognitive-behavioral group therapy for social phobia: Basic mechanisms and clinical strategies.* New York: Guilford Press.

Heimberg, R. G., Liebowitz, M. R., Hope, D. A., & Schneier, F. R. (Eds.). (1995). *Social phobia: Diagnosis, assessment, and treatment.* New York: Guilford Press.

Kessler, R. C., McGonagle, K. A., Zhao, S., Nelson, C. B., Hughes, M., Eshleman, S., Wittchen, H. U., & Kendler, K. S. (1994). Lifetime and 12-month prevalence of DSM-III-R psychiatric disorders in the United States: Results from the National Comorbidity Survey. *Archives of General Psychiatry, 51,* 8–19.

McNally, R. J. (1994). *Panic disorder: A critical analysis.* New York: Guilford Press.

Norton, G. R., Cox, B. J., Asmundson, G. J. G., & Maser, J. D. (1995). The growth of research on anxiety disorders in the 1980s. *Journal of Anxiety Disorders, 9,* 75–85.

Persons, J. B., Mennin, D. S., & Tucker, D. E. (2001). Common misconceptions about the nature and treatment of generalized anxiety disorder. *Psychiatric Annals, 31,* 501–508.

Rapee, R. M., & Heimberg, R. G. (1997). A cognitive-behavioural model of anxiety in social phobia. *Behaviour Research and Therapy, 35,* 741-756.

Starcevic, V., & Bogojevic, G. (1999). The concept of generalized anxiety disorder: Between the too narrow and too wide diagnostic criteria. *Psychopathology, 32,* 5–11.

Swinson, R. P., Antony, M. M., Rachman, S., & Richter, M. A. (Eds.). (1998). *Obsessive-compulsive disorder: Theory, research, and treatment.* New York: Guilford Press.

Twenge, J. M. (2000). The age of anxiety?: Birth cohort change in anxiety and neuroticism 1952–1993. *Journal of Personality and Social Psychology, 79,* 1007–1021.

Contents

PART III. Assessment and Treatment

PART IV. Special Populations

GENERALIZED ANXIETY DISORDER

PART I

Generalized Anxiety Disorder in the Clinic and in the Community

CHAPTER 1

Clinical Presentation and Diagnostic Features

DOUGLAS S. MENNIN
RICHARD G. HEIMBERG
CYNTHIA L. TURK

Anxiety disorders have received increasing attention in the clinical psychological and psychiatric literature (Cox, Wessel, Norton, Swinson, & Direnfeld, 1995; Norton, Cox, Asmundson, & Maser, 1995). However, as Dugas (2000) notes, relatively few of these investigations have focused on generalized anxiety disorder (GAD). One explanation for this paucity of research is that it has taken a great deal of time for the diagnosis of GAD to establish validity, given major shifts in how it has been defined. This has presented a challenge to our understanding and treatment of the condition. However, this situation is now changing in a positive direction.

This chapter reviews the development of GAD from a misunderstood and often maligned residual category to its current, more valid form, which has led to sizable advances in our understanding of its basic mechanisms. Specifically, this chapter covers (1) the history of GAD from Freud's early writings to the present diagnostic system; (2) the definition and distinctness of the construct of worry, especially as it relates to GAD; and (3) criticisms of the current diagnostic system, including suggestions for new directions.

THE NOSOLOGICAL HISTORY OF GAD

From Freud to DSM-II

Discussion of a generalized anxiety syndrome can be seen as early as Freud's writings on "anxiety neurosis" (e.g., Freud, 1920/1966). Freud distinguished between those who suffered from anxiety neurosis (which would include both GAD and panic disorder as currently defined) from those with "phobic neurosis" (which would include the current categories of agoraphobia, social phobia, and specific phobia). Rickels and Rynn (2001) note that Freud was the first to describe characteristics of worry, which he termed "anxious expectation." However, unlike the current conceptualization that emphasizes the cognitive load of worrying, Freud viewed the condition as typically presenting as diffuse and somatic, appearing as "free-floating anxiety" that often could not be readily identified by the patient. The first edition of the *Diagnostic and Statistical Manual of Mental Disorders* (DSM-I; American Psychiatric Association [APA], 1952) was heavily influenced by Freudian conceptualizations. Therefore, a patient with present-day GAD would probably have received a diagnosis of "anxiety reaction," and later, in DSM-II (APA, 1968), "anxiety neurosis" (Rickels & Rynn, 2001).

Neither early edition of the DSM separated generalized, chronic anxiety from more acute panic attacks. However, during the 1960s and 1970s, a number of events paved the way for the current form of diagnostic classification and, more specifically, for the appearance of GAD as a diagnostic category. First, Klein (1964) discovered that imipramine, a tricyclic antidepressant, was effective in treating acute panic but not more generalized anxiety—a discovery suggesting that these two types of anxiety may be distinct. Second, there was a growing movement away from theoretically based classification to more atheoretical, scientifically based diagnostic categories. Spitzer, Endicott, and Robins (1978) argued that much of the description provided in DSM-II was based on etiological conjecture rather than observable phenomena, and that without empirical validation of etiological factors, classification should be atheoretical and symptom-based (as in other areas of medicine). Spitzer and colleagues developed a classification system of mental disorders to be used in research with the aim of providing empirical support for these categories. This system, the Research Diagnostic Criteria (RDC), was the precursor to the diagnostic system in place today, which is largely symptom-based, atheoretical, and increasingly specific in its approach to classification.

DSM-III and DSM-III-R

DSM-III (APA, 1980) adopted the less theoretically biased and more empirical approach of the RDC, providing a specific descriptive nosology for the classification of anxiety disorders according to known or suspected differences in symptomatology, epidemiology, etiology, phenomenology, and treatment response. As a result, GAD and panic disorder/agoraphobia were separated. DSM-III also included phobic disorders, obsessive–compulsive disorder, and posttraumatic stress disorder. To meet criteria for a DSM-III diagnosis of GAD, one needed to qualify for symptoms in at least three of the following four categories: (1) symptoms reflecting tension, startle, and restlessness; (2) symptoms reflecting autonomic hyperactivity; (3) symptoms reflecting apprehensive expectation, including worry, fear, and rumination; and (4) symptoms reflecting hypervigilance. Furthermore, one needed to have met these criteria for at least 1 month, during which time no other disorder could be present.

Although this was the first instance in which GAD was considered a disorder in its own right, it would still be a long time until it would be accepted as an independent entity. DSM-III GAD was fraught with difficulty and was viewed with widespread skepticism in the psychiatric community. Early investigations into the reliability of GAD provided little support. In particular, interrater reliability was poor (kappa = .47; DiNardo, O'Brien, Barlow, & Waddell, 1983). This led some investigators to argue that GAD should not be considered a disorder in its own right (Breier, Charney, & Heninger, 1985).

Poor reliability of the diagnosis of GAD stemmed largely from the structure of the DSM-III. DSM-III provided a hierarchical system of diagnosis that minimized concurrent diagnoses. For example, anxiety disorders were not diagnosed in the presence of pathology presumed to be more pervasive, such as depressive disorders or schizophrenia. Furthermore, GAD was to be considered only when all other anxiety disorders had been ruled out (Spitzer & Williams, 1985). Thus GAD was a poorly defined residual category and tended to be assigned to those patients who experienced significant anxiety but did not evidence phobic avoidance or panic attacks. Given the nature of the DSM-III GAD criteria, it was unlikely to demonstrate specificity. As Barlow (1988, p. 567) noted, "the category of GAD in DSM-III produced so much confusion that few clinicians or investigators could agree on individuals who would meet this definition."

As a result of difficulties in differential diagnosis (including, but not limited to, GAD), the hierarchical rules for the assignment of concurrent diagnoses were modified in DSM-III-R (APA, 1987). Although a more pervasive disorder would take precedence if it shared symptoms with a less pervasive disorder, additional Axis I diagnoses could be assigned if the focus of the secondary concern was not related to the first disorder. One caveat was that the diagnosis of GAD could not be given if it occurred solely during the course of a mood disorder. Although this revision maintained the need for differential diagnosis, strict hierarchical rules had been lifted. The result was that GAD could be considered a disorder in its own right, even when other anxiety disorders were present.

In addition to the removal of hierarchical rules, the DSM-III-R diagnosis was more focused than its DSM-III predecessor. Whereas DSM-III largely retained Freud's notion of "free-floating anxiety," DSM-III-R made worry the central feature of GAD. In particular, to meet criteria for GAD, one had to demonstrate unrealistic and excessive worry or anxiety about two or more life circumstances (APA, 1987). In addition, anxiety and worry had to be present for at least 6 months (an increase from the less stringent criterion of 1 month in DSM-III). Data supported making worry the central feature of GAD. Sanderson and Barlow (1990) found that the presence of worry could be reliably diagnosed, with a kappa coefficient of .90. However, despite these changes, reliability for the DSM-III-R diagnosis of GAD remained moderate (kappa = .54; DiNardo, Moras, Barlow, Rapee, & Brown, 1993).

DSM-IV/DSM-IV-TR and ICD-10

One reason for the low reliability of DSM-III-R GAD may have been the fact that the associated symptom criteria remained diffuse. Although this list of symptoms was more detailed in DSM-III-R than in DSM-III (one needed to have 6 of 18 listed symptoms), the categories were still broad, including 4 symptoms of motor tension, 9 symptoms of autonomic hyperactivity, and 5 symptoms of vigilance and scanning. Most problematic was the inclusion of autonomic symptoms, which were found to be the least reliable aspect of the DSM-III-R diagnosis (Marten et al., 1993; Starcevic, Fallon, Uhlenhuth, & Pathak, 1994b). Marten and colleagues (1993) found that a reduced set of associated symptoms was more able to differentiate individuals with GAD from controls. As a result, DSM-IV adopted this reduced set of associated symptoms, which excluded autonomic symptoms but retained symptoms of tension and vigilance.

In addition, the worry criteria were modified to reflect a number of findings concerning components of the DSM-III-R diagnosis. First, investigations found that individuals with GAD were more likely than those without GAD to have difficulty controlling their worries (Craske, Rapee, Jackel, & Barlow, 1989), and difficulty controlling worry became one of the diagnostic criteria in DSM-IV. In contrast, content of worries appeared to have little ability to discriminate between individuals with GAD and controls (Abel & Borkovec, 1995). Specifically, whether worries were considered to be unrealistic or not had little discriminatory ability, and this was subsequently dropped from the criteria set. Furthermore, it was recognized that individuals with GAD could have pervasive worry regardless of how many different areas of their life were affected, and the requirement for two or more domains of worry was removed. Finally, overanxious disorder of childhood was subsumed under GAD (for a discussion of GAD in children, see Albano & Hack, Chapter 15, this volume).

These changes resulted in a diagnosis that has continued to gain in reliability with current assessments (see Turk, Heimberg, & Mennin,

Chapter 9, this volume, for a discussion of the reliability of DSM-IV diagnostic assessments). In sum, the essential feature of DSM-IV GAD is excessive worry occurring more days than not for at least 6 months. The worry may concern a number of different domains or activities (e.g., work, finances, family, and health) and must be difficult to control. In addition, the worry or anxiety must be associated with at least three (one for children) of the following six symptoms: (1) restlessness, (2) fatigue, (3) impaired concentration, (4) irritability, (5) muscle tension, and (6) sleep disturbance. As in all DSM-IV diagnoses, the worry must lead to significant distress or impairment and must not be due to another Axis I disorder, to a general medical condition, or to a substance use disorder (APA, 1994). Furthermore, DSM-IV maintained the requirement that GAD must not be present solely during the course of a mood disorder. The latest version of the DSM is a text revision of the DSM-IV (DSM-IV-TR; APA, 2000). DSM-IV-TR retained the DSM-IV diagnostic criteria set, but revised the text to reflect more recent investigations into the nature of GAD. In particular, prevalence rates and genetic studies reflecting the DSM-IV criteria were added.

DSM-IV diagnostic criteria were also modified to be more compatible with the 10th revision of the *International Classification of Diseases and Related Health Problems* (ICD-10; World Health Organization, 1992). One study reported a kappa of .86 for agreement between interviewers based on DSM-IV and ICD-10 (Starcevic & Bogojevic, 1999) criteria for comorbid GAD in a sample of patients with primary panic disorder and agoraphobia. However, substantial differences remain. ICD-10 does not require worry to be experienced as excessive or difficult to control. Furthermore, ICD-10 has retained the requirement of symptoms of autonomic hyperactivity and continues to disallow the diagnosis of GAD if major depression, a phobic disorder, panic disorder, or obsessive–compulsive disorder is present (similar to DSM-III). Finally, there is no requirement that the worry or anxiety be clinically impairing, as in DSM-IV. Indeed, Slade and Andrews (2001) found that approximately 50% of patients who met ICD-10 criteria for GAD did not also meet DSM-IV criteria, demonstrating that these two classification systems may detect different patients.

COMORBIDITY WITH OTHER DISORDERS

Although the DSM-IV/DSM-IV-TR diagnostic system allows more heterogeneous anxiety phenomenology within a diagnostic category, it also increases the likelihood that one will receive multiple diagnoses. "Comorbidity" refers to the occurrence of at least two different disorders in the same individual (Brown & Barlow, 1992). GAD has often been found to be comorbid, with approximately 60–90% of patients meeting criteria for another disorder (e.g., Brawman-Mintzer et al., 1993; Brown, Barlow, & Liebowitz, 1994; Sanderson & Barlow, 1990). In fact, "pure" presentations of GAD are rare, especially when diagnoses arc viewed longitudinally (e.g., Bruce, Machan, Dyck, & Keller, 2001).

Some have argued that, given the high rates of comorbidity in the anxiety disorders, these categories should not be viewed as distinct entities, but rather as different expressions of the same underlying diathesis (Andrews, 1996; Clark, Watson, & Mineka, 1994). Achenbach (1995) explains that other explanations for comorbidity are that the disorders reflect a higher-order taxon that includes both disorders; that the taxonomic borders between the disorders are not clearly specified; that the assessment materials do not clearly differentiate the disorders; or that a referral bias exists, in which cases with two disorders are more likely to be referred than individuals with only one disorder (commonly known as "Berkson's bias"). Kessler, Walters, and Wittchen (Chapter 2, this volume) argue that Berkson's bias may account for the high rates of comorbidity found in clinical samples. Nonetheless, it is clinically uncommon to see noncomorbid GAD; as such, the disorder often becomes difficult to detect when other disorders are present. In the remainder of this section, prevalence rates in clinical samples are reviewed (for rates in community samples, see Kessler et al., Chapter 2).

GAD appears to be the most common additional diagnosis among patients with social phobia (Barlow, Blanchard, Vermilyea, Vermilyea, & DiNardo, 1986; deRuiter, Rijken, Garssen, van Schaik, & Kraaimaat, 1989; Sanderson, DiNardo, Rapee, & Barlow, 1990; Turner, Beidel, Borden, Stanley, & Jacob, 1991), with rates as high as 33% (Turner et al., 1991) and as low as 17% (Moras, unpublished manuscript, cited in Brown & Barlow, 1992) reported in the literature. Social phobia is also diagnosed frequently in patients with GAD, with rates between 23% (Brawman-Mintzer et al., 1993) and 59% (Sanderson et al., 1990) reported. However, few studies have examined the characteristics of these disorders when they occur together. Mennin, Heimberg, and Jack (2000) examined GAD among patients with a principal diagnosis of social phobia. Patients with both social phobia and GAD demonstrated greater social anxiety and avoidance, general anxiety and negative mood, functional impairment, and overall psychopathology than patients with social phobia but without GAD.

Early studies of patients with GAD showed that these patients often experience panic attacks (Barlow, 1988). Rates of panic disorder have been found to range from 11% to 27% in patients with GAD (Brawman-Mintzer et al., 1993; Sanderson et al., 1990). Rates of GAD in patients with panic disorder have been found to range from 13% to 36% (Brown & Barlow, 1992; Sanderson et al., 1990). Obsessive–compulsive disorder can also occur in patients with GAD, although reported rates have been comparatively low (1–11%; Brawman-Mintzer et al., 1993; Brown, Moras, Zinbarg, & Barlow, 1993; Sanderson et al., 1990). Rates of GAD in obsessive–compulsive disorder are slightly higher, ranging between 6.5% (Brown et al., 1993) and 20% (Abramowitz & Foa, 1998). Nevertheless, there has been considerable controversy surrounding the conceptual separation of these disorders and their cognitive components—namely, worries and obsessions (see further discussion of this issue below).

GAD is often comorbid with mood disorders. Brawman-Mintzer and colleagues (1993) found that 42% of patients with GAD had a history of a past major depressive episode. GAD is also common in patients with major depressive disorder. Twenty percent of a sample of patients with major depressive disorder met criteria for GAD (Sanderson et al., 1990). DiNardo and Barlow (1990) reported unpublished findings showing a higher rate of GAD in major depression, with 45% meeting criteria. GAD has consistently been found to be the most common comorbid anxiety disorder among patients with dysthymic disorder. For example, Pini and colleagues (1997) found that 65% of patients with dysthymic disorder had GAD as a concurrent diagnosis, compared with 32% of patients with bipolar disorder and 37% of patients with major depressive disorder. Dysthymia is also a common secondary diagnosis in individuals with GAD, with rates as high as 50% reported (e.g., Garvey, Noyes, Anderson, & Cook, 1991).

Studies have recently begun to examine the occurrence of Axis II disorders in patients with anxiety disorders. GAD has been found to have a stronger relationship with personality disorders than panic disorder or agoraphobia, and this relationship is strengthened when major depression is also present (Reich et al., 1994). Sanderson, Wetzler, Beck, and Betz (1994) found that 49% of patients with GAD met criteria for at least one comorbid personality disorder. Sanderson and Wetzler (1991) found avoidant personality disorder and dependent personality disorder to be the most common Axis II diagnoses in 32 patients with GAD.

DIFFERENTIAL DIAGNOSIS

Do the high rates of comorbidity in clinical samples imply that GAD is not an entity in its own right? Should this disorder be subsumed under other diagnostic categories? Given the comorbidity rates presented above, one might expect GAD to have low levels of "specificity" (i.e., the extent to which its characteristics can be differentiated from those of other disorders). However, a number of studies have demonstrated the validity of the diagnosis by comparing symptom patterns with other diagnoses.

One examination found evidence for the specificity of GAD by demonstrating that the physical symptom criteria were endorsed at higher levels by these patients than by patients with other anxiety disorders (Ladouceur et al., 1999). Patients with GAD demonstrated higher levels of restlessness, insomnia, irritability, nausea, and headaches than patients with panic disorder (Nisita et al., 1990; Noyes et al., 1992). Conversely, patients with panic disorder had higher levels of trembling, rapid heartbeat, dizziness, faintness, dyspnea, chest pain, numbness, choking sensations, and derealization/depersonalization than patients with GAD (Nisita et al., 1990; Noyes et al., 1992). Noyes and colleagues (1992) concluded that GAD is characterized by central nervous system hyperarousal (e.g., muscle tension), whereas panic disorder is best characterized by autonomic arousal. (For a more detailed discussion of the distinctions between GAD and panic disorder, see Maser, 1998.)

A number of studies also suggest that social phobia and GAD can be reliably distinguished. For example, patients with social phobia reported higher levels of sweating, faintness, and palpitations than patients with GAD, and patients with GAD reported greater fear of dying and dizziness than those with social phobia (Reich, Noyes, & Yates, 1988). In addition, those with social phobia reported less frequent headaches and a higher frequency of dyspnea than patients with GAD (Reich et al., 1988). Insomnia has also been found to be more common in patients with GAD than in those with social phobia (Versiani, Mundim, Nardi, & Liebowitz, 1988). Gross, Oei, and Evans (1989) found that, similar to patients with panic disorder, patients with social phobia are more characterized by autonomic arousal than patients with GAD.

The research differentiating GAD from other anxiety disorders, such as panic disorder and social phobia, suggests that the removal of the autonomic hyperactivity symptom criteria in DSM-IV was warranted. A number of studies have found that, beyond worry, muscle tension and vigilance/scanning are the most commonly endorsed symptoms among patients with GAD (Abel & Borkovec, 1995; Brown, Marten, & Barlow, 1995; Marten et al., 1993; Starcevic, Fallon, Uhlenhuth, & Pathak, 1994a). In addition, these studies found that patients with GAD rarely endorsed autonomic symptoms. Laboratory studies using psychophysiological measurement have consistently found increases in electromyographic activity, suggesting elevated muscle tension (Hoehn-Saric, Hazlett, Pourmotabbed, & McLeod, 1997; Hoehn-Saric, McLeod, & Zimmerli, 1989). In particular, Hoehn-Saric and colleagues (1989) found that patients with GAD differed from controls on this measure of muscle tension, but not on physiological measures of autonomic activity. Finally, a number of studies have demonstrated that GAD could be distinguished from the other anxiety disorders based on presence of muscle tension (Brown, Antony, & Barlow, 1992; Joormann & Stöber, 1999). In fact, in a college sample, only muscle tension was uniquely associated with GAD (when the influence of depressive symptoms was controlled for; Joormann & Stöber, 1999). In contrast, the relationship between difficulty concentrating and GAD was reduced to a nonsignificant level when depressive symptoms were controlled for, suggesting that this symptom has comparably low levels of specificity in contributing to the detection of GAD versus major depression.

The results concerning muscle tension notwithstanding, the decision to make worry the central feature of GAD may be the strongest factor in the increase of reliability and validity of the DSM-IV diagnosis of GAD. In fact, Sanderson and Barlow (1990) found that excessive worry could be reliably diagnosed (kappa = .90). Although worry is common to all the anxiety disorders, it is present in greater amounts in GAD (Abel & Borkovec, 1995; Brown et al., 1993; Gross et al., 1989; Ladouceur et al., 1999). Borkovec (as reported in Brown et al., 1994) found that patients with GAD experienced a significantly greater degree of life interference due to their worry than patients with other anxiety disorders. Furthermore, there are substantial differences in the quality of this worry between patients with GAD and either patients with other disorders or non-disordered controls (Borkovec, Shadick, & Hopkins, 1991; Craske et al., 1989; Dugas et al., 1998; Starcevic, 1995).

Barlow and colleagues (1986) first suggested that the content of the cognitions in patients with GAD was different from the focused thoughts of physical or mental catastrophe found in patients with panic disorder. They found that persons who reported worry about multiple life circumstances were more often diagnosed as having GAD. Persons who had focused anxiety about having a panic attack were more often diagnosed as having panic disorder. A more recent study by Breitholtz, Johansson, and Öst (1999) found that patients with panic disorder had significantly more cognitions concerning physical danger, whereas patients with GAD were characterized by cognitions focusing on interpersonal conflicts and worry about significant others.

Sanderson and Barlow (1990) found that 91% of patients with GAD reported chronically worrying about minor events. This was significantly different from the 41% of patients with panic disorder who reported these same worries. This finding has been replicated in another study of GAD and panic disorder (Breitholtz et al., 1999), in a study comparing GAD and obsessive–compulsive disorder (Brown et al., 1993), and in a study comparing GAD and social phobia (Hoyer, Becker, & Roth, 2001). Dugas and colleagues (1998) found that patients with GAD worried more about the future than patients with other anxiety disorders. Ladouceur and colleagues (1999) found that patients with GAD scored higher than patients with other anxiety disorders on measures of problem-solving deficits and intolerance of uncertainty—two measures that have been shown to be related to worry. Also, Hoyer and colleagues (2001) found that higher frequency of worry, higher number of different worries, lower subjective controllability, and distress during worry differentiated patients with GAD from both controls and patients with social phobia. Furthermore, the number of excessive worries was found to differentiate GAD from anxiety disorder not otherwise specified (the actual residual category in DSM-IV) in a Hispanic sample (Street et al., 1997). In contrast, one study found that levels of worry could *not* be differentiated between patients with GAD and major depression (Starcevic, 1995). However, Diefenbach and colleagues (2001) found that patients with GAD did differ from patients with a mood disorder in the content of their reported worries. Whereas the patients with GAD were more likely to focus their worries on loss of control, the depressed patients' worry focused on an aimless future, lack of confidence, relationships, and financial concerns. This finding must be interpreted with caution, given that differences in worry content between disorders have often been found to be unreliable (see below; for a more in-depth discussion of the overlap of GAD and major depression, see Kessler et al., Chapter 2). Altogether, these findings demonstrate the importance of worry to GAD.

WORRY

Definition and History

Worry may characterize GAD, but how should worry be characterized? Worry is a universal experience, but a clear understanding of this phenomenon remains elusive. The word "worry" was first documented prior to the 12th century as a verb deriving from the Old English hunting term *wyrgan*, which meant "to kill by strangulation." *Wyrgan* is etymologically related to the Lithuanian word *vertzi*, which means "to constrict." These descriptions seem foreign to a modern understanding of the word "worry." However, the first definitions of the verb form of "worry," in the Merriam-Webster *WWWebster Dictionary*, are "to harass by tearing, biting, or snapping especially at the throat" and "to touch or disturb something repeatedly" (Merriam-Webster, 1999). Hallowell (1997) explains that just as a dog worries a bone by gnawing continually on it, people who worry chew and gnaw on a problem, devoting full attention to it.

Adam Phillips (1993) discusses these early definitions of worry in his book *On Kissing, Tickling, and Being Bored: Psychoanalytic Essays on the Unexamined Life*. He notes that, in addition to their obvious violent tone, these definitions illustrate that worry was something done unto another rather than unto oneself. The psychological sense of "worry" does not appear in the vernacular until the early 19th century when the noun form of the word arose. The *WWWebster Dictionary* defines the noun form of "worry" as "a mental distress or agitation resulting from concern usually for something impending or anticipated" (Merriam-Webster, 1999). Phillips points out that at a certain point in history, worrying became an act that people inflict on themselves rather than others. He explains, "What was once done by the mouths of the rapacious, the desirous, is now done, often with a relentless weariness, by the minds of the troubled" (p. 51).

Worry has only recently become a focus of psychological inquiry. In an attempt to define worry operationally, Challman (1974) echoed the focus on internal distress in the definitions given above when he described worry as "an unconsciously instigated mental activity that seeks to control fate through suffering" (p. 1141). As noted above, Sigmund Freud never wrote about worry per se, but he did write about the role of "anxious expectation" in the maintenance of anxiety. Davey and Tallis (1994) note that his account bears considerable resemblance to contemporary accounts of "anxious apprehension." Barlow (1988) notes that a cardinal feature of anxious apprehension is "intense worry" (p. 250).

Throughout the first half of the 20th century, few psychological investigators wrote about the nature of worry. Worry first received empirical attention in the test anxiety literature. Liebert and Morris (1967; Morris & Liebert, 1970) discovered that responses on a test anxiety questionnaire were composed of two distinct factors, which they labeled Worry and Emotionality. The Worry factor represented self-evaluative negative cognition about test performance. The Emotionality factor appeared to focus on awareness of feeling states and physiological activity. Worry has been found to have a stronger relationship than Emotionality to test performance (Deffenbacher & Deitz, 1978) and task-generated attentional interference (Deffenbacher, 1978).

Beginning in the early 1980s, research devoted to worry in its own right emerged. In examining the psychological aspects of insomnia, Borkovec (1979) noted that many individuals who had difficulty sleeping were engaged in excessive, negatively laden cognitive activity that could best be described as worrying. Since that time, Borkovec and colleagues (for a review, see Borkovec, Alcaine, & Behar, Chapter 4, this volume) have extensively examined the nature of the worry process. Borkovec, Robinson, Pruzinsky, and DePree (1983) developed a tentative definition of worry that closely resembles the current definition of the noun form of "worry" in the *WWWebster Dictionary*:

> Worry is a chain of thoughts and images, negatively affect-laden and relatively uncontrollable; it represents an attempt to engage in mental problem-solving on an issue whose outcome is uncertain but contains the possibility of one or more negative outcomes; consequently, worry relates closely to the fear process. (p. 10)

Borkovec (1994) has extended this definition by stating that worry involves predominantly thought activity rather than imagery. He notes, "Worry is a predominantly verbal–linguistic attempt to avoid future aversive events" (p. 7). Borkovec, Ray, and Stöber (1998) state that worry involves "talking to ourselves a lot about negative things, most often about negative events that we are afraid might happen in the future" (p. 562).

Differentiating Worry from Related Constructs

Similar to the suggestions of the early test anxiety literature, the definitions provided by Borkovec and colleagues describe worry as a cognitive phenomenon distinct from the physiological components of anxiety. However, they do not clarify how worry is to be differentiated from cognitive components of anxiety or from other conceptually similar cognitive processes, such as obsessions. As a result, a number of investigations have sought to explicate the distinctness of worry from these related constructs.

Worry and Anxiety

Prior to the study of worry in test anxiety, few investigators distinguished between the constructs of anxiety and worry (Breznitz, 1971). Clearly, a strong relationship between anxiety and worry exists. Had this not been the case, worry would not be considered central to the diagnosis of GAD. However, it remains unclear to what extent these constructs overlap, subsume each other, or are actually manifestations of the same underlying entity. Pruzinsky and Borkovec (1990) argue that distinguishing worry from anxiety is difficult because (1) worry may not in principle be distinguishable from anxiety except in artificial experimental situations; and (2) the elicitation of either cognitive or somatic components of an anxiety response in humans is likely to lead rather quickly to the other component.

O'Neill (1985) has criticized the independent use of the construct of worry. He argues, rather, that worry should be viewed solely as the cognitive component of anxiety. Using data from worry research, O'Neill builds a case that worry and anxiety share the same behavioral concomitants, and that changes in associated phenomena are reflected in similar changes in both worry and anxiety. Hence, in his view, the study of worry adds nothing substantial to the study of anxiety. Borkovec (1985) responds to this criticism by stating that, regardless of whether worry is or is not the cognitive component of anxiety, "we must next define the characteristics of that component and elucidate its functional relationships with other components and variables" (p. 481). Tallis, Eysenck, and Mathews (1991) argue that O'Neill presumes that the meaning of the term "anxiety" is widely agreed upon. In arguing to abandon the study of worry, O'Neill is suggesting that what is currently known about anxiety is satisfactory, is sufficient, and does not warrant further investigation into related cognitive elements. Tallis and colleagues assert that the investigation of cognitive processes such as worry furthers our understanding of anxiety.

Despite O'Neill's arguments, a number of examinations have demonstrated that worry and anxiety can be reliably differentiated. An early examination of worry and fear found that in response to a stressor, fear was a sufficient but not a necessary condition for worry (Levy & Guttman, 1976). In other words, worry can occur in the absence of fear. Correlations between worry and anxiety have been found to be somewhat high, with values approximating .70 (Davey, 1993; Davey, Hampton, Farrell, & Davidson, 1992; Russell & Davey, 1993). However, worry and anxiety demonstrated a significantly lower correlation in patients with GAD ($r = .18$; Meyer, Miller, Metzger, & Borkovec, 1990). Worry and trait anxiety accounted for unique variance in problem-solving skills and coping styles in a sample of college students (Davey et al., 1992). In addition, whereas worry was more associated with problem-focused coping styles, trait anxiety was often associated with an avoidant style of coping and lack of problem-solving confidence.

Induction of worry was found to produce a greater increase in negative cognitive intrusions than a neutral induction, whereas an anxiety induction did not (York, Borkovec, Vasey, & Stern, 1987). Stöber (1998) compared worried and anxious appraisals and found that, compared to worry, anxiety was more frequently focused on oneself than on others. Worry was more frequently associated with appraisals of others. Zebb and Beck (1998) found that worry was more highly associated with depression, confusion, lack of emotional control, and lack of control over problem solving than anxiety was. As described above, levels of worry cannot be differentiated between patients with GAD and patients with major depression (Starcevic, 1995). Furthermore, Andrews and Borkovec (1988) found that a worry induction produced both anxious and depressive affect. This effect was stronger than the effect of an anxiety induction on depressive affect or the effect of a depressive mood induction on anxious affect. These results suggest that worry may have a unique relationship to depressive affect beyond its common bond with anxiety.

Worry and Obsessions

The delineation of worry as a cognitive process increases its distinction from anxiety, but blurs its distinction from other cognitive processes. Colloquially, "worrying" and "obsessing" are often considered synonymous. In fact, many clients seen in clinical practice describe their worrying as obsessing. However, obsessions are operationally defined quite differently in clinical psychology and psychiatry than in common usage. DSM-IV (APA, 1994) provides a detailed definition of obsessions as "recurrent and persistent thoughts, impulses, or images that are experienced, at some time during the disturbance, as intrusive and inappropriate and that cause marked anxiety or distress" (p. 422).

Investigations have shown that obsessions differ from worry in their antecedents (Craske et al., 1989), content (Borkovec et al., 1991), form (Borkovec & Inz, 1990), and acceptability (Roemer & Borkovec, 1993). Brown and colleagues (1993) found that patients with obsessive–compulsive disorder and patients with GAD were distinguishable on the basis of their self-reported obsessions and worries, respectively. Also, Abramowitz and Foa (1998) found that indecisiveness, pathological responsibility, and worry about everyday topics distinguished patients with obsessive–compulsive disorder who had comorbid GAD from those who did not.

Examinations of worry and obsessions in nonclinical samples also lend support to their distinction. In a study by Coles, Mennin, and Heimberg (2001), items from measures of worry and obsession loaded on separate factors in an exploratory factor analysis. Wells and Morrison (1994), utilizing a diary methodology over a 2-week period, found worry to be reported as having more verbal content than obsessions, and obsessions to be more imagery-based. Worry was also rated as more realistic, more voluntary, harder to dismiss, more distracting, and of longer duration than obsessions. A recent set of studies (Langlois, Freeston, & Ladouceur, 2000a, 2000b) provided further evidence for the distinction between worries and obsessions. Results from these studies demonstrated that individuals differentiated these constructs on multiple dimensions, and that categorization errors (i.e., worry vs. obsession) were rare.

A number of associated cognitive process variables have also been shown to have stronger relationships with either obsessions or worry. Dugas, Gosselin, and Ladouceur (2001) found that intolerance of uncertainty (see Dugas, Buhr, & Ladouceur, Chapter 6, this volume, for a discussion of this construct) was more associated with worry than with obsessions or compulsions. Furthermore, Coles and colleagues (2001) found that "thought–action fusion" (Rassin, Merckelbach, Muris, & Spaan, 1999), a cognitive process in which thought and deed are confused, could differentiate obsessions and worries. Specifically, thought–action fusion was strongly related to obsessions after controlling for the effect of worry. Hazlett-Stevens, Zucker, and Craske (2002) found that thought–action fusion was weakly correlated with worry but unrelated to a diagnosis of GAD. Overall, these findings demonstrate that worry and obsessions, although related processes, are conceptually distinct.

Worry and Rumination

As described above, worry has been found to have a relationship to depression as well as to GAD (Diefenbach et al., 2001; Starcevic, 1995). Nolen-Hoeksema (1991) has found that rumination is related to the onset, maintenance, and severity of depression. Nolen-Hoeksema (1998, p. 216) defines "depressive rumination," a particular variety of rumination associated with depressed mood, as "focusing passively and repetitively on one's symptoms of distress and the meaning of those symptoms without taking action to correct the problems one identifies." The *WWWebster Dictionary* describes the etymology of "rumination" as deriving from the Latin *ruminatus,* which means "to chew repeatedly for an extended period of time" (Merriam-Webster, 1999). Similar to the derivation of worry, rumination refers to repetitive animal activity. In this case, cows are considered to ruminate food regurgitated from their multiple stomachs by chewing repeatedly. Research has linked depressive rumination to the onset of depression in nondepressed individuals (Just & Alloy, 1997), the exacerbation of depressed symptoms (Kuehner & Weber, 1999), and the increased chronicity of depressed symptoms (Nolen-Hoeksema, 2000).

Stöber (2000) has argued that worry and rumination represent different aspects of the same underlying process. However, despite descriptive overlap between these constructs, few studies have directly compared them. A recent study (Fresco, Frankel, Mennin, Turk, & Heimberg, 2002) found that worry and rumination were correlated ($r = .40$) with each other, but were demonstrated to be distinctive via factor-analytic methods. However, these processes were not at all distinctive in their relationships to anxiety and depression. Segerstrom, Tsao, Alden, and Craske (2000) found that worry and rumination loaded together on a higher-order factor, which they characterized as a maladaptive response set. However, a recent intriguing investigation into numerous forms of repetitive thought replicated the aggregation of worry and rumination (in a multidimensional scaling procedure) in a "negative valence repetitive thought" dimension, but also found that they did not aggregate on a dimension of "purpose of repetitive thought" (Segerstrom, Stanton, Alden, & Shortridge, in press). A general characterization of these constructs may be too broad in scope, and thus may obscure important differences between worry and rumination. Further examination into the relationship between these processes is necessary before any definitive conclusions can be reached.

Characteristics of Pathological Worry

When do worries become dysfunctional? Is worry always pathological? Bruhn (1990) offers that it is pathological

> when worry results in prolonged periods of introspection and social withdrawal; when the process of worry does not stimulate learning and extrapolation to other life situations; and when worry becomes so self-satisfying that it promotes a pattern of helplessness. (p. 561)

Anxiety is often considered to be an evolutionarily adaptive phenomenon. The Yerkes–Dodson law illustrates that at moderate levels, anxiety can improve performance. Indeed, it is difficult to imagine life without anxiety. Can the same be said of worry? Is it normal to worry? Worry may exist in nonpathological forms. Davey (1994) has criticized the definitions of worry reviewed above, stating that they focus on pathological forms of worry without addressing worry as a normal process. Hallowell (1997) suggests that worry can be helpful in motivating one to seek important goals. This view is reflected in an early account of worry by Janis (1958), who argued that when a situation contains a realistic difficulty, worry may help one cope in the long term. But worry is not always a response to realistic threat. In addition, worry can often become aversive and uncontrollable in itself. How should this pathological type of worry be differentiated from a normal adaptive response?

Some investigators have sought to differentiate the content of pathological worry from that of worry in nondisordered populations. Borkovec and colleagues (1983) examined domains of worry among college students. Whereas academic and interpersonal worries were rated as most frequent, concerns about physical harm were rated as least frequent. Wisocki (1988) found that among elderly individuals, health concerns were rated most highly, followed by interpersonal relations and finances. Craske and colleagues (1989) compared the content of worries in patients with GAD and nondisordered controls. They found that illness/health (31%) and family-related (28%) worries were most frequent, and worries about finances (3%) least frequent, in the group with GAD. The control participants in this study also reported worries about family-related issues (26%) as important, but rated work/school domains (30%) most frequently the objects of worry. For this group, illness/health worries (2%) were infrequent. Sanderson and Barlow (1990) also found that family-related concerns (79%) were frequent in patients with GAD. However, whereas Craske and colleagues found financial worries to be relatively infrequent in patients with GAD, Sanderson and Barlow (1990) found financial worries to be quite common (50%).

Borkovec and colleagues (1991) have also reported family and interpersonal concerns (31%) to be frequent in patients with GAD. However, control participants also had high levels of family and interpersonal worries (44%) and had higher levels of illness/health worries (25%) than the group with GAD (3%). Finally, Roemer, Molina, and Borkovec (1997) found that patients with GAD could only be differentiated from control participants by the presence of worry over minor matters. The results from these studies suggest that examinations of the content of worries provide little discrimination between individuals with pathological and nonpathological worries. In fact, domains of worry were found to be inconsistent within groups with GAD across studies.

Patients with GAD and individuals with nonpathological worries do not seem to differ in the content of their worries. However, these groups may differ in the severity and pervasiveness of their worries. In fact,

Mennin, Fresco, and Heimberg (1999) found that a dimensional measure of pathological worry had better sensitivity and specificity in identifying GAD than a measure of content domains of worry. This suggests that pathological worry may be a dimensionally more severe form of nonpathological worry. Indeed, one investigation utilizing taxometric analysis found that pathological worry and "normal" worry were actually dimensionally related rather than categorically distinct (Ruscio, Borkovec, & Ruscio, 2001). Furthermore, Craske and colleagues (1989) found that patients with GAD spent more time during the day worrying than did control participants. In addition, these patients were significantly less likely than control participants to recognize the precipitant of the worry and were significantly more likely to rate their worries as uncontrollable than control participants. Taken together, the research on worry demonstrates a specific relationship between pervasive levels of worry and GAD, and thus provides further validation of the current diagnostic classification.

CONCLUSIONS: LOOKING AHEAD TO DSM-V

A number of investigators continue to examine the viability of the DSM-IV-TR diagnosis and to determine what changes (if any) are necessary for the next edition of the diagnostic nomenclature, DSM-V. Some investigators have questioned the central focus on worry in the diagnosis of GAD (e.g., Rickels & Rynn, 2001). Bienvenu, Nestadt, and Eaton (1998) found that the associated six-symptom criteria set provided a better differentiation between individuals with and without GAD than the worry criteria did. However, it is important to note that this study utilized DSM-III-R criteria rather than the more refined DSM-IV criteria. Nonetheless, Rickels and Rynn (2001) argue that there is too great a focus on the worry component of GAD. They argue that chronic worrying does not always lead to a severe anxiety syndrome, given that many individuals with chronic worries do not meet criteria for GAD (Ruscio, 2002).

Other possible variables that have demonstrated a role in GAD beyond worry are beginning to receive attention. Intolerance of uncertainty has been shown to be a cognitive construct that is independent from worry and has discriminated GAD from other anxiety disorders (see Dugas et al., Chapter 6, for a discussion of this construct and related findings). Furthermore, Wells and Carter (2001) found that metacognitive beliefs about the detrimental nature of worry (i.e., worry about worrying) distinguished patients with GAD from those with other anxiety disorders when worry itself was controlled for. Finally, recent evidence suggests that emotion regulation deficits predict a diagnosis of GAD beyond the effects of worry, anxiety, and associated depression (Mennin, Heimberg, Turk, & Fresco, 2003). In particular, persons with GAD may experience emotions with greater intensity than persons with social phobia do (Turk, Heimberg, Luterek, Mennin, & Fresco, in press). Similarly, Roemer, Salters, Raffa, and Orsillo (in press) found unique associations between emotional avoidance and the severity of GAD when worry was controlled for.

Another criticism of the DSM-IV/DSM-IV-TR diagnosis of GAD is its placement on Axis I. A number of investigators have suggested that GAD may be better conceptualized as a personality or temperament disorder, given its chronicity, pervasiveness, and resistance to treatment (Akiskal, 1998; Rickels & Rynn, 2001; Sanderson & Wetzler, 1991). Another challenge to the current diagnostic criteria is reflected in studies finding that a 6-month duration requirement may be overly restrictive and miss significant cases of GAD (Maier et al., 2000; see Kessler et al., Chapter 2, this volume).

A recent paper also calls into question the mood disorder exclusionary criterion (in which one may not diagnose GAD if it fully overlaps with a mood disorder). Zimmerman and Chelminski (2003) compared patients with major depressive disorder and nonoverlapping GAD; patients with major depressive disorder and fully overlapping GAD (these patients would normally not receive a diagnosis of GAD, given the overlap); and patients without GAD or major depressive disorder. Both groups of depressed patients were found to have higher levels of suicidal ideation, social impairment, anxiety disorder comorbidity, eating disorders, somatoform disorders, and pathological worry, as well as a greater likelihood of a first-degree relative afflicted with GAD, than control patients. However, supporting the removal of this exclusionary criterion, the groups with GAD (i.e., overlapping vs. nonoverlapping) did not differ from each other.

Finally, Barlow and Wincze (1998) have suggested that the somatic symptom criteria set may require modification. Citing Brown and colleagues (1995), who found that many patients without GAD endorsed three of the six associated symptoms, they suggest raising the required number of symptoms to four. A number of other associated somatic symptoms, which are typically found in patients with GAD in clinical settings, may also be found to have a more specific relationship to GAD (e.g., tension headaches).

In summary, GAD has undergone major changes since its inception as a diagnosis over 20 years ago. Initially a "wastebasket" category that most mental health professionals viewed with a jaundiced eye, GAD is now widely considered a valid diagnostic category with significant associated disability. The reliability of the GAD diagnosis has improved substantially over this time, but continues to need improvement. More specific delineation of the central features of the disorder and proposed criteria are necessary as we begin to conceptualize changes for DSM-V. Consensus among researchers in operational definitions of each GAD criterion would further increases in reliability (given GAD's often variable and confusing diagnostic history). Nonetheless, in spite of high comorbidity rates, GAD can be reliably distinguished from other anxiety disorders. In particular, muscle tension and pervasive, excessive, and uncontrollable worry appear to be the most specific features of the condition. Finally, the study of worry has advanced our understanding of GAD. However, there are exciting new possible directions to expand our understanding of GAD, which may take us beyond the current focus on worry into the role of such factors as emotion dysregulation and interpersonal dysfunction. New investigations into these unexplored areas may help improve our understanding and treatment of GAD, thus providing further validation for this misunderstood diagnosis.

REFERENCES

Abel, J. L., & Borkovec, T. D. (1995). Generalizability of DSM-III-R generalized anxiety disorders to proposed DSM-IV criteria and cross-validation of proposed changes. *Journal of Anxiety Disorders, 9,* 303–315.

Abramowitz, J. S., & Foa, E. B. (1998). Worries and obsessions in individuals with obsessive–compulsive disorder with and without comorbid generalized anxiety disorder. *Behaviour Research and Therapy, 36,* 695–700.

Achenbach, T. (1995). Diagnosis, assessment, and comorbidity in psychosocial treatment research. *Journal of Abnormal Child Psychology, 23,* 45–65.

Akiskal, H. S. (1998). Toward a definition of generalized anxiety disorder as an anxious temperament type. *Acta Psychiatrica Scandinavica, 393*(Suppl.), 66–73.

American Psychiatric Association (APA). (1952). *Diagnostic and statistical manual of mental disorders.* Washington, DC: Author.

American Psychiatric Association (APA). (1968). *Diagnostic and statistical manual of mental disorders* (2nd ed.). Washington, DC: Author.

American Psychiatric Association (APA). (1980). *Diagnostic and statistical manual of mental disorders* (3rd ed.). Washington, DC: Author.

American Psychiatric Association (APA). (1987). *Diagnostic and statistical manual of mental disorders* (3rd ed., rev.). Washington, DC: Author.

American Psychiatric Association (APA). (1994). *Diagnostic and statistical manual of mental disorders* (4th ed.). Washington, DC: Author.

American Psychiatric Association (APA). (2000). *Diagnostic and statistical manual of mental disorders* (4th ed., text rev.). Washington, DC: Author.

Andrews, G. (1996). Comorbidity in neurotic disorders: The similarities are more important than the differences. In R. M. Rapee (Ed.), *Current controversies in the anxiety disorders* (pp. 3–20). New York: Guilford Press.

Andrews, V. H., & Borkovec, T. D. (1988). The differential effects of inductions of worry, somatic anxiety, and depression on emotional experience. *Journal of Behavior Therapy and Experimental Psychiatry, 19,* 21–26.

Barlow, D. H. (1988). *Anxiety and its disorders.* New York: Guilford Press.

Barlow, D. H., Blanchard, E. B., Vermilyea, J. A., Vermilyea, B. B., & DiNardo, P. A. (1986). Generalized anxiety and generalized anxiety disorder: Description and reconceptualization. *American Journal of Psychiatry, 143,* 40–44.

Barlow, D. H., & Wincze, J. (1998). DSM-IV and beyond: What is generalized anxiety disorder? *Acta Psychiatrica Scandinavica, 393*(Suppl.), 23–29.

Bienvenu, O. J., Nestadt, G., & Eaton, W. W. (1998). Characterizing generalized anxiety: Temporal and symptomatic thresholds. *Journal of Nervous and Mental Disease, 186,* 51–56.

Borkovec, T. D. (1979). Pseudo(experiential)-insomnia and idiopathic(objective) insomnia: Theoretical and therapeutic issues. *Advances in Behaviour Research and Therapy, 2,* 27–55.

Borkovec, T. D. (1985). Worry: A potentially valuable concept. *Behaviour Research and Therapy, 23,* 481–482.

Borkovec, T. D. (1994). The nature, functions, and origins of worry. In G. C. L. Davey & F. Tallis (Eds.), *Worrying: Perspectives on theory, assessment, and treatment* (pp. 5–33). Chichester, UK: Wiley.

Borkovec, T. D., & Inz, J. (1990). The nature of worry in generalized anxiety disorder: A predominance of thought activity. *Behaviour Research and Therapy, 28,* 153–158.

Borkovec, T. D., Ray, W. J., & Stöber, J. (1998). Worry: A cognitive phenomenon intimately linked to affective, physiological, and interpersonal behavioral processes. *Cognitive Therapy and Research, 22,* 561–576.

Borkovec, T. D., Robinson, E., Pruzinsky, T., & DePree, J. A. (1983). Preliminary exploration of worry: Some characteristics and processes. *Behaviour Research and Therapy, 21,* 9–16.

Borkovec, T. D., Shadick, R. N., & Hopkins, M. (1991). The nature of normal and pathological worry. In R. M. Rapee & D. H. Barlow (Eds.), *Chronic anxiety: Generalized anxiety disorder and mixed anxiety–depression* (pp. 29–51). New York: Guilford Press.

Brawman-Mintzer, O., Lydiard, R. B., Emmanuel, N., Payeur, R., Johnson, M., Roberts, J., Jarrell, M. P., & Ballenger, J. C. (1993). Psychiatric comorbidity in patients with generalized anxiety disorder. *American Journal of Psychiatry, 150,* 1216–1218.

Breier, A., Charney, D. S., & Heninger, G. R. (1985). The diagnostic validity of anxiety disorders and their relationship to depressive illness. *American Journal of Psychiatry, 142,* 787–797.

Breitholtz, E., Johansson, B., & Öst, L. G. (1999). Cognitions in generalized anxiety disorder and panic disorder patients: A prospective approach. *Behaviour Research and Therapy, 37,* 533–544.

Breznitz, S. (1971). A study of worrying. *British Journal of Social and Clinical Psychology, 10,* 271–279.

Brown, T. A., Antony, M. M., & Barlow, D. H. (1992). Psychometric properties of the Penn State Worry Questionnaire in a clinical anxiety disorders sample. *Behaviour Research and Therapy, 30,* 33–37.

Brown, T. A., & Barlow, D. H. (1992). Comorbidity among anxiety disorders: Implications for treatment and DSM-IV. *Journal of Consulting and Clinical Psychology, 60,* 835–844.

Brown, T. A., Barlow, D. H., & Liebowitz, M. R. (1994). The empirical basis of generalized anxiety disorder. *American Journal of Psychiatry, 151,* 1272–1280.

Brown, T. A., Marten, P. A., & Barlow, D. H. (1995). Discriminant validity of the symptoms constituting the DSM-III-R and DSM-IV associated symptom criterion of generalized anxiety disorder. *Journal of Anxiety Disorders, 9,* 317–328.

Brown, T. A., Moras, K., Zinbarg, R. E., & Barlow, D. H. (1993). Diagnostic and symptom distinguishability of generalized anxiety disorder and obsessive–compulsive disorder. *Behavior Therapy, 24,* 227–240.

Bruce, S. E., Machan, J. T., Dyck, I., & Keller, M. B. (2001). Infrequency of "pure" GAD: Impact of psychiatric comorbidity on clinical course. *Depression and Anxiety, 14,* 219–225.

Bruhn, J. G. (1990). The two sides of worry. *Southern Medical Journal, 83,* 557–562.

Challman, A. (1974). The empirical nature of worry. *American Journal of Psychiatry, 131,* 1140–1141.

Clark, L. A., Watson, D., & Mineka, S. (1994). Temperament, personality, and the mood and anxiety disorders. *Journal of Abnormal Psychology, 103,* 103–116.

Coles, M., Mennin, D. S., & Heimberg, R. G. (2001). Differentiating obsessions and worries: The role of thought–action fusion. *Behaviour Research and Therapy, 39,* 947–959.

Cox, B. J., Wessel, I., Norton, G. R., Swinson, R. P., & Direnfeld, D. M. (1995). Publication trends in anxiety disorders research: 1990–1992. *Journal of Anxiety Disorders, 9,* 531–538.

Craske, M. G., Rapee, R. M., Jackel, L., & Barlow, D. H. (1989). Qualitative dimensions of worry in DSM-III-R generalized anxiety disorder subjects and nonanxious controls. *Behaviour Research and Therapy, 27,* 397–402.

Davey, G. C. L. (1993). A comparison of three worry questionnaires. *Behaviour Research and Therapy, 31,* 51–56.

Davey, G. C. L. (1994). Pathological worrying as exacerbated problem-solving. In G. C. L. Davey & F. Tallis (Eds.), *Worrying: Perspectives on theory, assessment, and treatment* (pp. 35–59). Chichester, UK: Wiley.

Davey, G. C. L., Hampton, J., Farrell, J., & Davidson, S. (1992). Some characteristics of worrying: Evidence for worrying and anxiety as separate constructs. *Personality and Individual Differences, 13,* 133–147.

Davey, G. C. L., & Tallis, F. (Eds.). (1994). *Worrying: Perspectives on theory, assessment, and treatment.* Chichester, UK: Wiley.

Deffenbacher, J. L. (1978). Worry, emotionality, and task-generated interference in test anxiety: An empirical test of attentional theory. *Journal of Educational Psychology, 70,* 248–254.

Deffenbacher, J. L., & Deitz, S. R. (1978). Effects of test anxiety on performance, worry, and emotionality in naturally occurring exams. *Psychology in the Schools, 15,* 446–450.

deRuiter, C., Rijken, H., Garssen, B., van Schaik, A., & Kraaimaat, F. (1989). Comorbidity among the anxiety disorders. *Journal of Anxiety Disorders, 3,* 57–68.

Diefenbach, G. J., McCarthy-Larzelere, M. E., Williamson, D. A., Mathews, A., Manguno-Mire, G. M., & Bentz, B. G. (2001). Anxiety, depression, and the content of worries. *Depression and Anxiety, 14,* 247–250.

DiNardo, P. A., & Barlow, D. H. (1990). Syndrome and symptom comorbidity in the anxiety disorders. In J. D. Maser & C. R. Cloninger (Eds.), *Comorbidity in anxiety and mood disorders* (pp. 205–230). Washington, DC: American Psychiatric Press.

DiNardo, P. A., Moras, K., Barlow, D. H., Rapee, R. M., & Brown, T. A. (1993). Reliability of DSM-III-R anxiety disorder categories: Using the Anxiety Disorders Interview Schedule—Revised (ADIS-R). *Archives of General Psychiatry, 50,* 251–256.

DiNardo, P. A., O'Brien, G. T., Barlow, D. H., & Waddell, M. T. (1983). Reliability of DSM-III anxiety disorder categories using a new structured interview. *Archives of General Psychiatry, 40,* 1070–1074.

Dugas, M. J. (2000). Generalized anxiety disorder publications: So where do we stand? *Journal of Anxiety Disorders, 14,* 31–40.

Dugas, M. J., Freeston, M. H., Ladouceur, R., Rheaume, J., Provencher, M., & Boisvert,

J.-M. (1998). Worry themes in primary GAD, secondary GAD, and other anxiety disorders. *Journal of Anxiety Disorders, 12,* 253–261.

Dugas, M. J., Gosselin, P., & Ladouceur, R. (2001). Intolerance of uncertainty and worry: Investigating specificity in a nonclinical sample. *Cognitive Therapy and Research, 25,* 551–558.

Fresco, D. M., Frankel, A. N., Mennin, D. S., Turk, C. L., & Heimberg, R. G. (2002). Distinct and overlapping features of rumination and worry: The relationship of cognitive production to negative affective states. *Cognitive Therapy and Research, 26,* 179–188.

Freud, S. (1966). Anxiety. In J. Strachey (Ed. & Trans.), *Introductory lectures on psychoanalysis* (pp. 487–511). New York: Norton. (Original work published 1920)

Garvey, M. J., Noyes, R., Anderson, D., & Cook, B. (1991). Examination of comorbid anxiety in psychiatric inpatients. *Comprehensive Psychiatry, 32,* 277–282.

Gross, P. R., Oei, T. P., & Evans, L. (1989). Generalized anxiety symptoms in phobic disorders and anxiety states: A test of the worry hypothesis. *Journal of Anxiety Disorders, 3,* 159–169.

Hallowell, E. M. (1997). *Worry: Hope and help for a common condition.* New York: Ballantine Books.

Hazlett-Stevens, H., Zucker, B. G., & Craske, M. G. (2002). The relationship of thought-action fusion to pathological worry and generalized anxiety disorder. *Behaviour Research and Therapy, 40,* 1199–1204.

Hoehn-Saric, R., Hazlett, R. L., Pourmotabbed, T., & McLeod, D. R. (1997). Does muscle tension reflect arousal?: Relationship between electromyographic and electroencephalographic recordings. *Psychiatry Research, 71,* 49–55.

Hoehn-Saric, R., McLeod, D. R., & Zimmerli, W. D. (1989). Somatic manifestations in women with generalized anxiety disorder: Psychophysiological responses to psychological stress. *Archives of General Psychiatry, 46,* 1113–1119.

Hoyer, J., Becker, E. S., & Roth, W. T. (2001). Characteristics of worry in GAD patients, social phobics, and controls. *Depression and Anxiety, 13,* 89–96.

Janis, I. (1958). *Psychological stress.* New York: Wiley.

Joormann, J., & Stöber, J. (1999). Somatic symptoms of generalized anxiety disorder for the DSM-IV: Associations with pathological worry and depression symptoms in a nonclinical sample. *Journal of Anxiety Disorders, 13,* 491–503.

Just, N., & Alloy, L. B. (1997). The response styles theory of depression: Tests and an extension of the theory. *Journal of Abnormal Psychology, 106,* 221–229.

Klein, D. (1964). Delineation of two drug-responsive anxiety syndromes. *Psychopharmacologica, 5,* 397–408.

Kuehner, C., & Weber, I. (1999). Responses to depression in unipolar depressed patients: An investigation of Nolen-Hoeksema's response styles theory. *Psychological Medicine, 29,* 1323–1333.

Ladouceur, R., Dugas, M. J., Freeston, M. H., Rhéaume, J., Blais, F., Boisvert, J. M., & Thibodeau, N. (1999). Specificity of generalized anxiety disorder symptoms and processes. *Behavior Therapy, 30,* 191–208.

Langlois, F., Freeston, M. H., & Ladouceur, R. (2000a). Differences and similarities between obsessive intrusive thoughts and worry in a non-clinical population: Study 1. *Behaviour Research and Therapy, 38,* 157–173.

Langlois, F., Freeston, M. H., & Ladouceur, R. (2000b). Differences and similarities between obsessive intrusive thoughts and worry in a non-clinical population: Study 2. *Behaviour Research and Therapy, 38,* 175–189.

Levy, S., & Guttman, L. (1976). Worry, fear, and concern differentiated. *Israel Annals of Psychiatry and Related Disciplines, 14,* 211–228.

Liebert, R. M., & Morris, L. W. (1967). Cognitive and emotional components of test anxiety: A distinction and some initial data. *Psychological Reports, 20,* 975–978.

Maier, W., Gransicke, M., Freyberger, H. J., Linz, M., Heun, R., & Lecrubier, Y. (2000). Generalized anxiety disorder (ICD-10) in primary care from a cross-cultural perspective: A valid diagnostic entity? *Acta Psychiatrica Scandinavica, 101,* 29–36.

Marten, P. A., Brown, T. A., Barlow, D. H., Borkovec, T. D., Shear, M. K., & Lydiard, R. B. (1993). Evaluation of the ratings comprising the associated symptom criterion of DSM-III-R generalized anxiety disorder. *Journal of Nervous and Mental Disease, 181,* 676–682.

Maser, J. D. (1998). Generalized anxiety disorder and its comorbidities: Disputes at the boundaries. *Acta Psychiatrica Scandinavica, 393*(Suppl.), 12–22.

Mennin, D. S., Fresco, D. M., & Heimberg, R. G. (1999, November). *Determining when worry becomes clinically significant: A receiver operating characteristic (ROC) analysis approach.* Paper presented at the annual meeting of the Association for the Advancement of Behavior Therapy, Toronto.

Mennin, D. S., Heimberg, R. G., & Jack, M. S. (2000). Comorbid generalized anxiety disorder in primary social phobia: Symptom severity, functional impairment, and treatment response. *Journal of Anxiety Disorders, 14,* 325–343.

Mennin, D. S., Heimberg, R. G., Turk, C. L., & Fresco, D. M. (2003). *Preliminary evidence for an emotion regulation deficit model of generalized anxiety disorder: Testing a theoretical model.* Manuscript submitted for publication.

Merriam-Webster. (1999). *WWWebster Dictionary* [Online]. Available: http://www.m-w.com

Meyer, T. J., Miller, M. L., Metzger, R. L., & Borkovec, T. D. (1990). Development and validation of the Penn State Worry Questionnaire. *Behaviour Research and Therapy, 28,* 487–495.

Morris, L. W., & Liebert, R. M. (1970). Relationship of cognitive and emotional components of test anxiety to physiological arousal and academic performance. *Journal of Consulting and Clinical Psychology, 35,* 332–337.

Nisita, C., Petracca, A., Akiskal, H. S., Galli, L., Gepponi, I., & Cassano, G. B. (1990). Delimitation of generalized anxiety disorder: Clinical comparisons with panic and major depressive disorders. *Comprehensive Psychiatry, 31,* 409–415.

Nolen-Hoeksema, S. (1991). Responses to depression and their effects on the duration of depressive episodes. *Journal of Abnormal Psychology, 100,* 569–582.

Nolen-Hoeksema, S. (1998). The other end of the continuum: The costs of rumination. *Psychological Inquiry, 9,* 216–219.

Nolen-Hoeksema, S. (2000). Further evidence for the role of psychosocial factors in depression chronicity. *Clinical Psychology: Science and Practice, 7,* 224–227.

Norton, G. R., Cox, B. J., Asmundson, G. J. G., & Maser, J. D. (1995). The growth of research on anxiety disorders in the 1980s. *Journal of Anxiety Disorders, 9,* 75–85.

Noyes, R., Jr., Woodman, C., Garvey, M. J., Cook, B. L., Suelzer, M., Clancy, J., & Anderson, D. J. (1992). Generalized anxiety disorder vs. panic disorder: Distinguishing characteristics and patterns of comorbidity. *Journal of Nervous and Mental Disease, 180,* 369–379.

O'Neill, G. W. (1985). Is worry a valuable concept? *Behaviour Research and Therapy, 23,* 479–480.

Phillips, A. (1993). *On kissing, tickling, and being bored: Psychoanalytic essays on the unexamined life.* Cambridge, MA: Harvard University Press.

Pini, S., Cassano, G. B., Simonini, E., Savino, M., Russo, A., & Montgomery, S. A. (1997). Prevalence of anxiety disorders comorbidity in bipolar depression, unipolar depression and dysthymia. *Journal of Affective Disorders, 42,* 145–153.

Pruzinsky, T., & Borkovec, T. D. (1990). Cognitive and personality characteristics of worriers. *Behaviour Research and Therapy, 28,* 507–512.

Rassin, E., Merckelbach, H., Muris, P., & Spaan, V. (1999). Thought–action fusion as a causal factor in the development of intrusions. *Behaviour Research and Therapy, 37,* 231–237.

Reich, J. H., Noyes, R., & Yates, W. (1988). Anxiety symptoms distinguishing social phobia from panic and generalized anxiety disorders. *Journal of Nervous and Mental Disease, 176,* 510–513.

Reich, J. H., Perry, J. C., Shera, D., Dyck, I., Vasile, R., Goisman, R. M., Rodriguez-Villa, F., Massion, A. O., & Keller, M. (1994). Comparison of personality disorders in different anxiety disorder diagnoses: Panic, agoraphobia, generalized anxiety, and social phobia. *Annals of Clinical Psychiatry, 6,* 125–134.

Rickels, K., & Rynn, M. A. (2001). What is generalized anxiety disorder? *Journal of Clinical Psychiatry, 62*(Suppl. 11), 4–12.

Roemer, L., & Borkovec, T. D. (1993). Worry: Unwanted cognitive activity that controls unwanted somatic experience. In D. M. Wegner & J. W. Pennebaker (Eds.), *Handbook of mental control* (pp. 220–238). Englewood Cliffs, NJ: Prentice-Hall.

Roemer, L., Molina, S., & Borkovec, T. D. (1997). An investigation of worry content among generally anxious individuals. *Journal of Nervous and Mental Disease, 185,* 314–319.

Roemer, L., Salters, K., Raffa, S., & Orsillo, S. M. (in press). Fear and avoidance of internal experiences in GAD: Preliminary tests of a conceptual model. *Cognitive Therapy and Research.*

Ruscio, A. M. (2002). Delimiting the boundaries of generalized anxiety disorder: Differentiating high worriers with and without GAD. *Journal of Anxiety Disorders, 16,* 377–400.

Ruscio, A. M., Borkovec, T. D., & Ruscio, J. (2001). A taxometric investigation of the latent structure of worry. *Journal of Abnormal Psychology, 110,* 413–422.

Russell, M., & Davey, G. C. (1993). The relationship between life event measures and anxiety and its cognitive correlates. *Personality and Individual Differences, 14,* 317–322.

Sanderson, W. C., & Barlow, D. H. (1990). A description of patients diagnosed with DSM-III-R generalized anxiety disorder. *Journal of Nervous and Mental Disease, 178,* 588–591.

Sanderson, W. C., DiNardo, P. A., Rapee, R. M., & Barlow, D. H. (1990). Syndrome comorbidity in patients diagnosed with a DSM-III-R anxiety disorder. *Journal of Abnormal Psychology, 99,* 308–312.

Sanderson, W. C., & Wetzler, S. (1991). Chronic anxiety and generalized anxiety disorder: Issues in comorbidity. In R. M. Rapee & D. H. Barlow (Eds.), *Chronic anxiety: Generalized anxiety disorder and mixed anxiety–depression* (pp. 119–135). New York: Guilford Press.

Sanderson, W. C., Wetzler, S., Beck, A. T., & Betz, F. (1994). Prevalence of personality disorders among patients with anxiety disorders. *Psychiatry Research, 51,* 167–174.

Segerstrom, S. C., Stanton, A. L., Alden, L. E., & Shortridge, B. E. (in press). A multidimensional structure for repetitive thought: What's on your mind, and how, and how much? *Journal of Personality and Social Psychology.*

Segerstrom, S. C., Tsao, J. C. I., Alden, L. E., & Craske, M. G. (2000). Worry and rumination: Repetitive thought as a concomitant and predictor of negative mood. *Cognitive Therapy and Research, 24,* 671–688.

Slade, T., & Andrews, G. (2001). DSM-IV and ICD-10 generalized anxiety disorder: Discrepant diagnoses and associated disability. *Social Psychiatry and Psychiatric Epidemiology, 36,* 45–51.

Spitzer, R. L., Endicott, J., & Robins, E. (1978). Research Diagnostic Criteria: Rationale and reliability. *Archives of General Psychiatry, 35,* 773–782.

Spitzer, R. L., & Williams, J. B. W. (1985). Proposed revisions in the DSM-III classification of anxiety disorders based on research and clinical experience. In J. D. Maser & A. H. Tuma (Eds.), *Anxiety and the anxiety disorders* (pp. 759–773). Hillsdale, NJ: Erlbaum.

Starcevic, V. (1995). Pathological worry in major depression: A preliminary report. *Behaviour Research and Therapy, 33,* 55–56.

Starcevic, V., & Bogojevic, G. (1999). The concept of generalized anxiety disorder: Between the too narrow and too wide diagnostic criteria. *Psychopathology, 32,* 5–11.

Starcevic, V., Fallon, S., Uhlenhuth, E. H., & Pathak, D. (1994a). Comorbidity rates do not support distinction between panic disorder and generalized anxiety disorder. *Psychopathology, 27,* 269–272.

Starcevic, V., Fallon, S., Uhlenhuth, E. H., & Pathak, D. (1994b). Generalized anxiety disorder, worries about illness, and hypochondriacal fears and beliefs. *Psychotherapy and Psychosomatics, 61,* 93–99.

Stöber, J. (1998). Reliability and validity of two widely-used worry questionnaires: Self-report and self-peer convergence. *Personality and Individual Differences, 24,* 887–890.

Stöber, J. (2000). Worry, thoughts, and images: A new conceptualization. In U. von Hecker, S. Dutke, & G. Sedak (Eds.), *Generative mental processes and cognitive resources: Integrative research on adaptation and control* (pp. 223–244). Dordrecht, The Netherlands: Kluwer.

Street, L. L., Salman, E., Garfinkle, R., Silvestri, J., Carrasco, J., Cardenas, D., Zinbarg, R., Barlow, D. H., & Liebowitz, M. R. (1997). Discriminating between generalized anxiety disorder and anxiety disorder not otherwise specified in a Hispanic population: Is it only a matter of worry? *Depression and Anxiety, 5,* 1–6.

Tallis, F., Eysenck, M., & Mathews, A. (1991). Elevated evidence requirements and worry. *Personality and Individual Differences, 12,* 21–27.

Turk, C. L., Heimberg, R. G., Luterek, J. A., Mennin, D. S., & Fresco, D. M. (in press). Delineating emotion regulation deficits in generalized anxiety disorder: A comparison with social anxiety disorder. *Cognitive Therapy and Research.*

Turner, S. M., Beidel, D. C., Borden, J. W., Stanley, M. A., & Jacob, R. G. (1991). Social phobia: Axis I and II correlates. *Journal of Abnormal Psychology, 100,* 102–106.

Versiani, M., Mundim, F. D., Nardi, A. E., & Liebowitz, M. R. (1988). Tranylcypromine in social phobia. *Journal of Clinical Psychopharmacology, 8,* 279–283.

Wells, A., & Carter, K. (2001). Further tests of a cognitive model of generalized anxiety disorder: Metacognitions and worry in GAD, panic disorder, social phobia, depression, and nonpatients. *Behavior Therapy, 32,* 85–102.

Wells, A., & Morrison, A. P. (1994). Qualitative dimensions of normal worry and normal obsessions: A comparative study. *Behaviour Research and Therapy, 32,* 867–870.

Wisocki, P. A. (1988). Worry as a phenomenon relevant to the elderly. *Behavior Therapy, 19,* 369–379.

World Health Organization. (1992). *International classification of diseases and related health problems* (10th rev.). Geneva: Author.

York, D., Borkovec, T. D., Vasey, M. W., & Stern, R. (1987). Effects of worry and somatic anxiety induction on thoughts, emotion and physiological activity. *Behaviour Research and Therapy, 25,* 523–526.

Zebb, B. J., & Beck, J. G. (1998). Worry versus anxiety: Is there really a difference? *Behavior Modification, 22,* 45–61.

Zimmerman, M., & Chelminski, I. (2003). Generalized anxiety disorder in patients wtih major depression: Is DSM-IV's hierarchy correct? *American Journal of Psychiatry, 160,* 504–512.

CHAPTER 2

Epidemiology

RONALD C. KESSLER
ELLEN E. WALTERS
HANS-ULRICH WITTCHEN

Although the notion of persistent pathological anxiety has been a central concept in psychiatry since the founding of the discipline in the 19th century, the American Psychiatric Association (APA) did not introduce the diagnosis of generalized anxiety disorder (GAD) in its *Diagnostic and Statistical Manual of Mental Disorders* (DSM) until slightly over two decades ago, with the publication of the third edition (DSM-III; APA, 1980). Prior to that time, GAD was conceptualized as one of the two main components of anxiety neurosis, the other component being panic (APA, 1968). The recognition that these two syndromes, though often occurring together, are sufficiently independent empirically to be considered distinct disorders caused the separation of panic disorder and GAD in DSM-III. However, DSM-III conceptualized GAD as the residual diagnosis in the pair and saw the clinical significance of GAD as fairly minor.

The DSM-III definition of GAD required uncontrollable and diffuse (i.e., not focused on a single major life problem) anxiety or worry that was excessive or unrealistic in relation to objective life circumstances, and that persisted for 1 month or longer. A number of psychophysiological symptoms were required to occur with the anxiety or worry. Early clinical studies evaluating DSM-III GAD in clinical samples found that the disorder seldom occurred in the absence of some other comorbid anxiety or mood disorder (Breier, Charney, & Heninger, 1985; Breslau, 1985). This led some commentators to suggest that GAD might better be conceptualized as a prodrome, residue, or severity marker than as an independent disorder (Breslau & Davis, 1985b; Clayton et al., 1991; Noyes et al., 1992). Comorbidity between GAD and major depression was found to be lower as the duration of GAD increased (Breslau & Davis, 1985a), leading the DSM-III-R committee on GAD to require 6 months of symptoms for a diagnosis, rather than the 1 month required in DSM-III (APA, 1987). Further changes in the definition of excessive worry and the required number of associated symptoms were made in DSM-IV (APA, 1994).

PREVALENCE

Changing definitions of GAD have made it difficult to collect long-term data on the prevalence and course of the disorder. Nonetheless, a critical mass of data has become available over the past decade showing that in the United States the general population lifetime prevalence of DSM-III and DSM-III-R GAD is between 4% and 7%; the 1-year prevalence is between 3% and 5%; and the current prevalence is between 1.5% and 3% (Blazer, Hughes, George, Swartz, & Boyer, 1991; Kessler, Dupont, Berglund, & Wittchen, 1999; Wittchen, Zhao, Kessler, & Eaton, 1994). Community epidemiological surveys of DSM-III-R GAD carried out in other parts of the world have found similar prevalences (e.g., Bijl, Ravelli, & Van Zessen, 1998; Offord et al., 1996). These prevalence estimates are considerably lower than the estimated prevalences of major depression, social phobia, or specific phobia, but are quite comparable to those of panic disorder, agoraphobia without panic disorder, and dysthymia.

It should be noted that the prevalence estimates given above are based on DSM criteria. Whereas the DSM-III and DSM-III-R definitions of GAD required the worry to be excessive or unrealistic, and the DSM-IV definition requires the worry to be excessive, no such requirement exists in the *International Classification of Diseases and Related Health Problems*, 10th revision (ICD-10). One would consequently expect that the prevalence of GAD would be higher, possibly considerably higher, when ICD-10 criteria are used than when DSM-IV criteria are used. However, we are aware of no general population epidemiological research that has investigated this issue.

General population surveys that evaluate the core dimensions of personality consistently find that substantial proportions of the population report anxious personality characteristics, such as persistent tension, worry, nervousness, and restlessness, in assessments of neuroticism (Heath, Neale, Kessler, Eaves, & Kendler, 1992; Zuckerman, 1991). The rates of GAD found in psychiatric epidemiological surveys, however, are much lower. This suggests that the DSM definitions of GAD exclude a substantial proportion of people with clinically significant chronic anxiety (i.e., neuroticism). The reason for this exclusion is unclear, but one possibility is that many people who score high on personality scales of neuroticism have brief recurrent episodes of anxiety that do not meet the requirement of occurring more days than not for 6 months. Another possibility is that the anxiety of people with high neuroticism scores is not associated with the full range of psychophysiological symptoms required for a DSM diagnosis of GAD.

A recent report from the World Health Organization (WHO) study on Psychological Problems in Primary Care (Ustun & Sartorius, 1995) investigated these possibilities (Maier et al., 2000). The authors of this report attempted to validate the ICD-10 (WHO, 1990) requirements of a 6-month duration and four associated symptoms for a diagnosis of GAD. Their attempt compared levels of role impairment associated with GAD-like syndromes among "pure" cases (i.e., cases without other comorbid mental disorders) as a function of duration and number of associated symptoms. They found no evidence that impairment increased more after a duration of 6 months than at any other arbitrarily specified duration. In fact, revising the duration requirement to 1 month and lowering the number of required associated symptoms yielded the best discrimination between cases and noncases in terms of impaired role functioning.

Because this investigation examined a primary care sample, it is unknown how much the estimated population prevalence of GAD would increase if these changes in diagnostic criteria were evaluated in a general population sample. The increase in prevalence would probably be substantial. From these results, it must be concluded that uncertainty exists about the true population prevalence of the GAD syndrome. Taking available studies of neurotic personality traits as a guide, the true current prevalence of the clinically significant component of the GAD syndrome could be as high as 5–8% of the general population, compared to the 1.5–3.0% found in epidemiological studies of DSM GAD.

ONSET AND COURSE

Retrospective reports from respondents in community epidemiological surveys (e.g., Burke, Burke, Rae, & Regier, 1991; Kendler, Neale, Kessler, Heath, & Eaves, 1992a) and from patients in clinical studies (e.g., Barlow, Blanchard, Vermilyea, Vermilyea, & DiNardo, 1986; Rogers et al., 1999) consistently suggest that GAD typically begins in the decade between the late teens and the late 20s. Only a small number of first onsets occur subsequent to the mid-30s. Examination of comparative Kaplan–Meier age-at-onset curves in epidemiological samples suggests that specific phobia and social phobia are the only two anxiety or mood disorders with earlier age-at-onset distributions than GAD (Burke et al., 1991). It is noteworthy that childhood-onset cases of GAD are classified in some research as overanxious disorder of childhood rather than GAD, leading to a reduction in the estimated prevalence of GAD and an increase in the estimated age at onset.

Retrospective reports from respondents in community epidemiological surveys (e.g., Angst & Vollrath, 1991; Blazer et al., 1991) and from patients in clinical studies (Mancuso, Townsend, & Mercante, 1993; Noyes, Holt, & Woodman, 1996) also suggest that GAD is a very chronic condition, with episodes commonly persisting for a decade or longer. Prospective data show the same. The richest prospective data of this sort come from the Harvard/Brown Anxiety Research Program (HARP) (Warshaw, Keller, & Stout, 1994; Yonkers, Massion, Warshaw, & Keller, 1996). HARP is a prospective naturalistic study of patients with anxiety who were recruited initially from psychiatric clinics and hospitals in the Boston metropolitan area. In addition to obtaining detailed retrospective history data from these patients at baseline, HARP has thus far reported results for patients followed for 5 years (at 6-month intervals for the first 2 years and annually thereafter) to observe the natural history of their disorders. Only 15% of respondents with baseline GAD had a full remission for 2 months or longer at any time in the first year after baseline. This proportion increased to only 25% in the 2 years after baseline (Yonkers et al., 1996) and to 38% after 5 years (Yonkers, Dyck, Warshaw, & Keller, 2000).

One would expect the course of GAD to be more persistent among patients in treatment than in the general population. It is noteworthy, therefore, that the community epidemiological data collected in the Epidemiologic Catchment Area (ECA) study (Blazer et al., 1991) are consistent with the results of the HARP study. Both show that the duration of DSM-III GAD is typically chronic. An indirect confirmation of this same conclusion can be obtained by examining the ratio of current prevalence to lifetime prevalence in community epidemiological surveys. These ratios are typically in the range between 40% and 60% (e.g., Bijl et al., 1998; Offord et al., 1994). Although these ratios cannot distinguish the effects of chronicity from recurrence, such high ratios clearly imply that people with a history of GAD spend a substantial proportion of their subsequent lifetimes with the disorder.

SOCIODEMOGRAPHIC CORRELATES OF ONSET AND COURSE

Epidemiological surveys show that the lifetime prevalence of GAD is more common among women than men, among unmarried than married people, among racial/ethnic minorities than members of majority groups, and among respondents with low socioeconomic status (SES) than middle- or high-SES respondents (Blazer et al., 1991; Brawman-Mintzer & Lydiard, 1996; Wittchen et al., 1994). However, prospective analyses show that none of these sociodemographic variables is a significant predictor of the course of GAD (Yonkers et al., 2000). Consistent with this finding, unpublished analyses of cross-sectional epidemiological data from the WHO's International Consortium in Psychiatric Epidemiology (ICPE, 2000) show that none of these sociodemographic predictors is significantly related to the current prevalence of GAD among respondents with a lifetime history of the disorder, after age at onset and time since onset are controlled for.

In the case of acquired statuses like SES and marital status, where significant associations exist with lifetime prevalence, the absence of significant associations with course could be due to selection processes; that is, GAD or its determinants might influence subsequent SES or marital status. For example, whereas low SES may predispose an individual to excessive worry, excessive worry in some cases may lead to increased diligence that promotes increased education and occupational achievement, leading to a canceling of an association between SES and course of GAD. In the case of ascribed statuses that do not change over time, such as gender and race/ethnicity, a more plausible interpretation is that these statuses or their correlates do not affect the course of GAD, though they are etiologically significant for onset.

A complex nonlinear cross-sectional association also exists between GAD and age, with the highest current prevalences in the middle age groups (Wittchen et al., 1994). Decomposition shows that this association is caused by the joint occurrence of significant cohort effects (i.e., increasing prevalences among people born in more recent years, presumably due to the increase in environmental risk factors) and differential recurrence risk as a function of age (i.e., increasing risk of GAD's becoming persistent, related to increasing age). The cohort effect is inferred from comparisons of retrospective age-at-onset reports in cross-sectional community epidemiological surveys. These analyses suggest that the lifetime prevalence of GAD has been on the rise in successive cohorts born over the past half century. At least part of this presumed increase may be due to differential recall failure with age. However, the fact that the strength of the retrospectively reported intercohort difference in GAD is greater than for other disorders of comparable impairment argues against recall bias as a complete explanation. Once onset occurs, risk of current prevalence is inversely related to age but not to age at onset. Consequently, the highest current prevalence is in the middle years of life, due to a comparatively high lifetime risk (cohort effect) and a comparatively low rate of remission.

Perhaps the most intriguing of the sociodemographic correlates of GAD involves SES. This association has special interest because of preliminary evidence from the ICPE surveys that the association is stronger when ICD criteria are used instead of DSM criteria. The reason for this is that ICD, unlike DSM, does not require that persistent worry be excessive in order to qualify for a diagnosis of GAD. As one might expect, socioeconomically disadvantaged people are much more likely than other people to experience chronic life situations that lead to clinically significant persistent anxiety (e.g., housing instability or neighborhood violence). Because these anxieties are often justified (i.e., not excessive in light of objective life circumstances), DSM criteria rule out a diagnosis of GAD, dampening the association between SES and GAD.

COMORBIDITY

As noted at the beginning of the chapter, early clinical studies documented very high rates of comorbidity among patients with DSM-III GAD. This led to an expansion of the duration requirement from 1 month to 6 months in subsequent editions of the DSM. However, clinical studies using DSM-III-R criteria found that comorbidity remained quite high even with the 6-month duration requirement (e.g., Noyes et al., 1992; Roy-Byrne, 1996). This led to continued suggestions that GAD is not an independent disorder (Brawman-Mintzer et al., 1993; Gorman, 1996).

It is important to appreciate, though, that this evidence of high comorbidity comes almost entirely from clinical samples. Studies of GAD comorbidity carried out in community samples suggest that the initial concern about extremely high comorbidity in GAD was misplaced. Wittchen et al. (1994) first documented this in an analysis of a large community epidemiological survey, which showed that the proportion of people with DSM-III-R GAD and one or more other comorbid diagnoses was not dramatically higher than the rate of comorbidity among people with other anxiety or mood disorders. Wittchen and his colleagues explained the discrepancy between this result and earlier clinical findings by showing that comorbidity was a powerful predictor of help seeking among people with GAD. This suggests that the extremely high comorbidity in GAD is an artifact of treatment sample selection bias rather than an inherent feature of GAD.

A similar result regarding comorbidity in GAD is found by looking at lifetime comorbidity rather than episode comorbidity. Table 2.1 illustrates this result by presenting data from the U.S. National Comorbidity Survey (NCS) (Kessler et al., 1994), a large nationally representative survey of the U.S. household population. Table 2.1 shows the proportions of NCS respondents with particular lifetime DSM-III-R disorders who also met criteria for at least one other lifetime DSM-III-R comorbid disorder. As shown in the table, proportional lifetime comorbidity in GAD was not meaningfully higher than in dysthymia or panic disorder and was considerably lower than in mania.

Before we assume that this finding shows that comorbidity in GAD is no higher than in other anxiety or mood disorders, it is important to consider comparative comorbidities in terms of bivariate associations (e.g., sim-

TABLE 2.1. Proportions of National Comorbidity Survey (NCS) DSM-III-R Disorders with Lifetime Comorbidity

Mood disorders	
Major depressive episode	83.1%
Dysthymia	91.3%
Mania	99.4%
Any mood disorder	82.2%
Anxiety disorders	
Generalized anxiety disorder	91.3%
Panic disorder	92.2%
Social phobia	81.0%
Simple phobia	83.4%
Agoraphobia	87.3%
Posttraumatic stress disorder	81.0%
Any anxiety disorder	74.1%

Note. Disorders are operationalized without diagnostic hierarchy rules. Reprinted from Table 2-1 in "The Prevalence of Psychiatric Comorbidity" (p. 28) by R. C. Kessler, 1997, in S. Wetzler & W. C. Sanderson (Eds.), *Treatment Strategies for Patients with Psychiatric Comorbidity.* Copyright 1997 by John Wiley & Sons, Inc. This material was used by permission of John Wiley & Sons, Inc.

ple Pearson correlations, tetrachoric correlations, or odds ratios [ORs]) rather than in terms of conditional probabilities (i.e., conditional risks of one disorder, given the existence of another disorder). This is important, because conditional probabilities are influenced by differential prevalences. Analyzing the data in Table 2.1 this way reveals bivariate lifetime and 12-month comorbidities, expressed as ORs for GAD (with an average OR of 12.0) that are no larger than those for major depression (with an average OR of 12.5) or panic disorder (with an average OR of 12.0) (Kessler, 1995). An OR of 12 means that the odds of having versus not having one of the disorders in the pair are 12 times as high among people who have the other disorder than among those who do not have the other disorder.

SYMPTOM SPECIFICITY

An issue of special importance in the evaluation of comorbidity is whether the symptoms of a presumably distinct disorder form separate empirical clusters from symptoms of other disorders in representative samples (Robins & Guze, 1970). Maier and his colleagues (2000) evaluated this issue in the WHO study on Psychological Problems in Primary Care. They found that the associated psychophysiological symptoms of GAD specified in ICD-10 strongly clustered with the core symptoms of persistent worry and anxiety.

Comorbidity between GAD and major depression has been the focus of special interest, based on evidence that this is the most common type of anxiety–mood comorbidity (Kessler, 1997). One reason for this high comorbidity is presumably that the two disorders share a number of common symptoms. Therefore, it is noteworthy that investigations of comorbidity carried out at the symptom level rather than at the diagnostic level are able to find differentiation of GAD and major depression. Brown, Chorpita, and Barlow (1998) tested several models of structural relationships among symptoms of GAD and major depression, and found separate latent factors of positive affectivity, negative affectivity, and autonomic suppression (related to GAD). This finding strongly argues that GAD and major depression can be distinguished, despite the overlap of some core symptoms.

Consistent with this finding, analyses of twin data using an additive behavior-genetic model conclude that the environmental determinants of GAD and major depression are distinct (Kendler, Neale, Kessler, Heath, & Eaves, 1992b). In turn, this result is consistent with the finding in epidemiological research that GAD and major depression have significantly different sociodemographic predictors (Skodal, Schwartz, Dohrenwend, Levav, & Shrout, 1994). For example, SES is much more strongly related to major depression than to GAD. It is noteworthy that twin studies also suggest that the genes for GAD and major depression are the same (Kendler et al., 1992b), raising the possibility that the two syndromes are different manifestations of the same underlying disorder. However, the model on which this conclusion is based assumes that the joint effects of genes and environment are additive—in other words, that the impact of environmental determinants is not influenced by the presence or absence of genes. This is implausible. A more realistic interactive specification, which cannot be identified with conventional twin data, might well show differentiation of genetic effects. Consistent with this possibility, studies show differential aggregation of mental disorders in the families of patients with GAD and major depression (Reich, 1993); this finding suggests strongly that GAD and major depression are distinct disorders (Reich, 1995).

TEMPORAL PRIORITIES IN LIFETIME COMORBID GAD

Another important issue in evaluating comorbid conditions concerns the distinction between primary and secondary disorders. Although the primary–secondary distinction is defined in a number of ways, one of the most simple and intuitive of these definitions compares ages of onset. Based on NCS data, Table 2.2 shows the proportion of lifetime cases of specific DSM-III-R disorders that were temporally primary—that is, the proportion in which the disorder in question was the earliest lifetime dis-

TABLE 2.2. Proportions of Temporally Primary Cases among NCS DSM-III-R Disorders

Mood disorders	
Major depressive episode	41.1%
Dysthymia	37.7%
Mania	20.2%
Anxiety disorders	
Generalized anxiety disorder	37.0%
Panic disorder	23.3%
Social phobia	63.1%
Simple phobia	67.6%
Agoraphobia	45.2%
Posttraumatic stress disorder	52.1%

Note. Disorders are operationalized without diagnostic hierarchy rules. Reprinted from Table 2-3 in "The Prevalence of Psychiatric Comorbidity" (p. 32) by R. C. Kessler, 1997, in S. Wetzler & W. C. Sanderson (Eds.), *Treatment Strategies for Patients with Psychiatric Comorbidity.* Copyright 1997 by John Wiley & Sons, Inc. This material was used by permission of John Wiley & Sons, Inc.

order ever experienced by the respondent, according to retrospective age-at-onset reports. In cases where two or more disorders reportedly started at the same age and before any other disorders, both were coded as temporally primary.

The results are surprising in showing that simple phobia, social phobia, and posttraumatic stress disorder were the only DSM-III-R anxiety or mood disorders for which the majority of lifetime cases were temporally primary. In general, anxiety disorders are more likely than mood disorders to be temporally primary. The proportion temporally primary for GAD (37.0%) was comparable to the percentages for the mood disorders (20.2–41.1%) and slightly higher than for panic disorder (23.3%). Although not reported here, more detailed analyses of these data have shown that GAD was typically the temporally primary disorder in relation to depression among people with comorbid anxious–depression (Kessler et al., 1996).

PREDICTIVE PRIORITIES IN LIFETIME COMORBID GAD

It is a mistake to think of temporal priority as equivalent to causal priority. The easiest way to make this clear is to note that it is possible to have a pair of comorbid disorders in which the prior occurrence of Disorder *A* is not a significant predictor of the subsequent onset of Disorder *B*, even though Disorder *A* occurs before Disorder *B* in the vast majority of cases (Kessler & Price, 1993). This situation can occur when the base rates of the two disorders differ substantially, as with comorbidity between GAD and major depression (where major depression is much more common than GAD).

A more useful way to think about priorities in comorbidity is to investigate prediction: whether one disorder in a particular pair, when it is temporally primary, is a significant predictor of the subsequent first onset of the other disorder. The NCS examined this by using retrospective age-at-onset reports for each disorder to estimate a series of bivariate survival models, in which prior onset of one disorder was treated as a time-varying covariate of another disorder (Kessler, 1997). For ease of comparison, these models constrained the effects of temporally primary disorders to be constant across ages of onset, times since onset, and age at onset of the earlier disorders. All temporally primary anxiety and mood disorders were statistically significant predictors of the subsequent first onset of other anxiety and mood disorders. GAD did not stand out in any particular way in comparison to the other disorders—either in the magnitude of the effects of GAD in predicting later onset of other disorders, or in the magnitude of the effects of other temporally primary disorders in predicting first onset of GAD. This means that any questioning of the validity of GAD as a diagnostic entity on the basis of data about predictive priority in comorbidity would apply equally to major depression, panic disorder, social phobia, and all the other anxiety and mood disorders considered in this analysis.

PREDICTIVE PRIORITIES INVOLVING SEVERITY AND COURSE

NCS analyses also investigated whether comorbidity is associated more strongly with the severity or course of GAD than of other anxiety or mood disorders (Kessler, 2000). The rationale was that if GAD is a prodrome, residue, or severity marker of other disorders, the severity and course of GAD should be much more strongly affected by comorbidity than those of other anxiety or mood disorders. The results showed that comorbidity was generally associated with increased severity and persistence for all anxiety and mood disorders. Although the patterns involving GAD were generally similar to those for the other disorders considered in the analysis, there was one important exception. GAD was the only anxiety or mood disorder in which persistence, as indirectly indicated by recency (with age at onset and time since onset controlled for), was unrelated to comorbidity.

Yonkers and colleagues (2000) reported a similar result in an analysis of the prospective study of the predictors of the clinical course of GAD in the HARP study. The HARP data also showed that the course of comorbid GAD was unrelated to whether the GAD was primary or secondary (Rogers et al., 1999). Other studies arrived at different conclusions about the effects of comorbidity on the course of GAD (Angst & Vollrath, 1991; Durham, Allan, & Hackett, 1997; Mancuso et al., 1993). However, the inconsistency of this evidence—in conjunction with the clear and consistent evidence that comorbidity is significantly related to the course of other anxiety and mood disorders—means that, if anything, GAD behaves more like an independent disorder in this respect than do other anxiety or mood disorders.

This finding is relevant to the hierarchy requirement in DSM-IV that periods of generalized anxiety occurring exclusively within episodes of major depression do not qualify for a diagnosis of GAD. It is noteworthy that there is no symmetrical hierarchy rule in DSM-IV that periods of depression occurring exclusively within episodes of generalized anxiety do not qualify for a diagnosis of major depression. Given that GAD is usually temporally primary to major depression, and that episodes of GAD generally persist much longer than episodes of major depression, the number of people with GAD whose anxiety occurs exclusively within episodes of major depression is quite small. However, a sizable number of people with major depression may have episodes of depression that occur exclusively within longer episodes of anxiety. It would be useful for future research to investigate subtypes of depression along this dimension.

THE IMPAIRMENTS ASSOCIATED WITH PURE AND COMORBID GAD

As previously noted, Wittchen and his associates found the false appearance of high comorbidity in GAD in early clinical studies to be due to an exceptionally strong help-seeking bias among people with comorbid GAD. People in the general population with GAD had extremely low rates of help seeking in the absence of some other comorbid mental disorder. There are at least two plausible interpretations of this finding. One is that pure GAD is not seriously impairing in itself; only when GAD co-occurs with other anxiety or mood disorders does the level of distress in GAD motivate people with the disorder to seek treatment. If this is the case, it could be argued that GAD may be an independent disorder, but it is only clinically significant when it is part of a comorbid cluster in which the comorbid disorders should be the focus of clinical attention. The other plausible interpretation is that people with GAD worry about a great many things, but seldom perceive that their worrying is a problem without the presence of other comorbid disorders that are more easily recognized as pathological. The distinction between these two possibilities is of considerable importance in evaluating whether GAD should be considered a clinically significant disorder in its own right.

Three recent studies focused on pure and comorbid GAD in primary care samples and obtained results relevant to this issue (Olfson et al., 1997; Ormel et al., 1994; Schonfeld et al., 1997). All three studies found that "pure" GAD, defined as a current episode of this disorder in the absence of any of the other mood, anxiety, or substance use disorders assessed in the primary care samples, was associated with meaningful levels of impairment in a number of life domains. In the largest of these studies, Ormel and colleagues (1994) found that mean numbers of disability days in the past month were much higher among primary care patients with pure GAD (4.4) than among patients with none of the psychiatric disorders assessed in their survey (1.7). Schonfeld and colleagues (1997) found that mean age- and sex-adjusted scores on the 0–100 Short Form-36 scale of social functioning (Stewart, Hays, & Ware, 1988) were much lower (with a high score indicating good functioning) among primary care patients with pure GAD (71.0) than among those with none of the psychiatric disorders assessed in their survey (83.6).

Given the importance placed on major depression in previous studies of comorbid GAD, it is noteworthy that the impairment associated with pure major depression was greater and more varied than that associated with pure GAD in two of these studies (Olfson et al., 1997; Schonfeld et al., 1997). However, the reliability of these findings can be called into question, based on the fact that the numbers of patients with pure disorders in these studies were quite small: only between 4 and 14 cases of pure GAD, and only between 25 and 54 cases of pure depression. Differences in the magnitude of impairment associated with pure GAD versus pure depression were much smaller in the study carried out by Ormel and colleagues (1994), which included considerably larger numbers of respondents with pure GAD ($n = 272$) and pure depression ($n = 438$). Aggregate impairments of GAD and major depression were also found to be quite similar to each other in a large primary care study conducted by Spitzer and colleagues (1995) that did not distinguish between pure and comorbid cases.

It is important to note that the evaluations of comorbidity in all these primary care studies included other psychiatric disorders in addition to GAD and depression. Given the higher prevalence of comorbidity between GAD and depression than of other types of anxiety–mood comorbidity (Kessler, 1997), more focused general population data are necessary to evaluate the separate and joint effects of these two disorders, as well as to evaluate the effects of broader comorbidities in the general population. This was recently done in a comparative analysis of pure and comorbid GAD and depression in two large nationally representative epidemiological surveys in the United States (Kessler et al., 1999).

Table 2.3 presents data reproduced from the investigation on the associations between 12-month GAD without depression and 12-month major depression without GAD and impairment, adjusted for other comorbid disorders and for sociodemographic variables. The first two columns report associations involving GAD without depression. All six of these coefficients show that GAD was associated with higher impairments than found among respondents who did not have GAD (three of the six were statistically significant). The next two columns report associations involving major depression without GAD. All of these coefficients show that depression was associated with significantly higher impairment than found among respondents who did not have depression. Finally, comparison of the impairment associated with GAD without depression versus depression without GAD is reported in the last two columns of the table. None of these differences was statistically significant. Data from the same report found that anxiety–depression was associated with higher impairment than found among respondents with only one of the two disorders. This report also noted that the magnitude of this impairment did not differ depending on which of the two disorders was temporally primary, either on a lifetime basis or in terms of episode onset.

TABLE 2.3. The Effects (Odds Ratios) of 12 Month GAD without Major Depression (MD) and MD without GAD in Predicting Impairments in Two U.S. National Surveys,[a] Controlling for Sociodemographics and Other 12-Month DSM-III-R Disorders[b]

	GAD without MD		MD without GAD		GAD without MD vs. MD without GAD	
	Survey 1	Survey 2	Survey 1	Survey 2	Survey 1	Survey 2
Fair/poor perceived mental health	6.0[*]	4.8[*]	3.3[*]	5.2[*]	1.6	0.8
High work impairment	3.5	3.5	3.5[*]	8.5[*]	0.9	0.5
High social impairment	2.5[*]	1.2	2.0[*]	1.6[*]	1.5	1.0

Note. Reprinted from Table 2 in "Impairment in Pure and Comorbid Generalized Anxiety Disorder and Major Depression at 12 Months in Two National Surveys" by R. C. Kessler, R. L. DuPont, P. Berglund, & H. U. Wittchen, 1999, *American Journal of Psychiatry, 156,* p. 1919. Copyright 1999, the American Psychiatric Association. Reprinted by permission.
[a]The two surveys indicated here are the NCS (Survey 1; Kessler et al., 1994) and the Midlife Development in the U.S. Survey (Survey 2; Kessler et al., 1999).
[b]Results are based on separate regression equations evaluating the effect of either GAD or major depression in predicting one of the impairment measures in one of the samples while controlling for sociodemographic variables (age, gender, education, race/ethnicity, employment status, marital status, and urbanicity) and other 12-month DSM-III-R disorders. Models in the first two columns evaluate the effect of 12-month GAD on the subsample of respondents who did not have 12-month MD. Models in the middle two columns evaluate the effect of 12-month MD on the subsample of respondents who did not have 12-month GAD. Models in the last two columns evaluate the relative impairments of GAD without MD versus MD without GAD in analyses that are confined to respondents in those two subsamples.
[*]Significant at the .05 level (two-sided test).

PATTERNS OF TREATMENT SEEKING

As noted earlier in the chapter, the NCS data showed clearly that comorbidity was a powerful predictor of help seeking among people with GAD (Wittchen et al., 1994). It is important to appreciate that this finding was not obtained because pure GAD is not severe enough to motivate help-seeking efforts. The results presented in the preceding section have shown that pure GAD is as impairing as pure major depression. Why, then, do a much higher proportion of people with pure depression than with pure GAD seek professional help? One plausible explanation for this difference is that GAD often starts so early in life and has such an insidious onset, often associated with underlying personality pathology (Blashfield et al., 1994), that many people with GAD do not realize that they have an emotional problem until they develop secondary disorders.

Olfson, Kessler, Berglund, and Lin (1998) contributed one piece of evidence that is indirectly consistent with this interpretation. They documented that speed of initial treatment contact after first onset of GAD was inversely related to age at onset of the disorder in general population samples in both the United States and Ontario. Figure 2.1 presents the aggregate speed of contact curves for GAD reported by Olfson and colleagues, while Table 2.4 presents the effects of age at onset. As shown in Figure 2.1, approximately one-third of people with GAD sought treatment in the year of onset of the disorder, whereas the average delay in initial treatment contact was more than a decade among people who delayed beyond the first year. This was true not only in the United States, where there are financial barriers to seeking mental health treatment, but also in Ontario, where such barriers are substantially lower. This result argues against the notion that financial barriers to treatment are an important determinant of treatment delays. The finding that age at onset was associated with speed of help seeking, as shown in Table 2.4, can most plausibly be attributed to an increased recognition of anxiety as a problem with increasing age at onset. The especially strong age-at-onset effect for seeking treatment in the year of onset is consistent with the finding of Hoehn-Saric, Hazlett, and McLeod (1993) that the vast majority of people with early-onset GAD reported an insidious onset, while people with later-onset GAD were more likely to report an acute onset associated with a precipitating stressful event.

These pervasive delays in help seeking are especially upsetting, in light of the fact that effective cognitive-behavioral (Barlow, 2002) and pharmacological (Hackett, 2000) therapies exist for the treatment of GAD. There is also promising evidence regarding the efficacy of psychodynamic treatments for GAD (Crits-Christoph, Connolly, Azarian, Crits-Christoph, & Shappell, 1996). Perhaps even more upsetting is the fact that only a small proportion of people with GAD get treatment, even though

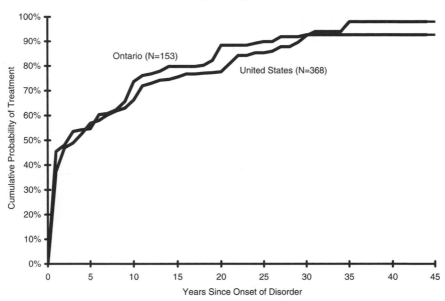

FIGURE 2.1. Speed-of-contact curves for the probability of initial treatment contact after first onset of GAD in the United States and Ontario. Reprinted from Part 2 of Figure 1 in "Psychiatric Disorder Onset and First Treatment Contact in the United States and Ontario" by M. Olfson, R. C. Kessler, P. A. Berglund, & E. Lin, 1998, *American Journal of Psychiatry, 155,* p. 1416. Copyright 1998, the American Psychiatric Association. Reprinted by permission.

the majority of them come into frequent contact with the primary care system. Indeed, GAD is the most commonly found anxiety disorder in primary care settings, both in the United States (Barrett, Oxman, & Gerber, 1988) and in many other parts of the world (Ustun & Sartorius, 1995). This is due to the fact that people with GAD frequently present for treatment with complaints of minor physical problems. The problem is that their anxiety is seldom taken as a focus of treatment, because primary care patients with GAD seldom include anxiety among their presenting complaints, and primary care physicians seldom recognize anxiety in their patients unless it is a presenting complaint (Ormel et al., 1990). This lack of recognition of the underlying psychological problem leads to frustrations on the part of patients, who typically are not relieved of the secondary psychophysiological symptoms that are usually their presenting complaints (Katon et al., 1990; Lin et al., 1991). Patient screening and demand management initiatives are currently being evaluated in an effort to increase recognition and treatment of GAD among these patients.

Another source of considerable concern regarding treatment of GAD is that research shows that a substantial proportion of patients in treat-

TABLE 2.4. The Effects of Age at Onset on Speed of First Treatment Contact for GAD in the United States and Ontario

| | Odds ratios[a] for treatment contact | | | |
| | In the year of onset of GAD | | In subsequent years | |
Age at onset	U.S.	Ontario	U.S.	Ontario
≤12	1.0	1.0	1.0	1.0
13–19	22.5	7.5	1.4	1.3
20–29	73.6	35.8[*]	2.0	2.0
≥ 30	92.5	21.2[*]	5.6[*]	2.3

Note. Adapted from Tables 1 and 2 in "Psychiatric Disorder Onset and First Treatment Contact in the United States and Ontario" by M. Olfson, R. C. Kessler, P. A. Berglund, & E. Lin, 1998, *American Journal of Psychiatry, 155*, pp. 1417–1418. Copyright 1998, the American Psychiatric Association. Adapted by permission.
[a]These odds ratios were obtained by exponentiating logistic regression coefficients (in the model to predict contact in the year of onset of GAD) and by discrete-time survival coefficients (in the model to predict contact in subsequent years) from a model that included controls for cohort (in both) and time since onset (in the model to predict contact in subsequent years). There were 368 cases of GAD in the U.S. sample and 153 in the Ontario sample.
[*]Significant at the .05 level (two-sided test).

ment receive inadequate treatment. In a follow-up of the HARP sample, Goisman, Warshaw, and Keller (1999) showed that as of 1996, dynamic psychotherapy remained the most commonly used form of talk therapy for patients with GAD. They found that only a small number of patients received cognitive-behavioral therapies, even though treatment trials have documented the effectiveness of cognitive-behavioral therapies for GAD, whereas no such data exist yet for psychodynamic therapies. In a parallel analysis of the HARP data, Salzman, Goldenberg, Bruce, and Keller (2001) showed that up to one-third of patients seeking medical treatment for GAD in 1996 were unmedicated at the time of interview. An unspecified additional proportion were undermedicated. Consistent with these results, Wang, Berglund, and Kessler (2000), analyzed data from a large U.S. national telephone–mail survey conducted in 1996–1997 and found that the majority of patients in treatment for anxiety or mood disorders during those years received treatments that did not meet the minimum standards for effectiveness stipulated in published treatment guidelines.

OVERVIEW

This chapter shows that GAD is a commonly occurring mental disorder that typically has an early age at onset, a chronic course, and a high degree of comorbidity with other anxiety and mood disorders. Comorbid

GAD is often temporally primary, especially in relation to mood disorders. The weight of evidence reviewed here argues against the view that GAD is better conceptualized as a prodrome, residue, or severity marker of other disorders than as an independent disorder in its own right. Recent community epidemiological studies and primary care studies show consistently that comorbidity in GAD is no greater than in most other anxiety or mood disorders when comorbidities are evaluated in unrestricted samples. Furthermore, the data reviewed here show that pure GAD is associated with impairments comparable in magnitude to the impairments associated with other clinically significant anxiety and mood disorders. In addition, the clinical course of GAD is less consistently related to comorbidity than is the course of other anxiety and mood disorders. These findings argue that the status of GAD as an independent disorder is at least as strongly supported by available evidence as are other anxiety or mood disorders.

The chapter has also shown that there is considerable uncertainty regarding even very basic epidemiological characteristics of the GAD syndrome. Lingering concerns about the independence of GAD have conspired to exacerbate this problem by promoting repeated changes in the diagnostic criteria for GAD from DSM-III to DSM-III-R and to DSM-IV. These successive changes have made it difficult to amass consistent long-term data on the natural history of GAD. Available evidence on diagnostic thresholds for GAD raises questions about whether the requirements of a 6-month minimum duration and the specific number of psychophysiological symptoms are optimal for capturing all of the people in the general population who suffer from a clinically significant generalized anxiety syndrome. An additional source of potential bias in this regard is the fact that the DSM system requires anxiety to be "excessive" to qualify as GAD. It is interesting to note that there is no comparable DSM requirement that dysphoria must be excessive to qualify as major depression. These uncertainties as to the most appropriate diagnostic threshold regarding duration and number of symptoms, and the discrepancy between the diagnostic requirements for anxiety and depression, make it very difficult to gain a clear understanding of the true breadth and depth of the GAD syndrome in the population. Future work is needed, ideally in unbiased epidemiological samples, to resolve these basic uncertainties.

Given the strong comorbidity between GAD and major depression, the fact that the majority of people with this type of comorbidity report that the onset of GAD occurred prior to the onset of depression, and the fact that temporally primary GAD significantly predicts the subsequent onset of depression and other secondary disorders, a question can be raised as to whether early intervention and treatment of primary GAD might be effective in preventing the subsequent first onset of secondary anxiety and depression. Unfortunately, little is known about this possibility, due to the fact (noted above) that very few people with pure GAD seek treatment. We do not understand why this is so. Given the early onset of GAD and its strong effects in predicting the subsequent onset, severity, and persistence of other disorders, efforts are needed to collect epidemiological data on the reasons for low help seeking in pure GAD, and to develop outreach strategies that might be able to correct this situation.

ACKNOWLEDGMENTS

Preparation of this chapter was supported by U.S. Public Health Service Grant No. U01-MH60220 and by the Global Research on Anxiety and Depression Network (GRAD), through an unrestricted educational grant from Wyeth-Ayerst Pharmaceuticals (http://www.gradnetwork.com). The helpful comments of Sergio Aguilar-Gaxiola, Kathleen Merikangas, and Bedirhan Ustun are gratefully acknowledged.

REFERENCES

American Psychiatric Association (APA). (1968). *Diagnostic and statistical manual of mental disorders* (2nd ed.). Washington, DC: Author.

American Psychiatric Association (APA). (1980). *Diagnostic and statistical manual of mental disorders* (3rd ed.). Washington, DC: Author.

American Psychiatric Association (APA). (1987). *Diagnostic and statistical manual of mental disorders* (3rd ed., rev.). Washington, DC: Author.

American Psychiatric Association (APA). (1994). *Diagnostic and statistical manual of mental disorders* (4th ed.). Washington, DC: Author.

Angst, J., & Vollrath, M. (1991). The natural history of anxiety disorders. *Acta Psychiatrica Scandinavica, 141*, 446–452.

Barlow, D. H. (2002). *Anxiety and its disorders* (2nd ed.). New York: Guilford Press.

Barlow, D. H., Blanchard, R. B., Vermilyea, J. B., Vermilyea, B. B., & DiNardo, P. A. (1986). Generalized anxiety and generalized anxiety disorder: Description and reconceptualization. *American Journal of Psychiatry, 143*, 40–44.

Barrett, J., Oxman, T. E., & Gerber, P. D. (1988). The prevalence of psychiatric disorders in primary care practice. *Archives of General Psychiatry, 45*, 1100–1106.

Bijl, R. V., Ravelli, R., & Van Zessen, G. (1998). Prevalence of psychiatric disorder in the general population: Results of the Netherlands Mental Health Survey and Incidence Study (NEMESIS). *Social Psychiatry and Psychiatric Epidemiology, 33*, 587–595.

Blashfield, R., Noyes, R., Reich, J., Woodman, C., Cook, B. L., & Garvey, M. (1994). Personality disorder traits in generalized anxiety and panic disorder patients. *Comprehensive Psychiatry, 35*, 329–334.

Blazer, D. G., Hughes, D., George, L. K., Swartz, M., & Boyer, R. (1991). Generalized anxiety disorder. In L. N. Robins & D. A. Regier (Eds.), *Psychiatric disorders in America* (pp. 180–203). New York: Free Press.

Brawman-Mintzer, O., & Lydiard, R. B. (1996). Generalized anxiety disorder: Issues in epidemiology. *Journal of Clinical Psychiatry, 57*(Suppl. 7), 3–8.

Brawman-Mintzer, O., Lydiard, R. B., Emmanuel, N., Payeur, R., Johnson, M., Roberts, J., Jarrell, M. P., & Ballenger, J. C. (1993). Psychiatric comorbidity in patients with generalized anxiety disorder. *American Journal of Psychiatry, 150,* 1216–1218.

Breier, A., Charney, D. S., & Heninger, G. R. (1985). The diagnostic validity of anxiety disorders and their relationship to depressive illness. *American Journal of Psychiatry, 142,* 787–797.

Breslau, N. (1985). Depressive symptoms, major depression and generalized anxiety: A comparison of self-reports on CES-D and results from diagnostic interviews. *Psychiatry Research, 15,* 219–229.

Breslau, N., & Davis, G. C. (1985a). DSM-III generalized anxiety disorder: An empirical investigation of more stringent criteria. *Psychiatry Research, 15,* 231–238.

Breslau, N., & Davis, G. C. (1985b). Further evidence on the doubtful validity of generalized anxiety disorder [Letter]. *Psychiatry Research, 16,* 177–179.

Brown, T. A., Chorpita, B. F., & Barlow, D. H. (1998). Structural relationships among dimensions of the DSM-IV anxiety and mood disorders and dimensions of negative affect, positive affect, and autonomic arousal. *Journal of Abnormal Psychology, 107,* 179–192.

Burke, K. C., Burke, J. D., Jr., Rae, D. S., & Regier, D. A. (1991). Comparing age at onset of major depression and other psychiatric disorders by birth cohorts in five U.S. community populations. *Archives of General Psychiatry, 48*(9), 789–795.

Clayton, P. J., Grove, W. M., Coryell, W., Keller, M. B., Hirschfeld, R., & Fawcett, J. (1991). Follow-up and family study of anxious depression. *American Journal of Psychiatry, 148,* 1512–1517.

Crits-Christoph, P., Connolly, M. B., Azarian, K., Crits-Christoph, K., & Shappell, S. (1996). An open trial of brief supportive–expressive psychotherapy in the treatment of generalized anxiety disorder. *Psychotherapy, 33,* 418–430.

Durham, R. C., Allan, T., & Hackett, C. A. (1997). On predicting improvement and relapse in generalized anxiety disorder following psychotherapy. *British Journal of Clinical Psychology, 36,* 101–119.

Goisman, R. M., Warshaw, M. G., & Keller, M. B. (1999). Psychosocial treatment prescriptions for generalized anxiety disorder, panic disorder, and social phobia, 1991–1996. *American Journal of Psychiatry, 156,* 1819–1821.

Gorman, J. M. (1996). Comorbid depression and anxiety spectrum disorders. *Depression and Anxiety, 4,* 160–168.

Hackett, D. (2000). Venlafaxine XR in the treatment of anxiety. *Acta Psychiatrica Scandinavica, 406,* 30–35.

Heath, A. C., Neale, M. C., Kessler, R. C., Eaves, L. J., & Kendler, K. S. (1992). Evidence for genetic influences on personality from self-reports and informant ratings. *Journal of Personality and Social Psychology, 63*(1), 85–96.

Hoehn-Saric, R., Hazlett, R. L., & McLeod, D. R. (1993). Generalized anxiety disorder with early and late onset of anxiety symptoms. *Comprehensive Psychiatry, 34,* 291–298.

International Consortium of Psychiatric Epidemiology (ICPE). (2000). Cross-national comparisons of the prevalences and correlates of mental disorders: Results from the WHO International Consortium in Psychiatric Epidemiology. *Bulletin of the World Health Organization, 78,* 413–426.

Katon, W., von Korff, M., Lin, E., Lipscomb, P., Russo, J., Wagner, E., & Polk, E. (1990). Distressed high utilizers of medical care: DSM-III-R diagnoses and treatment needs. *General Hospital Psychiatry, 12,* 355–362.

Kendler, K. S., Neale, M. C., Kessler, R. C., Heath, A. C., & Eaves, L. J. (1992a). Generalized anxiety disorder in women: A population based twin study. *Archives of General Psychiatry, 49,* 267–272.

Kendler, K. S., Neale, M. C., Kessler, R. C., Heath, A. C., & Eaves, L. J. (1992b). Major depression and generalized anxiety disorder: Same genes, (partly) different environments? *Archives of General Psychiatry, 49,* 716–722.

Kessler, R. C. (1995). The epidemiology of psychiatric comorbidity. In M. Tsuang, M. Tohen, & G. E. P. Zahner (Eds.), *Textbook of psychiatric epidemiology* (pp. 179–197). New York: Wiley.

Kessler, R. C. (1997). The prevalence of psychiatric comorbidity. In S. Wetzler & W. C. Sanderson (Eds.), *Treatment strategies for patients with psychiatric comorbidity* (pp. 23–48). New York: Wiley.

Kessler, R. C. (2000). The epidemiology of pure and comorbid generalized anxiety disorder: A review and evaluation of recent research. *Acta Psychiatrica Scandinavica, 406,* 7–13.

Kessler, R. C., Dupont, R. L., Berglund, P., & Wittchen, H.-U. (1999). Impairments in pure and comorbid generalized anxiety disorder and major depression at 12 months in two national surveys. *American Journal of Psychiatry, 156,* 1915–1923.

Kessler, R. C., McGonagle, K. A., Zhao, S., Nelson, C. B., Hughes, M., Eshleman, S., Wittchen, H.-U., & Kendler, K. S. (1994). Lifetime and 12–month prevalence of DSM-III-R psychiatric disorders in the United States: Results from the National Comorbidity Survey. *Archives of General Psychiatry, 51,* 8–19.

Kessler, R. C., Nelson, C. B., McGonagle, K. A., Liu, J., Swartz, M. S., & Blazer, D. G. (1996). Comorbidity of DSM-III-R major depressive disorder in the general population: Results from the U.S. National Comorbidity Survey. *British Journal of Psychiatry, 168,* 17–30.

Kessler, R. C., & Price, R. H. (1993). Primary prevention of secondary disorders: A proposal and agenda. *American Journal of Community Psychology, 21,* 607–633.

Lin, E., Katon, W., von Korff, M., Bush, T., Lipscomb, P., Russo, J., & Wagner, E. (1991). Frustrating patients: Physician and patient perspectives among distressed high users of medical services. *Journal of General Internal Medicine, 6,* 241–246.

Maier, W., Gansicke, M., Freyberger, H. J., Linz, M., Heun, R., & Lecrubier, Y. (2000). Generalized anxiety disorder (ICD-10) in primary care from a cross-cultural perspective: A valid diagnostic entity? *Acta Psychiatrica Scandinavia, 101,* 29–36.

Mancuso, D. M., Townsend, M. H., & Mercante, D. E. (1993). Long-term follow-up of generalized anxiety disorder. *Comprehensive Psychiatry, 34,* 441–446.

Noyes, R., Holt, C. S., & Woodman, C. L. (1996). Natural course of anxiety disorders. In M. Mavissakalian & R. F. Prien (Eds.), *Long-term treatments of anxiety disorders* (pp. 1–48). Washington, DC: American Psychiatric Press.

Noyes, R., Jr., Woodman, C., Garvey, M. J., Cook, B. L., Suelzer, M., Clancy, J., & Anderson, D. J. (1992). Generalized anxiety disorder vs. panic disorder: Distinguishing characteristics and patterns of comorbidity. *Journal of Nervous and Mental Disease, 180,* 369–379.

Offord, D. R., Boyle, M. H., Campbell, D., Goring, P., Lin, E., Wrong, M., & Racine, A. (1996). One year prevalence of psychiatric disorder in Ontarians 15 to 64 years of age. *Canadian Journal of Psychiatry, 41,* 559–563.

Offord, D. R., Campbell, D., Cochrane, J., Goering, P. N., Lin, E., Rhodes, A., & Wong, M. (1994). *Mental health in Ontario: Selected findings from the Mental Health Supplement to the Ontario Health Survey.* Toronto: Queen's Printer for Ontario.

Olfson, M., Fireman, B., Weissman, M. M., Leon, A. C., Sheehan, D. V., Kathol, R. G.,

Hoven, C., & Farber, L. (1997). Mental disorders and disability among patients in a primary care group practice. *American Journal of Psychiatry, 154,* 1734–1740.

Olfson, M., Kessler, R. C., Berglund, P. A., & Lin, E. (1998). Psychiatric disorder onset and first treatment contact in the United States and Ontario. *American Journal of Psychiatry, 155,* 1415–1422.

Ormel, J., Van den Brink, W., Koeter, M. W., Giel, R., Van Der Meer, K., Van De Willige, G., & Wilmink, F. W. (1990). Recognition, management and outcome of psychological disorders in primary care: A naturalistic follow-up study. *Psychiatric Medicine, 20,* 909–923.

Ormel, J., Von Korff, M., Ustun, B., Pini, S., Korten, A., & Oldehinkel, T. (1994). Common mental disorders and disability across cultures: Results from the WHO Collaborative Study on Psychological Problems in General Health Care. *Journal of the American Medical Association, 272,* 1741–1748.

Reich, J. (1993). Distinguished mixed anxiety/depression from anxiety and depressive groups using the family history method. *Comprehensive Psychiatry, 34,* 285–290.

Reich, J. (1995). Family psychiatric histories in male patients with generalized anxiety disorder and major depressive disorder. *Annals of Clinical Psychiatry, 7,* 71–78.

Robins, E., & Guze, S. B. (1970). Establishment of diagnostic validity in psychiatric illness: Its application to schizophrenia. *American Journal of Psychiatry, 126,* 983–987.

Rogers, M. P., Warshaw, M. G., Goisman, R. M., Goldenberg, I., Rodriguez-Villa, F., Mallya, G., Freeman, S. A., & Keller, M. B. (1999). Comparing primary and secondary generalized anxiety disorder in a long-term naturalistic study of anxiety disorders. *Depression and Anxiety, 10,* 1–7.

Roy-Byrne, P. P. (1996). Generalized anxiety and mixed anxiety–depression: Association with disability and health care utilization. *Journal of Clinical Psychiatry, 57,* 86–91.

Salzman, C., Goldenberg, I., Bruce, S. E., & Keller, M. B. (2001). Pharmacologic treatment of anxiety disorders in 1989 versus 1996: Results from the Harvard/Brown Anxiety Disorders Research Program. *Journal of Clinical Psychiatry, 62,* 149–152.

Schonfeld, W. H., Verboncoeur, C. J., Fifer, S. K., Lipschutz, R. C., Lubeck, D. P., & Bueschinf, D. P. (1997). The functioning and well-being of patients with unrecognized anxiety disorders and major depressive disorder. *Journal of Affective Disorders, 43,* 105–119.

Skodal, A. E., Schwartz, S., Dohrenwend, B. P., Levav, I., & Shrout, P. E. (1994). Minor depression in a cohort of young adults in Israel. *Archives of General Psychiatry, 51,* 542–551.

Spitzer, R. L., Kroenke, K., Linzer M., Hahn, S. R., Williams, J. B., deGruy, F. V., III, Brody, D., & Davies, M. (1995). Health-related quality of life in primary care patients with mental disorders. *Journal of the American Medical Association, 274,* 1511–1517.

Stewart, A. L., Hays, R. D., & Ware, J. E., Jr. (1988). The MOS short-form general health survey: Reliability and validity in a patient population. *Medical Care, 26,* 724–735.

Ustun, T. B., & Sartorius, N. (Eds.). (1995). *Mental illness in general health care: An international study.* Chichester, UK: Wiley.

Wang, P. S., Berglund, P., & Kessler, R. C. (2000). Recent care of common mental disorders in the United States: Prevalence and conformance with evidence-based recommendations. *Journal of General Internal Medicine, 15,* 284–292.

Warshaw, M. G., Keller, M. B., & Stout, R. L. (1994). Reliability and validity of the longitudinal interval follow-up evaluation for assessing outcome of anxiety disorders. *Journal of Psychiatric Research, 28*(6), 531–545.

Wittchen, H.-U., Zhao, S., Kessler, R. C., & Eaton, W. W. (1994). DSM-III-R generalized anxiety disorder in the National Comorbidity Survey. *Archives of General Psychiatry, 51*, 355–364.

World Health Organization (WHO). (1990). *International classification of diseases and related health problems (10th rev.): Classification of mental and behavioral disorders. Diagnostic criteria for research.* Geneva: Author.

Yonkers, K. A., Dyck, I. R., Warshaw, M., & Keller, M. B. (2000). Factors predicting the clinical course of generalized anxiety disorder. *British Journal of Psychiatry, 176*, 544–549.

Yonkers, K. A., Massion, A., Warshaw, M., & Keller, M. B. (1996). Phenomenology and course of generalized anxiety disorder. *British Journal of Psychiatry, 168*, 308–313.

Zuckerman, M. (1991). *Psychobiology of personality.* New York: Cambridge University Press.

CHAPTER 3

From Anxious Temperament to Disorder

An Etiological Model

JENNIFER L. HUDSON
RONALD M. RAPEE

Despite the recent increase in the theoretical and empirical literature devoted to generalized anxiety disorder (GAD), surprisingly few publications have examined the potential etiological pathways to the disorder. Instead, the focus has been on the nature and treatment of GAD (Dugas, 2000). For a fuller understanding of the disorder, a complete picture that includes etiology is required. An awareness of the pathways to the disorder will, in turn, have important implications for the prevention and treatment of GAD.

The current chapter reviews the available evidence regarding the development of GAD and presents a model that can be used as a guide for future etiological research.[1] Of course, this model must be considered preliminary, as etiological research in the anxiety disorders remains in its infancy. Further limiting this quest is the small number of studies that have specifically examined the development of GAD. Most relevant research has either focused on other anxiety disorders (see Hudson & Rapee, 2000) or taken a broader perspective, examining the development of the anxiety disorders as a whole.

---

[1]The model presented here is a modification of previously presented ideas (see Rapee, 2001).

Much of the research on GAD has suffered from the frequent and major changes in nosology across the editions of the American Psychiatric Association's *Diagnostic and Statistical Manual of Mental Disorders* (DSM; see Mennin, Heimberg, & Turk, Chapter 1, this volume). As a result, the few studies that have examined specific etiological factors in GAD have used a variety of different criteria, making it difficult to obtain a cohesive understanding of the ever-changing construct that is GAD.

Despite these nosological changes, one view of GAD is that it is synonymous with elevated levels of trait anxiety (Rapee, 1991). Other researchers have also argued this point, suggesting that GAD represents a more fundamental type of anxiety that may underlie the other anxiety disorders (Barlow, 2002; Brown, Barlow, & Liebowitz, 1994). As a result, the model that we present is considered applicable to anxiety disorders in general. As etiological research advances, a more refined model that incorporates specific pathways to the individual disorders may be possible. The pathways to the anxiety disorders and more specifically to GAD are likely to be varied. Thus the model presented allows for a complex array of potential pathways. The research examining these potential pathways is explored. This chapter covers (1) genetic factors; (2) temperamental factors; and (3) environmental influences (including environmental support of avoidance, the effects of the social environment, and external environmental events).

GENETIC CONTRIBUTION

Perhaps the most widely studied etiological component of anxiety is genetics. There has been a multitude of studies consistently showing that there is a significant genetic contribution to the variance in anxiety symptomatology and disorders (Andrews, Stewart, Allen, & Henderson, 1990; Andrews, Stewart, Morris-Yates, Holt, & Henderson, 1990; Jardine, Martin, & Henderson, 1984; Kendler, Neale, Kessler, Heath, & Eaves, 1992; Torgersen, 1983; Tyrer, Alexander, Remington, & Riley, 1987). Overall, these studies have suggested that genetics account for approximately 30–40% of the variance in anxiety symptomatology and disorders.

Evidence from twin studies has tended to suggest that what is inherited is a general predisposition toward anxiety and depression rather than any specific genetic factor (Andrews, Stewart, Morris-Yates, et al., 1990; Torgersen, 1983). For example, Andrews, Stewart, Morris-Yates, and colleagues (1990) carried out a large twin study of anxiety and depressive disorders. There was no evidence for the specific heritability of individual anxiety disorders; rather, the data supported a notion that what is inherited is a general propensity toward neurosis. A more recent child study examining covariance between anxious and depressive symptoms in a sample of 490 twin pairs aged 8–16 years also showed that shared genetics accounted for a large proportion of the variance (Eley, 1997).

A slightly different picture has emerged from two twin studies of GAD, major depression, and other anxiety disorders, suggesting the possibility of two genetic factors (Kendler et al., 1995; Scherrer et al., 2000). Kendler and colleagues (1995) assessed 2,163 female twins for the presence of psychiatric disorders and showed that GAD and major depression were largely influenced by the same genetic factor (Factor 1). The study also showed a shared genetic risk for panic disorder, phobia, and bulimia nervosa (Factor 2). Although anxiety and depressive disorders loaded (to some extent) on both factors, the results indicated that there may be two somewhat separate genetic pathways for these disorders. That is, an individual may inherit a general predisposition toward (1) GAD and depression or (2) panic and phobia. In a similar study of male–male twin pairs, Scherrer and colleagues (2000) examined the degree to which liability for GAD and panic disorder was due to common genetic factors. This analysis showed that whereas 22.6% of the variance in symptoms was shared between GAD and panic disorder, a unique genetic influence (i.e., not shared with GAD) accounted for 21.2% of the variance in liability for panic disorder. Although the authors argued that it made no difference to the final model, diagnosis of GAD was based on liberal criteria, which included worry for at least 1 month, rather than the more conservative DSM-IV (American Psychiatric Association, 1994) criterion of 6 months. The 1-month criterion was used because of the low prevalence rates of GAD in the sample when the 6-month criterion was employed.

Although the findings of Kendler and colleagues (1995) and Scherrer and colleagues (2000) suggest the presence of multiple genetic factors, their findings also provide continued support for a general genetic vulnerability toward anxiety and depression. At this stage, it would be premature to draw definite conclusions about the existence of more than one distinct genetic factor. Nevertheless, the evidence points to a general predisposition toward anxiety and depression rather than a specific heritability for GAD.

Evidence from family studies of anxiety suggests that the environment, not genetics, is primarily responsible for the development of a specific anxiety disorder. In addition to providing evidence for a strong familial component to anxiety, the results of family studies suggest that this component may be largely disorder-specific. For example, Noyes, Clarkson, Crowe, Yates, and McChesney (1987) showed that first-degree relatives of individuals with GAD had an increased risk for GAD, but not panic disorder, in comparison to control families. Family studies of other anxiety disorders have also produced evidence for familial transmission of specific disorders (Fyer, Mannuzza, Chapman, Martin, & Klein, 1995; Last, Hersen, Kazdin, Orvaschel, & Perrin, 1991). Although genetics may be heavily involved in an increased general risk for anxiety and depression, the development of specific disorders may be largely the result of the environment (Eley, 1997).

THE ROLE OF TEMPERAMENT

One area of research that may help to answer the question of what is inherited is the study of temperament. "Temperament," defined as an "intrinsic behavioral characteristic of a child" (Sanson, Prior, Garino, Oberklaid, & Sewell, 1987, p. 97), is likely to represent inherited qualities to some extent. Although definitions of temperament vary among theorists, it is generally agreed that temperament has a biological and genetic basis (Derryberry & Rothbart, 1984; Prior, Sanson, Oberklaid, & Northam, 1987; see Prior, 1992). Examining the link between certain temperamental patterns and later anxiety disorders may have important implications for understanding the manifestation of genetic heritability.

Several researchers have identified dimensions of temperament. For example, Thomas and Chess (1985) identified three different patterns of temperament: (1) "easy" temperament, (2) "difficult" temperament, and (3) "slow-to-warm-up" temperament. For example, a classification of a difficult temperament was given to children who displayed a negative approach response to new situations, irregular eating and sleeping, frequent crying and tantrums, and slowness in adapting to change. Another example of dimensions of temperament comes from research using the Revised Infant Temperament Questionnaire (Carey & McDevitt, 1978). This questionnaire assesses nine temperamental factors: "approach," "activity/reactivity," "food fussiness," "rhythmicity," "cooperation/manageability," "placidity," "threshold," "irritability," and "persistence." Buss and Plomin (1984) also refer to three factors of temperament: "sociability," "activity," and "emotionality."

One area of temperament research that has gained much attention in recent times is the study of "behavioral inhibition" (BI). BI is a temperamental category defined in terms of reactions of withdrawal, wariness, avoidance, and shyness in novel situations, and is assessed following a series of laboratory observations of the child's behavior in novel situations (Garcia Coll, Kagan, & Reznick, 1984; Reznick et al., 1986). Kagan (1989) suggests that approximately 15% of a normal sample of infants may be classified as exhibiting BI.

Of relevance to the current review is the degree to which these temperamental dimensions and categories are related to later anxiety symptoms and disorders. Research that has examined this potential link has been carried out by examining (1) retrospective reports of anxious adults regarding their temperament as children; (2) temperament and anxiety symptoms in infants and children; (3) temperament in children at risk of developing anxiety disorders; or (4) temperament and its longitudinal association with later anxiety symptoms and disorders. Again, much of this research, with the exception of some of the BI studies, has broadly examined anxiety symptoms and disorders rather than GAD specifically.

Retrospective Reports from Anxious Adults

The retrospective report of anxious adults has indicated that anxious behaviors may be identifiable from an early age. For example, adults with GAD commonly report being anxious all of their lives (Rapee, 1991). Studies of other anxiety disorders have also shown that anxious adults report higher levels of anxiety symptoms or anxiety-related behaviors as children in comparison to control groups (Lipsitz et al., 1994; Rapee & Melville, 1997).

Temperament and Anxiety in Children

In research at the Child and Adolescent Anxiety Clinic at Macquarie University, mothers of clinically anxious children (n = 95) were more likely to report retrospectively that their children were "difficult" in the first year of life (crying, difficulties sleeping, pain, and gas) than mothers of children who were not clinically anxious (n = 75) (Rapee & Szollos, 1997). Differences between these groups were also evident in later years, with the mothers of anxious children reporting that their children had more fears in the second year of life, greater difficulties settling into day care and school, and greater difficulties adjusting to babysitters. Interestingly, children with specific anxiety disorders did not differ on these measures.

Temperament Studies of At-Risk Children

Several studies have examined temperament in children at risk for developing an anxiety disorder. Merikangas, Avenevoli, Dierker, and Grillon (1999) measured temperament and psychophysiology in children of parents with an anxiety disorder. Children of anxious parents were not shown to differ from children of nonanxious parents on questionnaire measures of temperament. However they did differ on several psychophysiological measures that may reflect differences in arousal. Thus it is possible that the differences in psychophysiology may reflect a difference in vulnerability to anxiety in these children.

Slightly different results were found in an examination of children of parents with panic disorder and agoraphobia and/or major depressive disorder (Rosenbaum et al., 1988). Children of parents with panic disorder and agoraphobia with or without comorbid depression were more

likely to be classified as BI than children of parents without panic disorder and agoraphobia.

Longitudinal Studies

One of the most informative methods of examining the link between temperament and anxiety disorder is longitudinal research. Several studies
have examined temperament and anxiety using this method (Biederman
et al., 1993, 2001; Caspi, Henry, McGee, Moffitt, & Silva, 1995; Rende,
1993; Rubin, 1993). For example, Rende (1993) followed 1- to 4-year-old
children until the age of 7 years. Mothers' reports of temperament were
assessed with the Emotionality, Activity, and Sociability Scale (Buss &
Plomin, 1984), and mothers' reports of the child's internalizing and
externalizing symptoms were assessed with the Child Behavior Checklist
(CBCL; Achenbach & Edelbrock, 1979). Supporting the notion of a temperamental component in the development of anxiety, the study showed
that anxiety and depressive symptoms at age 7 were related to (1) higher
levels of emotionality in infancy and early childhood for both boys and
girls, and (2) lower levels of sociability for girls only.

Perhaps the most impressive body of longitudinal data relates to BI.
The findings from a 3-year follow-up of infants with and without BI suggest that an inhibited child is significantly more likely than an uninhibited
child to have DSM-III-R avoidant disorder of childhood, separation anxiety disorder, or agoraphobia at baseline measurement, and also more
likely to develop avoidant disorder and separation anxiety disorder over
the following 3-year period (Biederman et al., 1993). Children with stable
BI over the 3-year period were more likely than children with unstable BI
or without BI to develop an anxiety disorder. This result suggests that the
stability of BI may be an important factor in the development of anxiety.
In another study, 164 children identified at 4 months of age as either
"high-reactive" (high levels of motor activity, high levels of crying) or "low-
reactive" (low levels of motor activity/crying) were followed for 7 years
(Kagan, Snidman, Zentner, & Peterson, 1999). In support of the previous
findings, a greater number of high-reactive infants than of low-reactive infants (45% vs. 15%) exhibited anxious symptoms at age 7.

Taken together, the results of retrospective and prospective studies
support a link between early temperamental styles and anxiety. More specifically, temperamental styles of high arousal, emotionality, and BI are
likely to place a child at risk for developing later anxiety symptoms and
disorders. Although research has identified temperamental factors associated with later anxiety, it is important to note that not all temperamentally
vulnerable children develop an anxiety disorder. This finding suggests
that there must be other factors—probably environmental—that affect
whether a vulnerable child ultimately develops an anxiety disorder. There

has been much focus in the literature on potential environmental factors involved in the development of anxiety disorders.

ENVIRONMENTAL INFLUENCES

In addition to providing information on heritability, behavior-genetic studies provide evidence for the instrumental role of the environment in the development of anxiety disorders. Results from *adult* twin studies indicate a fundamental role for nonshared environmental factors (experiences specific to the individual) in the development of anxiety disorders, while shared environmental factors (experiences common to siblings in a family) have been shown to play a minimal role (Jardine et al., 1984; Kendler et al., 1995). Some researchers have argued that the family is only likely to be important in the development of psychopathology when it is part of a child's nonshared environment (Pike & Plomin, 1996; Rowe, 1997). In contrast, the results emerging from several recent twin studies of *children* demonstrate that shared environmental factors account for a significant amount of variance in both anxiety symptoms and disorders (Edelbrock, Rende, Plomin, & Thompson, 1995; Eley, 1997; Thapar & McGuffin, 1995; Topolski et al., 1997). In fact, in one study, shared environment was the only significant predictor of variance in self-reported anxiety symptoms in a sample of adolescent twins recruited from the community (Thapar & McGuffin, 1995). Although these results may seem to portray an exaggerated account of the role of shared environment, the overall results from child twin studies indicate a more important role for shared environment than is indicated by adult studies.

Recently, however, Kendler (2001) has argued that two limitations of the twin study methodology may cause the results to underrepresent the role of the family environment. First, Kendler has argued that the twin modeling studies define the "family environment" as those experiences shared between siblings that contribute to similarity. When a child responds to a family event (such as divorce or parental discipline) differently from his or her sibling, this would be defined by twin studies as part of the child's individual environment and not as part of the shared environment. Second, Kendler argues that twin studies have limited statistical power to assess the family environment, and large samples are required to detect even a moderate effect. Thus the twin modeling methodology may not provide an accurate assessment of the family environment.

So in what way may one's environment shape the development of GAD? Three sources of environmental influence that may be of importance in the development of anxiety disorders are (1) environmental support of avoidance, (2) transmission of threat and coping information, and (3) external environmental events.

Environmental Support of Avoidance

Avoidance of threatening stimuli has been clearly identified as an integral factor in the maintenance of anxiety disorders. It is our belief that environmental support of avoidance behavior promotes the development of anxiety disorders by further fueling an anxious vulnerability. An inhibited child may select from his or her environment components that foster the child's tendency to avoid novel/threatening stimuli. In turn, this continual avoidance may further shape the child's temperamental vulnerability to pathology. In the early years, a child's parents form the primary environment and therefore the greatest opportunity for supporting this avoidant style of interacting with the world. Through the years, the influence of siblings and peers may become increasingly important.

Parental Support of Avoidance

Despite some behavior geneticists' argument that the family environment is not important in the development of anxiety disorders, the potential role of parenting in the development of psychopathology has received much attention in the literature. In a review of parenting and the anxiety disorders, Rapee (1997) concluded that despite the multitude of methodological problems limiting the research in this area, there are surprisingly consistent findings linking controlling and overprotective parenting with the anxiety disorders. The ultimate consequence of these parenting behaviors may be the limitation of a child's interaction with the environment. That is, a parent's behavior may support a child's avoidance.

Although much of this research has been retrospective in nature, several studies of anxious children and their parents have allowed a more thorough testing of this association (e.g., Barrett, Rapee, Dadds, & Ryan, 1996; Chorpita, Albano, & Barlow, 1996; Hirshfeld, Biederman, Brody, Faraone, & Rosenbaum, 1997; Hudson & Rapee, 2001; Siqueland, Kendall, & Steinberg, 1996).

Barrett and colleagues (1996) examined the responses of anxious children aged 7–14 years to a hypothetical situation of ambiguous threat before and after a discussion of the situation with their parents. Anxious children reported more avoidant coping responses after the discussion of the situation with their parents than before. In contrast, children with oppositional defiant disorder and control children showed a decrease in avoidant responses following the family discussion. Further analysis of the family discussion revealed that parents of anxious children supported avoidant responses by their child to the situation (Dadds, Barrett, Rapee, & Ryan, 1996).

To further examine the parenting of anxious children, we designed a task that would enable the measurement of involvement and help-giving behaviors in mothers of anxious children (Hudson & Rapee, 2001). Children were given a moderately stressful puzzle task, and their mothers' behavior during the task was assessed. Clear differences were identified in degree of involvement between mothers of anxious children and mothers of nonanxious children. Mothers of children with anxiety disorders gave more help and were more intrusive with their help during the task than were mothers of nonanxious children. These results further indicate that parents of anxious children may be attempting to prevent the children from experiencing distress by rushing in to help, rather than allowing the children to solve the problem on their own.

Using a similar design, we examined parent–child interactions in the siblings of anxious children in order to determine whether overinvolved parenting was specific to the anxious children. We predicted that nonanxious siblings of anxious children would not experience the same amount of parental involvement during the task as the anxious children would. Our hypotheses were developed from theories of "child effects" on parenting; that is, parenting behaviors do not occur in isolation, but rather are influenced to some extent by a child's temperament (e.g., Bell, 1977). Although the preliminary results of this study (Hudson & Rapee, 1998) supported our hypothesis, the final results showed a nonsignificant difference in parental involvement during the task for anxious children and their siblings (Hudson & Rapee, 2002). Compared to mothers of nonanxious children, mothers of anxious children were more involved during interactions with both the anxious children and the siblings of the anxious children. If, as the results of this study suggest, parental overinvolvement does not occur specifically in response to an anxious child, it is possible that factors such as parental anxiety or personality contribute to the development of an overprotective, overinvolved parenting style (Levy, 1943; Parker, 1983; Parker & Lipscombe, 1981).

The majority of studies that have examined the relationship between parenting behavior and anxiety disorders have been limited by their inability to test causality and the direction of potential effect. One study that has employed longitudinal methods has indicated an interaction effect between parenting and temperament. In home observations of high- and low-reactive infants, Arcus (cited in Kagan, Snidman, Arcus, & Reznick, 1994) showed that the degree to which mothers held their infants when the infants did not need help predicted the children's fear approximately a year later. However, this effect was found only for high-reactive infants. One possible explanation of these results is that parental overprotection on its own may not be sufficient to cause increased anxiety; however, when it occurs in the presence of inhibited temperament, it does so.

Conclusions regarding the reciprocal relationship between temperament and parental behavior need to be postponed until further longitudinal inquiry of the relationship is carried out. Nevertheless, research so far has established that parental overinvolvement—that is, behavior supporting a child's restricted exposure to his or her environment—is linked with moderate consistency to the anxiety disorders in general. The research has not indicated a unique relationship between parenting and GAD.

There has also been a substantial amount of literature and research on an infant's attachment to his or her caregiver. According to Bowlby (1969/1974, 1973), an infant's attachment or bond with his or her caregiver serves an evolutionary function to bring the infant into closer proximity with the caregiver. Ainsworth, Blehar, Waters, and Wall (1978) proposed that a securely attached infant uses the mother (or other primary caregiver) as a secure base from which to explore the environment. Ainsworth's "Strange Situation" allows an infant's behavior in relation to the mother to be categorized into one of four main attachment classifications: (1) avoidant, (2) secure, (3) ambivalent, or (4) disorganized (Ainsworth et al., 1978; Main & Solomon, 1986). An infant with an avoidant attachment tends to minimize distress during separation from and reunion with the caregiver. The baby resists contact with the caregiver throughout the situation and displays obvious avoidance of the caregiver on reunion. Parents of avoidant infants have been described as rejecting and insensitive to their children's needs (Ainsworth et al., 1978). Secure infants seek proximity and contact with their caregivers, particularly on reunion. These infants may become distressed when mothers separate from them, but are easily soothed when the caregivers return. Mothers of secure infants have been described as sensitive to their children's needs (Ainsworth et al., 1978). Conversely, children with ambivalent attachments maximize their distress following separation and reunion. They have extreme difficulty separating from their caregivers and have difficulty being soothed on reunion. Such a baby may demonstrate anger toward the caregiver or may appear passive. Mothers of ambivalent infants tend to be less rejecting than mothers of avoidant babies; nevertheless, they display less affectionate behavior than mothers of secure infants (Ainsworth et al., 1978). Children with disorganized attachments tend to have no systematic strategy for responding to their caregivers. This fourth category was introduced by Main and Solomon (1986) as a means of classifying infants whose behavior did not obviously fall into the other three categories. Infants with disorganized attachments are more likely to come from maltreated samples and are at greatest risk for social, biological, and developmental problems (Carlson, Cichetti, Barnett, & Braunwald, 1989; Cummings & Cicchetti, 1990; Main & Solomon, 1990).

Only two studies have examined the relationship of attachment in infancy to the presence of anxiety disorders in childhood or adolescence (Shaw, Keenan, Vondra, Delliquadri, & Giovannelli, 1997; Warren, Huston, Egeland, & Sroufe, 1997). Warren and colleagues (1997) examined the attachment classifications of 172 infants at 12 months of age and followed them into adolescence. Only the first three attachment categories were examined (avoidant, secure, and ambivalent). Of the infants classified as having ambivalent attachments at 12 months, 28% were diagnosed with an anxiety disorder in adolescence, compared to 12% of securely attached infants and 16% of infants with avoidant attachments. Ambivalent attachment was associated with increased risk of developing an anxiety disorder in adolescence even after a mother's anxiety and a child's temperament were accounted for.

Similarly, Shaw and colleagues (1997) followed a sample of 12-month-old infants from low-income families for 4 years. In this study, all four categories of attachment were assessed. Disorganized attachment at 12 months significantly predicted the child's internalizing symptoms as measured by the CBCL (Achenbach & Edelbrock, 1979) at 5 years of age. However, on closer examination, the withdrawal items of the CBCL significantly correlated with disorganized attachment, whereas no significant association was found between attachment and items measuring depression or anxiety. These results suggest that although disorganized attachment may predict symptoms of withdrawal later in life, it does not necessarily predict symptoms of anxiety or depression.

Maternal anxiety has also been identified as a factor contributing to the development of insecure attachment. For example, Manassis, Bradley, Goldberg, Hood, and Swinson (1994) showed that in a sample of 18 anxiety-disordered mothers of preschool-age children, 80% of the children were identified as insecurely attached (note that specific types of insecure attachments were not examined in this study). Thus children with anxious mothers may be more likely than children of nonanxious mothers to develop insecure attachments. As anxious children are more likely to have anxious parents (Last, Hersen, Kazdin, Francis, & Grubb, 1987), these results have important implications for children with anxiety disorders.

Finally, Rapee and colleagues have recently shown that attachment style and temperament may interact in the production of anxious symptoms. Preschool children aged about 4 years were assessed both in the laboratory to determine inhibition and in a standard Strange Situation assessment with their mother (Shamir-Essakow, Ungerer, & Rapee, 2002). Anxiety diagnoses were determined via structured interview with the mothers. Ambivalent attachment style was associated with anxiety diagnoses in the children, but this was mediated by a strong correlation between ambivalent attachment and BI. On the other hand, avoidant attachment interacted with BI to predict anxiety diagnoses. Specifically, children who were showed both BI and avoidant attachment were much more likely to have received anxiety diagnoses than children in the other quadrants.

In summary, the evidence from the attachment literature provides information that mother–child bonds at an early age may be predictive of later anxiety disorders. So far, one study has shown that infants with insecure (ambivalent) attachments appear to be at greater risk of developing an anxiety disorder. However, it is possible that this is a result of shared variance with an inhibited temperament. On the other hand, there is emerging evidence that an avoidant attachment style may interact with inhibition to produce anxious symptomatology, although further longitudinal studies are needed.

Nonparental Support of Avoidance

In a similar manner to spending time with parents, spending time with peers or siblings who are also anxious, introverted, or hesitant to take risks may further exacerbate an anxious child's temperament by limiting those activities that could potentially allow habituation of his or her fears. This is an understudied area, and there is very limited empirical evidence to support these hypotheses. More recently, however, there has been a trend in the literature toward investigating the influence of peers in the development of personality and psychopathology. For example, some recent research has pointed to the possible importance of the peer group in maintaining attitudes related to weight concerns and dieting (Paxton, Schutz, Wertheim, & Muir, 1999). Some authors have even argued for the importance of the peer group to the virtual exclusion of parental influence (Harris, 1995). Although it is unlikely that peer influence exceeds the impact of other environmental factors, this is nevertheless an important area of investigation.

Transmission of Threat and Coping Information

The environment can also be influential in the development of anxiety through the transmission of threat and coping information. This transmission may occur via modeling (Bandura & Rosenthal, 1966) or through the direct provision of threat or coping information. An individual may learn to be fearful or anxious in certain situations by watching the behavior of others. Although this method of learning has been less clearly defined for GAD, several studies using both animal and human subjects have demonstrated the pivotal role of modeling in the acquisition of phobias (Cook & Mineka, 1989; Muris, Steerneman, Merckelbach, & Meesters, 1996; Ollendick & King, 1991). For example, Cook and Mineka (1989) found that rhesus monkeys developed a fear of toy snakes by observing a videotape of other monkeys demonstrating fear responses to toy snakes. Furthermore, in a community study of 1,092 children, Ollendick and King (1991) showed that 56% of the children attributed the onset of their fears to vicarious conditioning experiences, and 39% of these children attributed the acquisition of their fear to being told stories about the feared object by parents, teachers, friends, or acquaintances.

In a recent study, Gerull and Rapee (2002) investigated whether mothers' modeling of fearful responses affected their infants' approach–avoidance behavior. Mothers from the community and their infants aged 15–20 months were shown two novel threatening stimuli (a rubber snake and a spider). The mothers were instructed to reveal the object to the children and respond with a happy or fearful facial expression and tone. After 1- and 10-minute delays, the infants were presented with the stimuli again. This time, the mothers' expressions were neutral. Observation of their behavior on the second and third trials showed that children were more likely to avoid the object when it was initially paired with a fearful expression.

These results suggest that infants' approach–avoidance behavior toward a novel object can be affected for up to 10 minutes following a single pairing with mothers' facial expressions. The potential effect of repeated and extended modeling of anxious behavior in novel situations is likely to be more long-lasting. Even more dramatic effects may occur for inhibited children who already exhibit avoidance behavior in novel situations. The parents' own anxiety may also contribute to the degree to which modeling shapes their children's responses to novel objects. The more anxious a parent, the more likely he or she would be to demonstrate fearful or anxious behavior. The combination of an anxious parent and a vulnerable child is likely to augment the effect of modeling on the child's behavior. Although these data refer to learning of specific fears, there is little doubt that GAD consists of fears of many specific situations and events. It might be speculated that if a young child is exposed to an anxious parent who displays fearfulness in response to a wide variety of cues, the child will eventually learn to generalize the reflected fearfulness and will eventually internalize a more general rule, such as "The world is a dangerous place."

Children model their behavior not only on their parents' behavior, but also on that of others, such as peers and siblings. As the children grow older, their behavior is more likely to be influenced by the opinions and behaviors of peers than by those of their parents. Adults too may model and learn from the anxious behavior of spouses/partners, peers, colleagues, or society. These sources of influence, though potentially important in shaping an anxious individual, have received far less attention in the literature than has the influence of parents.

External Environmental Events

Contributing significantly to an understanding of the etiology of anxiety disorders is the awareness of the impact of external environmental events. This includes both the impact of stressful life events and the learning of particular associations through conditioning experiences. Positive experiences or learning of safety cues may also act as protective factors.

The experience of stressful events during childhood has been clearly linked to an increased risk for the development of anxiety disorders (Tiet et al., 1998). Retrospective reports of adults and children provide further support for this link (Brown & Harris, 1993; Brown, Harris, & Eales, 1993; Faravelli, Webb, Amboentti, Fonnescu, & Sessarego, 1985; Rapee & Szollos, 1997). For example, parents of clinically anxious children reported that their children experienced a greater number of stressful events in their early years, in comparison to the reports of mothers of nonanxious children (Rapee & Szollos, 1997).

Specific research examining the occurrence of traumatic events in the lives of both adults and children with GAD also supports this link. Adults with GAD (clinical and undergraduate samples) were more likely than nonanxious adults to report exposure to a potentially traumatic event (Roemer, Molina, Litz, & Borkovec, 1997). Torgersen (1986) compared individuals with GAD to patients with panic disorder, showing that patients with GAD were more likely to report the death of a parent before age 16. In a sample of children with anxiety disorders, Manassis and Hood (1998) found that psychosocial adversity predicted the degree of impairment in children with GAD, but did not predict impairment in children with phobic disorders. Taken together, these findings provide preliminary evidence that traumatic events may play a significant role in the development of anxiety disorders, particularly GAD.

Early adverse events have also been shown to have a significant and lasting effect on an individual's physiology. More specifically, there is evidence that early stressful events can lead to increased activity of corticotropin-releasing factor neurons and to changes in the functioning of the hypothalamic–pituitary–adrenal axis (see Dienstbier, 1989; Heim & Nemeroff, 1999; Sapolsky, 1989). These changes in physiology may place a child at greater risk of developing an anxiety disorder by increasing his or her sensitivity to stress.

Research with anxious adults has indicated that the number of stressful events is not related to the onset of anxiety. Rather, the impact of the negative events may be mediated by the individual's vulnerability to anxiety. Rapee, Litwin, and Barlow (1990) asked clinically anxious adults (including those with GAD) and nonanxious adults to report on the number and impact of stressful life events in the 6 months preceding onset of their disorder. Raters who were unaware of participants' anxiety status examined each of the stressors, providing an objective rating of the event's negativity. There were no differences between the two groups in the number of stressful events or in the objective ratings of negativity. Despite this, clinically anxious adults reported a greater negative impact of the events than nonanxious adults, leading the authors to conclude that the impact of the negative life events was influenced by the individuals' prior vulnerability to anxiety. That is, when an individual vulnerable to anxiety is faced with a negative life event, the event is likely to be experienced as more distressing.

One factor that is considered integral in understanding the effects of stressful events is controllability (Chorpita & Barlow, 1998). Chorpita and Barlow (1998) hypothesize that early experience of reduced control over one's environment will increase a child's vulnerability to anxiety disorder. They propose that an environment of reduced control leads to an increased probability of interpreting future situations as uncontrollable. This may involve dramatic experiences of uncontrollability, such as chronic abuse or neglect, as well as chronically impoverished environments. But more commonly, it is likely to reflect more subtle effects—such as overcontrolling parenting, in which the child is limited in his or her degree of decision making (e.g., see Rapee, 1997). Low perceptions of control are said to increase the individual's underlying inhibition (Gray, 1987; Kagan, Reznick, & Snidman, 1987) and may also result in a general sense of lack of safety (e.g., Woody & Rachman, 1994).

Some of the strongest support for this model comes from research with infant rhesus monkeys. Monkeys reared in an environment in which they had complete control over the delivery of food, water, and treats displayed significantly less fear and more exploratory behavior in novel environments than monkeys reared in situations of limited control (Mineka, Gunnar, & Champoux, 1986). These results support the hypothesis that control over one's environment may be causally associated with lower levels of fearfulness.

In summary, adverse life events, particularly uncontrollable events, may place an individual at greater risk of developing an anxiety disorder. Stressful, uncontrollable events early in life may alter the individual's ability to respond to future stressors by increasing physiological arousal and sensitivity to future stressors. Although some stressors may be severe and traumatic enough to lead directly to the onset of an anxiety disorder, the impact of external environmental events is more likely to be the result of an interaction between the individual's temperament and the stressor.

A MODEL OF THE DEVELOPMENT OF GAD

From this review of the etiological research, it is obvious that many pathways may lead an individual to develop anxiety disorders such as GAD. These pathways are not yet fully understood, and so far only a partial picture can be offered. The model, presented in Figure 3.1, is partly speculative because of the limited research available on the etiology of GAD. The model depicts six main factors that have been discussed throughout this chapter: (1) genetic factors, (2) anxious vulnerability (manifested by temperament), (3) parental anxiety, (4) environmental support of avoidance, (5) transmission of threat and coping information, and (6) external environmental effects.

It is clear that there is a strong genetic component contributing to the

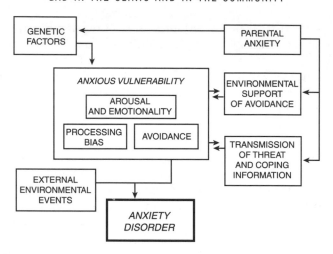

FIGURE 3.1. An etiological model of anxiety. From Rapee (2001). Copyright 2001 by Oxford University Press. Adapted by permission.

anxiety disorders, although the specific manifestation of these genetic factors is not yet clear. What is clear is that GAD shares much of its genetic variance with both depression and the other anxiety disorders. There has been some evidence that there may also be a unique genetic contribution to individual anxiety disorders, although this is still far from clear. A child who inherits a genetic predisposition toward anxiety is likely to exhibit an anxious vulnerability, manifested partly as increased sensitivity, greater emotionality, and greater physiological arousal to threat. These temperamental variables are likely to contribute to the maintenance of the child's vulnerability to anxiety. Greater emotionality and greater physiological arousal may give rise to an increased tendency to interpret situations as threatening, as well as a more avoidant coping style. An inhibited child who avoids novel stimuli is prevented from habituating to potentially fearful stimuli. The child's restriction of exposure to the world increases the child's sensitization to novel stimuli. This behavior may also lead to the limited development of social skills and coping skills, further contributing to the impact the disorder will have on the individual's life. Initially, the child may be rewarded for avoidance of novel situations by the reduction of distress and attention from others in the environment. This maladaptive pattern may further serve to promote the child's avoidance. In addition to behavioral avoidance, Borkovec, Alcaine, and Behar (Chapter 4, this volume) argue that worry, a key feature of GAD (Barlow, 2002; Rapee, 1991), reflects a strategy of cognitive avoidance. Borkovec and colleagues argue that worry serves to suppress processing of threat information and lower physiological arousal. Despite the fact that GAD is characterized by above-average arousal, worry serves to restrict physiological arousal (Brown, Chorpita, & Barlow, 1998).

It is possible that the child's anxious temperament allows selection of behaviors from others in his or her environment (parents, siblings, teachers, peers) that provide support for the child's style of interacting with the world. The relationship between the child's anxious vulnerability and environmental support of avoidance is represented in Figure 3.1 with bidirectional arrows. The parents of a child with an anxious temperament may be more likely to become overinvolved with their child in an effort to reduce and prevent the child's distress. This maladaptive pattern of parental overinvolvement in turn may reinforce the child's vulnerability to anxiety by increasing the child's perception of threat, reducing the child's perceived control over threat, and ultimately increasing the child's avoidance of threat. That is, parents who protect their child from stressful experiences or who take control in stressful situations may teach their child that the world is a dangerous place from which the child needs protection and over which he or she has no control. In terms of adult models of GAD, the child may thus be directed into an ongoing search for safety (Woody & Rachman, 1994) or may be left with a low illusion of control (Barlow, 2002). Conversely, parents who encourage their child's independence and encourage their child to face difficult situations may reduce the likelihood of their child's developing an anxiety disorder. Other significant persons (such as peers, siblings, spouse/partner, teachers, and colleagues) may also help to support and maintain this maladaptive style.

In addition to supporting the individual's natural avoidant coping style, various aspects of the social environment may provide an individual with new behaviors and attitudes. Foremost among these would be verbal instructions or modeling of anxious behaviors, which are likely to further shape an individual's vulnerability toward disorder. This relationship is also likely to be of a bidirectional nature. An individual may model the anxious behavior of other significant persons in his or her environment (parents, peers, siblings) and learn how to behave in the face of fearful or ambiguous stimuli by observing these persons. To some extent, these socialization experiences may occur independently of the child's anxious temperament. However, an anxious child is likely to choose an environment that increases the likelihood of being exposed to anxious modeling of behavior. For example, temperamentally anxious children may associate with anxious peers. In addition to transmission of information via modeling and verbalizations, cultural and social influences may provide the individual with anxious behaviors.

Given the familial basis of anxiety (Last et al., 1991; Silverman, Cerny, & Nelles, 1988), parents of anxious children are also likely to be anxious and to exhibit a cognitive bias toward threat. Therefore, an anxious parent may be more likely to overprotect his or her child, due to an increased perception of danger and an increased sensitivity to the child's distress. The model depicts the contribution parental anxiety makes not only through the genetic transmission of anxiety, but also through the increased likelihood of modeling of anxious behavior and support of avoidant behavior.

An individual who is vulnerable to anxiety may also experience stressful events that still further increase the individual's vulnerability. Research has suggested that one of the integral factors in determining the impact of the stressful event is the controllability of the event: The more uncontrollable the environment, the greater the anxiety (Chorpita & Barlow, 1998). Furthermore, research has indicated that events related to danger, and not loss, are more likely to trigger anxiety than depression (Finlay-Jones & Brown, 1981). We predict that the experience of uncontrollable threat events interacts with the individual's vulnerability to produce an episode of disorder. Given a sufficiently vulnerable individual, little or no environmental trigger may be necessary to produce an anxiety disorder. Similarly, given an environmental event of sufficient magnitude, even low-vulnerability individuals may develop a disorder (e.g., posttraumatic stress disorder). But in most cases, we expect a combination of more or less vulnerability interacting with more or less severe stressors to be involved in the development of an anxiety disorder. In the case of GAD, we would predict that the typical picture would be of greater input from temperamental vulnerability and little or no input from objectively dramatic life events.

The distinction between vulnerability and disorder is a fine one. In fact, some studies have been unable to differentiate between individuals high in trait anxiety and clinically anxious individuals (e.g., see Ladouceur, Blais, Freeston, & Dugas, 1998). The difference between vulnerability and disorder, however, is likely to represent a difference in severity and interference of anxiety symptoms. With increasing severity and interference, the individual moves along a pathway from vulnerability to disorder. This progression may occur in response to specific or non-specific threat experiences; as a result, the onset of disorder may occur gradually with accumulating stressors, or dramatically in the case of a specific threat experience. The increase in "usual" levels of anxiety is accompanied by increased avoidance behavior, decreased perceptions of control and increased perceptions of threat, thereby maintaining the increased severity and interference of anxiety symptoms (see Rapee, 1991; Woody & Rachman, 1994) and maintaining the presence of disorder.

The onset of disorder may also be influenced by the individual's developmental level. For example, an inhibited, emotional child may not develop GAD until he or she reaches school age. At school, the child is presented with increased stressors, such as separation from parents, homework, performance situations, and formal schedules. There is a noticeable developmental shift in the foci of children's fear from early childhood to adolescence (see Schniering, Hudson, & Rapee, 2000). In young children, fears tend to be more concrete, while in adolescence, anxiety is more likely to focus on social-evaluative concerns and more abstract worries. The child's cognitive and emotional development is likely to have an impact on the transition from vulnerability to disorder.

In conclusion, the model presented here is tentative. The etiological research has been far from conclusive about direct pathways to GAD. The model is intended as a guide for future research and highlights those areas that have received limited attention. The model also provides preliminary direction for research into the prevention of anxiety disorders. From the information available on the etiology of anxiety disorders, only a general model of anxiety disorders can truly be presented. It is hoped that in the future a clearer understanding of pathways to specific disorders will be possible.

REFERENCES

Achenbach, T. M., & Edelbrock, C. S. (1979). The Child Behavior Profile: 2. Boys aged 12–16 and girls aged 6–11 and 12–16. *Journal of Consulting and Clinical Psychology, 47,* 223–233.

Ainsworth, M. D. S., Blehar, M. C., Waters, E., & Wall, S. (1978). *Patterns of attachment: A study of the Strange Situation.* Hillsdale, NJ: Erlbaum.

American Psychiatric Association. (1994). *Diagnostic and statistical manual of mental disorders* (4th ed.). Washington, DC: Author.

Andrews, G., Stewart, G. W., Allen, R., & Henderson, A. S. (1990). The genetics of six neurotic disorders: A twin study. *Journal of Affective Disorders, 19,* 23–29.

Andrews, G., Stewart, G. W., Morris-Yates, A., Holt, P., & Henderson, A. S. (1990). Evidence for a general neurotic syndrome. *British Journal of Psychiatry, 157,* 6–12.

Bandura, A., & Rosenthal, T. (1966). Vicarious classical conditioning as a function of arousal level. *Journal of Personality and Social Psychology, 3,* 54–62.

Barlow, D. H. (2002). *Anxiety and its disorders: The nature and treatment of anxiety and panic* (2nd ed.). New York: Guilford Press.

Barrett, P. M., Rapee, R. M., Dadds, M. R., & Ryan, S. (1996). Family enhancement of cognitive style in anxious and aggressive children. *Journal of Abnormal Child Psychology, 24,* 187–203.

Bell, R. Q. (1977). Socialization findings reexamined. In R. Q. Bell & L. V. Harper (Eds.), *Child effects on adults* (pp. 53–84). Hillsdale, NJ: Erlbaum.

Biederman, J., Rosenbaum, J. F., Bolduc-Murphy, E. A., Faraone, S. V., Chaloff, J., Hirshfeld, D. R., & Kagan, J. (1993). A 3–year follow-up of children with and without behavioral inhibition. *Journal of the American Academy of Child and Adolescent Psychiatry, 32,* 814–821.

Biederman, J., Hirshfeld-Becker, D. R., Rosenabum, J. F., Herot, C., Friedman, D., Snidman, N., Kagan, J., & Faraone, S. V. (2001). Further evidence of association between behavioral inhibition and social anxiety in children. *American Journal of Psychiatry, 158,* 1673–1679.

Bowlby, J. (1973). *Attachment and loss: Vol. 2. Separation.* London: Hogarth Press.

Bowlby, J. (1974). *Attachment and loss: Vol. 1. Attachment.* London: Hogarth Press. (Original work published 1969)

Brown, G. W., & Harris, T. O. (1993). Etiology of anxiety and depressive disorders in an inner-city population: 1. Early adversity. *Psychological Medicine, 23,* 143–154.

Brown, G. W., Harris, T. O., & Eales, M. J. (1993). Etiology of anxiety and depressive disorder in an inner-city population: 2. Comorbidity and adversity. *Psychological Medicine, 23,* 155–165.

Brown, T. A., Barlow, D. H., & Liebowitz, M. R. (1994). The empirical basis of generalized anxiety disorder. *American Journal of Psychiatry, 151,* 1272–1280.

Brown, T. A., Chorpita, B. F., & Barlow, D. H. (1998). Structural relationships among dimensions of the DSM-IV anxiety and mood disorders and dimensions of negative affect, positive affect, and autonomic arousal. *Journal of Abnormal Psychology, 107,* 179–192.

Buss, A. H., & Plomin, R. (1984). *Temperament: Early developing personality traits.* Hillsdale, NJ: Erlbaum.

Carey, W. B., & McDevitt, S. C. (1978). Revision of the Infant Temperament Questionnaire. *Pediatrics, 68,* 735–739.

Carlson, V., Cicchetti, D., Barnett, D., & Braunwald, K. (1989). Disorganized/disoriented attachment relationships in maltreated infants. *Developmental Psychology, 25,* 525–531.

Caspi, A., Henry, B., McGee, R. O., Moffitt, T. E., & Silva, P. A. (1995). Temperamental origins of child and adolescent behavior problems: From age three to age fifteen. *Child Development, 66,* 55–68.

Chorpita, B. F., Albano, A. M., & Barlow, D. H. (1996). Cognitive processing in children: Relation to anxiety and family influences. *Journal of Clinical Child Psychology, 25,* 170–176.

Chorpita, B. F., & Barlow, D. H. (1998). The development of anxiety: The role of control in the early environment. *Psychological Bulletin, 124,* 3–21.

Cook, M., & Mineka, S. (1989). Observational conditioning of fear to fear-relevant versus fear-irrelevant stimuli in rhesus monkeys. *Journal of Abnormal Psychology, 98,* 448–459.

Cummings, E. M., & Cicchetti, D. (1990). Toward a transactional model of relations between attachment and depression. In M. T. Greenberg, D. Cicchetti, & E. M. Cummings (Eds.), *Attachment in the preschool years: Theory, research and interventions* (pp. 339–372). Chicago: University of Chicago Press.

Dadds, M. R., Barrett, P. M., Rapee, R. M., & Ryan, S. (1996). Family process and child anxiety and aggression: An observational analysis. *Journal of Abnormal Child Psychology, 24,* 715–734.

Derryberry, D., & Rothbart, M. K. (1984). Emotion, attention and temperament. In C. Izard, J. Kagan, & R. Zajonc (Eds.), *Emotions, cognition, and behavior* (pp. 132–166). Cambridge, UK: Cambridge University Press.

Dienstbier, R. A. (1989). Arousal and physiological toughness: Implications for mental and physical health. *Psychological Review, 96,* 84–100.

Dugas, M. J. (2000). Generalized anxiety disorder publications: So where do we stand? *Journal of Anxiety Disorders, 14,* 31–40.

Edelbrock, C., Rende, R., Plomin, R., & Thompson, L. A. (1995). A twin study of competence and problem behavior in childhood and early adolescence. *Journal of Child Psychology and Psychiatry, 36,* 775–785.

Eley, T. C. (1997). General genes: A new theme in developmental psychopathology. *Current Directions in Psychological Science, 6,* 90–95.

Faravelli, C., Webb, T., Amboentti, A., Fonnescu, F., & Sessarego, A. (1985). Prevalence of traumatic early events in 31 agoraphobic patients with panic attacks. *American Journal of Psychiatry, 142,* 1493–1494.

Finlay-Jones, R., & Brown, G. W. (1981). Types of stressful life events and the onset of anxiety and depressive disorders. *Psychological Medicine, 11,* 803–815.

Fyer, A. J., Mannuzza, S., Chapman, T. F., Martin, L. Y., & Klein, D. F. (1995). Specificity in familial aggregation of phobic disorders. *Archives of General Psychiatry, 52,* 564–573.

Garcia Coll, C., Kagan, J., & Reznick, J. S. (1984). Behavioral inhibition in young children. *Child Development, 55,* 1005–1019.

Gerull, F. C., & Rapee, R. M. (2002). Mother knows best: Effects of maternal modelling on the acquisition of fear and avoidance behaviour in toddlers. *Behaviour Research and Therapy, 40,* 279–287.

Gray, J. A. (1987). *The psychology of fear and stress* (2nd ed.). Cambridge, UK: Cambridge University Press.

Harris, J. R. (1995). Where is the child's environment?: A group socialization theory of development. *Psychological Review, 102,* 458–489.

Heim, C., & Nemeroff, C. B. (1999). The impact of early adverse experiences on brain systems involved in the pathophysiology of anxiety and affective disorders. *Biological Psychiatry, 46,* 1509–1522.

Hirshfeld, D. R., Biederman, J., Brody, L., Faraone, S. V., & Rosenbaum, J. F. (1997). Associations between expressed emotion and child behavioral inhibition and psychopathology: A pilot study. *Journal of the American Academy of Child and Adolescent Psychiatry, 36,* 205–213.

Hudson, J. L., & Rapee, R. M. (1998, July). *Parenting of anxious children and their siblings.* Paper presented at the triennial meeting of the World Congress of Behavioral and Cognitive Therapies, Acapulco, Mexico.

Hudson, J. L., & Rapee, R. M. (2000). The origins of social phobia. *Behavior Modification, 24,* 102–129.

Hudson, J. L., & Rapee, R. M. (2001). Parent–child interactions and the anxiety disorders: An observational analysis. *Behaviour Research and Therapy, 39,* 1411–1427.

Hudson, J. L., & Rapee, R. M. (2002). Parent–child interactions in clinically anxious children and their siblings. *Journal of Clinical Child and Adolescent Psychology, 31*(4), 548–555.

Jardine, R., Martin, N. G., & Henderson, A. S. (1984). Genetic covariance between neuroticism and the symptoms of anxiety and depression. *Genetics Epidemiology, 1,* 89–107.

Kagan, J. (1989). Temperamental contributions to social behavior. *American Psychologist, 44,* 668–674.

Kagan, J., Reznick, J. S., & Snidman, N. (1987). The physiology and psychology of behavioral inhibition in children. *Child Development, 58,* 1459–1473.

Kagan, J., Snidman, N., Arcus, D., & Reznick, J. S. (1994). *Galen's prophecy: Temperament in human nature.* New York: Basic Books.

Kagan, J., Snidman, N., Zentner, M., & Peterson, E. (1999). Infant temperament and anxious symptoms in school age children. *Development and Psychopathology, 11,* 209–224.

Kendler, K. S. (2001). Twin studies of psychiatric illness: An update. *Archives of General Psychiatry, 58,* 1005–1014.

Kendler, K. S., Neale, M. C., Kessler, R. C., Heath, A. C., & Eaves, L. J. (1992). Major depression and generalized anxiety disorder: Same genes, (partly) different environments? *Archives of General Psychiatry, 49,* 716–722.

Kendler, K. S., Walters, E. E., Neale, M. C., Kessler, R. C., Heath, A. C., & Eaves, L. J.

(1995). The structure of the genetic and environmental risk factors for six major psychiatric disorders in women: Phobia, generalized anxiety disorder, panic disorder, bulimia, major depression, and alcoholism. *Archives of General Psychiatry, 52,* 374–383.

Ladouceur, R., Blais, F., Freeston, M. H., & Dugas, M. J. (1998). Problem solving and problem orientation in generalized anxiety disorder. *Journal of Anxiety Disorders, 12,* 139–152.

Last, C. G., Hersen, M., Kazdin, A., Francis, G., & Grubb, H. J. (1987). Psychiatric illness in the mothers of anxious children. *American Journal of Psychiatry, 144,* 1580–1583.

Last, C. G., Hersen, M., Kazdin, A., Orvaschel, H., & Perrin, S. (1991). Anxiety disorders in children and their families. *Archives of General Psychiatry, 48,* 928–935.

Levy, D. M. (1943). *Maternal overprotection.* New York: Columbia University Press.

Lipsitz, J. D., Martin, L. Y., Mannuzza, S., Chapman, T. F., Liebowitz, M. R., Klein, D. F., & Fyer, A. J. (1994). Childhood separation anxiety disorder in patients with adult anxiety disorders. *American Journal of Psychiatry, 151,* 927–929.

Main, M., & Solomon, J. (1986). Discovery of an insecure–disorganized/disoriented attachment pattern. In T. B. Brazelton & M. W. Yogman (Eds.), *Affective development in infancy* (pp. 95–124). Norwood, NJ: Ablex.

Main, M., & Solomon, J. (1990). Procedures for identifying infants as disorganized/disoriented during the Ainsworth Strange Situation. In M. Greenberg, D. Cicchetti, & E. M. Cummings (Eds.), *Attachment in the preschool years: Theory, research and intervention* (pp. 121–160). Chicago: University of Chicago Press.

Manassis, K., Bradley, S., Goldberg, S., Hood, J., & Swinson, R. P. (1994). Attachment in mothers with anxiety disorders and their children. *Journal of the American Academy of Child and Adolescent Psychiatry, 33,* 1106–1113.

Manassis, K., & Hood, J. (1998). Individual and familial predictors of impairment in childhood anxiety disorders. *Journal of the American Academy of Child and Adolescent Psychiatry, 37,* 428–434.

Merikangas, K. R., Avenevoli, S., Dierker, L., & Grillon, C. (1999). Vulnerability factors among children at risk for anxiety disorders. *Biological Psychiatry, 46,* 1523–1535.

Mineka, S., Gunnar, M., & Champoux, M. (1986). Control and early socioemotional development: Infant rhesus monkeys reared in controllable versus uncontrollable environments. *Child Development, 57,* 1241–1256.

Muris, P., Steerneman, P., Merckelbach, H., & Meesters, C. (1996). The role of parental fearfulness and modeling of children's fears. *Behaviour Research and Therapy, 34,* 265–268.

Noyes, R., Jr., Clarkson, C., Crowe, R. R., Yates, W. R., & McChesney, C. M. (1987). A family study of generalized anxiety disorder. *American Journal of Psychiatry, 144,* 1019–1024.

Ollendick, T. H., & King, N. J. (1991). Origins of childhood fears: An evaluation of Rachman's theory of fear acquisition. *Behaviour Research and Therapy, 29,* 117–123.

Parker, G. (1983). *Parental overprotection: A risk factor in psychosocial development.* Sydney: Grune & Stratton.

Parker, G., & Lipscombe, P. (1981). Influences on maternal protection. *British Journal of Psychiatry, 138,* 303–311.

Paxton, S. J., Schutz, H. K., Wertheim, E. H., & Muir, S. L. (1999). Friendship clique and peer influences on body image concerns, dietary restraint, extreme weight-loss behaviors, and binge eating in adolescent girls. *Journal of Abnormal Psychology, 108,* 255–266.

Pike, A., & Plomin, R. (1996). Importance of nonshared environment factors for childhood and adolescent psychopathology. *Journal of the American Academy of Child and Adolescent Psychiatry, 35*, 560–570.

Prior, M. (1992). Childhood temperament. *Journal of Child Psychology and Psychiatry, 33*, 249–279.

Prior, M., Sanson, A., Oberklaid, F., & Northam, E. (1987). Measurement of temperament on one to three year old children. *International Journal of Behavioural Development, 10*, 121–132.

Rapee, R. M. (1991). Generalized anxiety disorder: A review of clinical features and theoretical concepts. *Clinical Psychology Review, 11*, 419–440.

Rapee, R. M. (1997). The potential role of childrearing practices in the development of anxiety and depression. *Clinical Psychology Review, 17*, 47–67.

Rapee, R. M. (2001). The development of generalized anxiety. In M. W. Vasey & M. R. Dadds (Eds.), *The developmental psychopathology of anxiety* (pp. 481–503). New York: Oxford University Press.

Rapee, R. M., Litwin, E. M., & Barlow, D. H. (1990). Impact of life events on subjects with panic disorder and on comparison subjects. *American Journal of Psychiatry, 147*, 640–644.

Rapee, R. M., & Melville, L. F. (1997). Recall of family factors in social phobia and panic disorder: Comparison of mother and offspring reports. *Depression and Anxiety, 5*, 7–11.

Rapee, R. M., & Szollos, A. (1997, November). *Early life events in anxious children.* Paper presented at the 31st annual meeting of the Association for Advancement of Behavior Therapy, Miami, FL.

Rende, R. D. (1993). Longitudinal relations between temperament traits and behavioral syndromes in middle childhood. *Journal of the American Academy of Child and Adolescent Psychiatry, 32*, 287–290.

Reznick, J. S., Kagan, J., Snidman, N., Gersten, M., Baak, K., & Rosenberg, A. (1986). Inhibited and uninhibited children: A follow-up study. *Child Development, 54*, 361–368.

Roemer, L., Molina, S., Litz, B. T., & Borkovec, T. D. (1997). Preliminary investigation of the role of previous exposure to potentially traumatizing events in generalized anxiety disorder. *Depression and Anxiety, 4*, 134–138.

Rosenbaum, J. F., Biederman, J., Gersten., M., Hirshfeld, D. R., Meminger, S. R., Herman, J. B., Kagan, J., Reznick, J. S., & Snidman, N. (1988). Behavioral inhibition in children of parents with panic disorder and agoraphobia: A controlled study. *Archives of General Psychiatry, 45*, 463–470.

Rowe, D. C. (1997). As the twig is bent?: The myth of child-rearing influences on personality development. *Journal of Counseling and Development, 68*, 606–611.

Rubin, K. H. (1993). The Waterloo longitudinal project: Correlates and consequences of social withdrawal from childhood to adolescence. In K. H. Rubin & J. B. Asendorpf (Eds.), *Social withdrawal, inhibition, and shyness in children* (pp. 291–314). Hillsdale, NJ: Erlbaum.

Sanson, A., Prior, M., Garino, E., Oberklaid, F., & Sewell, J. (1987). The structure of infant temperament: Factor analysis of the Revised Infant Temperament Questionnaire. *Infant Behavior and Development, 10*, 97–104.

Sapolsky, R. M. (1989). Hypercortisolism among socially subordinate wild baboons originates at the CNS level. *Archives of General Psychiatry 46*, 1047–1051.

Scherrer, J. F., True, W. R., Xian, H., Lyons, M. J., Eisen, S. A., Goldberg, J., Lin, N., & Tsuang, M. T. (2000). Evidence for genetic influences common and specific to symptoms of generalized anxiety and panic. *Journal of Affective Disorders, 57*, 25–35.

Schniering, C. A., Hudson, J. L., & Rapee, R. M. (2000). Issues in the diagnosis and assessment of anxiety disorders in children and adolescents. *Clinical Psychology Review, 20,* 453–478.

Shamir-Essakow, G., Ungerer, J., & Rapee, R. M. (2002). *Attachment, behavioural inhibition, and anxiety problems in preschool children.* Manuscript submitted for publication.

Shaw, D. S., Keenan, K., Vondra, J. I., Delliquadri, E., & Giovannelli, B. S. (1997). Antecedents of preschool children's internalizing problems: A longitudinal study of low-income families. *Journal of the American Academy of Child and Adolescent Psychiatry, 36,* 1760–1767.

Silverman, W. K., Cerny, J. A., & Nelles, W. B. (1988). The familial influence in anxiety disorders: Studies on the offspring of patients with anxiety disorders. In B. B. Lahey & A. E. Kazdin (Eds.), *Advances in clinical child psychology* (pp. 223–248). New York: Plenum Press.

Siqueland, L., Kendall, P. C., & Steinberg, L. (1996). Anxiety in children: Perceived family environments and observed family interaction. *Journal of Clinical Child Psychology, 25,* 225–237.

Thapar, A., & McGuffin, P. (1995). Are anxiety symptoms in childhood heritable? *Journal of Child Psychology and Psychiatry, 36,* 439–447.

Thomas, A., & Chess, S. (1985). The behavioral study of temperament. In J. Strelau & F. H. Farley (Eds.), *The biological bases of personality and behavior: Vol. 1. Theories, measurement techniques and development* (pp. 213–225). Washington, DC: Hemisphere.

Tiet, Q. Q., Bird, H. R., Davies, M., Hoven, C., Cohen, P., Jensen, P. S., & Goodman, S. (1998). Adverse life events and resilience. *Journal of the American Academy of Child and Adolescent Psychiatry, 37,* 1191–1200.

Topolski, T. D., Hewitt, J. K., Eaves, L. J., Silberg, J. L., Meyer, J. M., Rutter, M., Pickles, A., & Simonoff, E. (1997). Genetic and environmental influences on child reports of manifest anxiety and overanxious disorders: A community-based twin study. *Behavior Genetics, 27,* 15–28.

Torgersen, S. (1983). Genetic factors in anxiety disorders. *Archives of General Psychiatry, 40,* 1085–1089.

Torgersen, S. (1986). Childhood and family characteristics in panic and generalized anxiety disorders. *American Journal of Psychiatry, 143,* 630–632.

Tyrer, P., Alexander, J., Remington, M., & Riley, P. (1987). Relationship between neurotic symptoms and neurotic diagnosis: A longitudinal study. *Journals of Affective Disorders, 13,* 13–21.

Warren, S. L., Huston, L., Egeland, B., & Sroufe, L. A. (1997). Child and adolescent anxiety disorders and early attachment. *Journal of the American Academy of Child and Adolescent Psychiatry, 36,* 637–644.

Woody, S., & Rachman, S. (1994). Generalized anxiety disorder (GAD) as an unsuccessful search for safety. *Clinical Psychology Review, 14,* 743–753.

PART II
Theoretical and Empirical Approaches

CHAPTER 4

Avoidance Theory of Worry and Generalized Anxiety Disorder

THOMAS D. BORKOVEC
OSCAR M. ALCAINE
EVELYN BEHAR

Worry is a pervasive human experience and is the defining characteristic of generalized anxiety disorder (GAD) (see Mennin, Heimberg, & Turk, Chapter 1, this volume). Determining what functions it serves in human anxiety may be critical to the development of therapeutic methods for ameliorating the suffering that it causes. Perhaps its most significant function resides in the likely use of the process as an internal avoidance response.

At one level of analysis, the claim that worry is a cognitive avoidance response to perceived threat would seem to be self-evident. If a human being is anticipating a significant problem, he or she will be highly motivated to solve (remove) the problem. Cognitive activity, including the ability to recall the past and think about or imagine possible futures and behaviors to adapt to such futures, is a highly sophisticated system for problem solving. In fact, modern cognitive theory posits that thought evolved precisely to anticipate the future and to identify ways to maximize good outcomes and minimize bad ones (e.g., McGuire & McGuire, 1991). Detecting threat creates a problem to be solved. Indeed, threat represents the most significant problem that organisms face, given that it relates to survival. Threat signals the need to find an effective way to avoid or minimize bad events. If behavioral avoidance cannot be employed to remove the threat and the problem remains unsolved, a solution to the threat must still be found for the sake of survival, and cognitive activity is the only device left available. Worry is thus an understandable cognitive attempt to solve the problem of possible future danger; it functions to avoid the occurrence of temporally distant bad events. To the extent that worry does indeed reduce aspects of the threat and/or is perceived to prevent bad events, worry should be negatively reinforced like any avoidance behavior. The extant literature suggests that worry does indeed function as a cognitive avoidance response (potentially in several different ways), and that the conditions necessary for negative reinforcement are frequently present.

The purpose of the present chapter is to review empirical literature relevant to the potential avoidance functions of worry; to describe the significant consequences of that process; and to suggest areas of possible therapeutic innovation for reducing chronic worry and GAD, based on what is known about its nature and functions. It is first useful, however, to provide a brief overview of the historical context within which scientific research on worry emerged.

A HISTORICAL CONTEXT FOR THE EMERGENCE OF INTEREST IN WORRY

The Two-Stage Theory of Anxiety

From an evolutionary perspective, fear is advantageous; it facilitates fight-or-flight responses to environments that threaten survival. Although fear can serve an adaptive function in this way, it can also be manifested in the pathological forms seen in the anxiety disorders, wherein the fear is excessive and/or leads to maladaptive behavior in response to situations that are not actually threatening. From a classic learning theory perspective, we humans develop anxiety as a response to nonthreatening situations because we have been punished in the past in the presence of those situations. Once such an emotional response is conditioned, we naturally seek to escape or avoid those situations because we do not wish to experience the punishment again. As long as we avoid the conditioned stimuli, however, extinction cannot occur, and the learned anxiety response will be maintained. This description is very familiar to the field of behavior therapy. A significant portion of its theoretical foundation, from which many of its exposure therapy methods have emerged, rests in Mowrer's (1947) two-stage theory of fear: Classically conditioned acquisition of fear is followed by operantly conditioned avoidance of fear cues, resulting in fear maintenance due to a lack of unreinforced exposure to those conditioned stimuli.

In the application of this perspective to human anxiety, motoric avoidance and external fear cues naturally received the greatest amount of attention in the early days of behavior therapy, given that field's initial emphasis on observable behaviors and on the understanding and treatment of circumscribed phobic disorders for which clearly identifiable environmental triggers existed. Despite significant therapeutic advances in the treatment of several of the anxiety disorders, these two early emphases were not very useful for attempts to address diffuse anxiety, or what eventually became GAD in the third edition of the *Diagnostic and Statistical Manual of Mental Disorders* (DSM-III; American Psychiatric Association [APA], 1980). This disorder was not characterized by specific, anxiety-provoking triggers, and behavioral avoidance was not an obvious symptomatic feature. Without specific external fear cues to use in exposure, and without an approach response to encourage to counteract avoidance of such cues, traditional exposure techniques seemed to have little relevance.

The Role of Cognition and the Conditioned Response in Anxiety Process

Two separate but related lines of thought were, however, emerging shortly after the beginnings of behavior therapy that ultimately provided a foundation for conceptual and therapeutic advances for GAD. First, with the advent of interest in cognitive processes potentially involved in psychological problems (Bandura, 1969), the possibility that humans might be capable of cognitively avoiding feared stimuli (and thus preserving anxious meanings despite repeated exposures and without behavioral avoidance) was eventually raised. In the most obvious example of this, the fact that phobic stimuli may be presented in daily life or in therapy does not guarantee that phobic individuals will attend to those stimuli; they may well avoid them by actively shifting their attention to something else. Second, with increasing awareness that the response-produced stimuli of the conditioned response might themselves be part of the conditioned stimulus complex, the possibility that exposure to internal anxiety responses might be important for effective and efficient exposure therapies was increasingly considered. Under this circumstance, avoidance of internal fear cues (either by covert or overt means) might well play a role in the maintenance of anxiety. The implications of the view that anxiety responses are part of the conditioned stimulus complex have historically been played out in various developments, such as the deliberate elicitation of fear in implosive therapy (Stampfl & Levis, 1967), the concept of "fear of fear" in agoraphobia (Goldstein & Chambless, 1978), and the use of interoceptive exposure in panic control treatment (Barlow, 1988). These emerging lines of thought regarding the role of cognitive processes in anxiety and the response-produced stimulus value of internal fear cues eventually culminated in Foa and Kozak's (1986) theoretical notion that accessing the full fear structure stored in memory (including its stimulus, response, and meaning propositions, based on Lang's [1985] bioinformational model of fear) and the provision of corrective information during repeated exposures are the central mechanisms of the extinction process.

Our own interest in cognitive avoidance dates back to the time of Thomas Borkovec's dissertation, which compared systematic desensitization, implosive therapy, and an avoidance response placebo in the treatment of analogue snake phobia (Borkovec, 1972, 1974). Because the theoretical underpinnings of both these exposure therapies were grounded in classic learning theory, the ideal control condition for them would logically involve the provision of the same amount of exposure to feared hierarchy scenes, but with the addition of the imagination of an avoidance response to each scene presentation. Based on Mowrer's (1947) theory, these are precisely the conditions assumed to occur in daily life exposures to anxiety-provoking stimuli that should maintain the anxiety. The fact that the avoidance response group failed to show outcome improvement on heart rate measures and displayed maintenance of heart rate arousal throughout the process of phobic scene exposures (in contrast to the declining heart rates of the two behavioral therapies) provided evidence that cognitive (imagined) avoidance, like behavioral avoidance, could function to preserve anxiety despite repeated confrontations with the feared situation. A subsequent investigation (Grayson & Borkovec, 1978) similarly found that imagining avoidance responses to phobic scenes resulted in greater progressive increases in subjective fear across hierarchy images than did a condition involving imagination of effective coping with the feared situation. Moreover, Grayson, Foa, and Steketee (1982) found that attention deployed toward or away from anxiety-provoking stimuli during exposure treatment significantly influences the rate of between-session extinction.

These findings suggested a cognitive–perceptual extension of Mowrer's two-stage theory (Borkovec, 1979), which posited that cognitive escape or avoidance might (1) contribute to the original development of anxious responding, (2) facilitate the maintenance of already established phobias, and (3) mitigate the otherwise ameliorating effects of repeated exposures occurring in the course of daily life or in therapy. The latter two effects were hypothetically due to the fact that such cognitive maneuvers would preclude the *functional* exposure necessary to promote extinction. Also contained within this theoretical position was an emphasis on the likelihood that the conditioned anxiety response itself might be a part of the conditioned stimulus complex, and therefore potentially a necessary ingredient for effective exposure treatment.

By the late 1980s, DSM-III-R (APA, 1987) changed its diagnostic criteria for GAD, making a cognitive process (worry) its central defining characteristic (see Mennin et al., Chapter 1, this volume). Since that time, although some progress had been made in applying traditional cognitive-behavioral techniques (e.g., relaxation training, generic cognitive therapy, and self-control desensitization techniques) to the treatment of the disorder (see Leahy, Chapter 11, this volume), it also became apparent that the development of effective therapies for GAD might well depend upon a better, more specific understanding of the nature and functions of worry. And the extension of theory to include cognitive avoidance and the importance of accessing all elements of the fear structure provided one of the useful bases for the search for such an understanding.

Worry as a Cognitive Process Relevant to Anxiety

Experimental interest in worry itself emerged mainly in the early 1970s within the test anxiety literature, where worry was defined as a cognitive component of anxiety distinct from its physiological elements. The fact that measures of worry predicted such things as test performance and grade point average, whereas measures of the physiological anxiety element did not, supported that distinction (see Deffenbacher, 1980). When Borkovec and colleagues began their experimental studies of worry, they were already convinced by this test anxiety research, by their interviews of individuals with chronic worry, and by their own introspective experiences that worry was closely related to fear and anxiety processes (see Borkovec, Robinson, Pruzinsky, & DePree, 1983). Indeed, empirical investigations found that anxiety was the predominant affective experience during worry and that worry, like fear, had incubating effects, generating an increase in negative thought intrusions after brief inductions compared to the decrease in intrusions after lengthy inductions (Borkovec, Robinson, et al., 1983; Pruzinsky & Borkovec, 1990). So Borkovec (1985) speculated that worry should also have some type of cognitive avoidance function, and his group was primed to recognize such functions, should they emerge in subsequent research.

Any theory proposing the central role of an avoidance behavior in pathological anxiety necessarily assumes the importance of threat detection; it is the perception of threat that initiates the anxiety process. As MacLeod and Rutherford (Chapter 5, this volume) comprehensively describe, worry and GAD are indeed characterized by a pervasive bias toward threat detection and interpretation. Our chapter focuses on worry as one of the significant ways in which human beings respond to perceived threat.

COGNITIVE AVOIDANCE THROUGH THE WORRY PROCESS

The Predominance of Thought Activity in the Worry Process

The first empirical hint that worry may function as an avoidance response emerged from an investigation of clients with GAD and nonanxious controls, from whom thought samples were collected during periods of self-relaxation and worry (Borkovec & Inz, 1990). During relaxation, the clients reported nearly equal amounts of thought and imagery, whereas the controls reported a predominance of imagery. During the subsequent worry period, thought predominated for both groups. Clients with GAD also rated the affective valence of their mentations as significantly more anxious than did the controls, even during the relaxation state. Importantly, both the thought–imagery ratios and the valence ratings normalized once the clients completed a trial of psychotherapy. This study and a replication (Freeston, Dugas, & Ladouceur, 1996) established that worry is phenomenologically experienced primarily as negative verbal/linguistic (as opposed to imaginal) activity. When we humans worry, we are talking to ourselves in anxious ways. Later psychophysiological evidence strengthened the conclusion of thought predominance; both GAD as a condition and worry as a state have been associated with increases in left frontal cortical activation (Borkovec, Ray, & Stöber, 1998; Carter, Johnson, & Borkovec, 1986; Heller, Nitschke, Etienne, & Miller, 1997; Tucker, Antes, Stenslie, & Barnhardt, 1978; Tyler & Tucker, 1982). Although the fact that imagery declined from relaxed states among nonanxious people to worrisome states among clients with GAD in the Borkovec and Inz (1990) study might merely have indicated that the excessive thought contained in worry allows for less imagery, Borkovec and Inz realized that this same outcome could alternately or additionally reflect the motivated use of worrisome thought in order to avoid negative images.

Further hints that this might be the case have come from Stöber's (1998; Stöber, Tepperwien, & Staak, 2000) work on the abstract nature of worry. Stöber and colleagues have found that nonworry topics are associated with more imagery than are worry topics, and that increased worry about any given topic is associated with lessened imagery. They have also found that whatever imagery does emerge from worry topics is objectively rated to be less concrete. Paivio (1986) has shown that forming images from abstract (as opposed to concrete) words and sentences requires a greater amount of time and produces images that are subsequently rated as more abstract and less vivid. Given what is known about the nature of worry, and given dual-coding theory, the findings of Stöber's group make sense. They suggest that the conceptual, verbal nature of worry largely limits conscious accessibility to parallel-processed images, and that even when occasional catastrophic images do occur in awareness, they are likely to be less vivid, intrusive, attention-grabbing, and emotionally distressing. Again, such conditions suggest the possibility of motivated cognitive avoidance.

If motivated cognitive avoidance is in fact involved in the above-described effects, what might be the imagery mechanisms that are susceptible to worry's mitigating influence? According to Kosslyn (1983), imagery involves both a retrieval mechanism and a refresher mechanism. Once an image is formed by retrieval from memory, a separate refreshing process is needed to maintain it. Worry probably primes the involuntary retrieval of periodic aversive images, but at the same time serves as a means of cognitive avoidance in response to them. Kosslyn would be likely to place the point of worry impact at the level of the refreshing mechanism. Shifting to worry upon each image occurrence would interfere with the refreshment of that image, and the image would fade away. During a worry episode, the spread of associations continues along the verbal/linguistic pathway until another catastrophic image is encountered and the same process occurs again. Such a process would reflect the classic operation of Mowrer's two-stage anxiety theory at the cognitive level.

The Suppression of Somatic Anxiety

Obviously, we believe that the predominance of thought in the worry process is crucial for understanding its nature and functions, and that the distinction between thought and imagery is fundamental to that understanding. Psychophysiological research on the differences between these two types of cognitive activity has contributed significantly to why we believe this to be true. Specifically, this literature has provided an answer to how worrisome thought might be used as an avoidance response—that is, as an immediate coping response to the anxiety generated by the perception of threat, and not solely as a cognitive attempt to solve the problem of perceived future danger. The answer resides in the fact that verbal articulation of fear material elicits little cardiovascular response, whereas imagination of a scene that represents the same material evokes considerable heart rate reaction (Vrana, Cuthbert, & Lang, 1986). Applying this fact to what is known about worry, one can speculate that when aversive images occur in the process of worry and/or when threatening environmental stimuli are detected, the shifting of attention to worrisome thinking upon each occurrence or detection results in the escape from or avoidance of the somatic element of the fear response to the aversive stimuli; internal fear cues would be muted, and part of Foa and Kozak's (1986) requirements for extinction are left unfulfilled. In this way, worry may be an attempt to suppress both the aversive images (e.g., via reduced concreteness) and the unpleasant somatic anxiety (Mowrer's "bad states") otherwise elicited by them. Such a process would need to continue throughout a worry episode. Thinking about worrisome concerns would necessarily prime catastrophic images related to those concerns, and thus tend to increase the frequency of such images (images and thought occur simultaneously and integratively in dual-coding theory; Paivio & Marschark, 1991). Upon each image occurrence, however, there is functional reason to shift immediately to thought activity in order to reduce the physiological/affective distress elicited by the images. Thus worry is hypothetically motivated both by the need to remove perceived threat (i.e., to find a solution to the problem) and by its suppression of certain (somatic) aspects of anxious experience.

Significantly, empirical research has documented that the presence of a worrisome state in fact suppresses an important type of somatic response to feared images—specifically, sympathetic (fight-or-flight) activation. Remarkably, this suppression has been found both for sympathetic activation that would otherwise occur in response to feared material and for sympathetic activation during the worry process itself.

Suppression in Response to Fear Material

Over 20 years ago, Tucker and Newman (1981) found that individuals spontaneously engage in verbalization as a strategy to achieve disengagement and emotional control while decreasing their sympathetic arousal to distressing, aversive information. Borkovec and Hu (1990) discovered several years later that speech-anxious participants who engaged in worrisome thought prior to each of several presentations of a phobic image showed very little cardiovascular response to those images, despite reporting heightened subjective anxiety. In contrast, participants who engaged in either relaxed thinking or neutral thinking showed strong heart rate reaction to the images (with declining reaction over repeated images in the relaxed-thinking group). In a partial replication of this effect, Borkovec, Lyonfields, Wiser, and Diehl (1993) found that this suppression of somatic response was linked to the amount of worrisome thinking that occurred and not merely the amount of thinking in general. Peasley-Miklus and Vrana (2000) also found lessened heart rate response to feared imagery following worrisome thinking than after relaxed thinking when the thinking periods were used as the baseline for measuring the imagery response (although the effect did not occur if the baseline was taken from prethought periods).

All three investigations indicated that the actual somatic reactions to images containing feared material are muted by preceding worry. Thus, throughout the process, worry periodically and immediately produces some removal of Mowrer's "bad states"; this is supportive of the notion that worry acts as a negatively reinforced avoidance activity. By so doing, worry will simultaneously preclude exposure to certain aspects of internal fear cues—a fact that will play a significant role when we discuss the implications of worry for the maintenance of anxiety, as well as for the development of therapeutic interventions for GAD.

One recent investigation (Hazlett-Stevens & Borkovec, 2001) qualifies the generality of this suppression effect. Preceding worry did not lessen physiological responding during repeated *in vivo* exposures to public speaking among speech-anxious participants. It did result in the greatest subjective anxiety experienced during the exposures compared to preceding neutral and relaxation conditions (in replication of the Borkovec & Hu [1990] investigation). Hazlett-Stevens and Borkovec argued that public speaking inherently generates a high degree of physiological activation, given its complex cognitive–motor demands, and that this may have overwhelmed any effects of the worrisome cognitive state. Despite the physiological evidence that the entire fear structure had been accessed in all conditions, they also argued that the greater subjective fear responses to the repeated speeches shown in the worry condition suggested a maintenance of anxious meaning and thus a preclusion of extinction, due instead to the possible absence of the second requirement in Foa and Kozak's (1986) model (i.e., the processing of corrective information). If one worries before and after exposure to a feared event, internal or external information that nothing bad is happening or has happened is less likely to be processed. Although investigation of the impact of worry on emotional processing during *in vivo* exposure to other anxiety-provoking situations is warranted, at present we can confidently conclude only that worry suppresses somatic responses to imaginal material.

Suppression during Worrisome Episodes

Although worry's specific inhibition of the sympathetic activation during images of feared material is a significant piece in the puzzle of worry mechanisms, it turns out that both GAD and worry are associated with a general suppression of sympathetic activity as well. The only peripheral psychophysiological measure shown to be elevated in GAD, both at rest and in response to challenge, has been muscle tension. Otherwise, despite their connection to anxiety, both the condition of GAD and the state of worry are not characterized very often by the sympathetic activation so prevalent in other anxiety disorders. Instead, they are associated with reduced autonomic variability, indicative of sympathetic inhibition and/or deficient parasympathetic tone (Hoehn-Saric & McLeod, 1988; Hoehn-Saric, McLeod, & Zimmerli, 1989; Lyonfields, Borkovec, & Thayer, 1995; Thayer, Friedman, & Borkovec, 1996). Clients with GAD even show this specific type of rigid autonomic functioning during resting states. Moreover, the induction of worry, even among those who do not habitually worry, causes similar effects during its occurrence. It is significant that several experimental tasks known to decrease autonomic variability (mental arithmetic, recall of a past aversive event, threat of shock, and isometric grip; Grossman, Stemmler, & Meinhardt, 1990; Grossman & Svebak, 1987) involve processes that are decidedly and tonically characteristic of clients with GAD. Paralleling these physiological data, Marten and colleagues (1993) found that only symptoms significantly mediated by the central nervous system (restlessness or feeling keyed up or on edge, disturbed sleep, muscle tension, irritability, being easily fatigued, and difficulty concentrating) were frequently and reliably reported by clients with GAD, whereas symptoms mediated by the autonomic nervous system were less common. As a result of this empirical observation, the former symptoms were retained and the latter were deleted from the associated symptom checklist for GAD in DSM-IV (APA, 1994). It is also significant that reduced parasympathetic tone, characteristic of GAD, is implicated in attentional control mechanisms (see Porges, 1992)—possibly providing a basis for the attentional difficulties and biases documented in this disorder (see MacLeod & Rutherford, Chapter 5).

What mechanisms might be responsible for worry's specific suppressing effects on somatic reactions to phobic imagery and/or its effects on sympathetic activity in general? Although the answer remains speculative, a few possibilities appear reasonable. First, because worry absorbs attentional and other cognitive resources, it may be difficult to shift attention away from the worry process to some other stimulus (such as a phobic image). Second, Gray's (1982) neurophysiological theory of anxiety suggests that this emotion will occur when information received from the environment is aversive and/or when it differs from the information expected. Notice that in the phobic imagery studies, a preceding period of worrying creates an internal state in which the external information matches significant elements of the content of the worrying. Under this circumstance, there is a reduction in the degree of mismatch between information received and information expected, removing one of the anxiety-eliciting conditions in Gray's theory. Third, if worry is primarily thought, and if thought is less closely tied to efferent command than is imagery (Lang, 1985) or real-life events, then some sympathetic suppression, both in general and in response to threat, derives from the very (thinking) nature of worry. Whatever mechanisms are at work to explain why thought is not strongly connected to efferent command (and therefore to affect, physiology, and behavior) should reside within the neuroanatomy of cortical and subcortical functioning. But it is at least clear that evolution was wise to create a conceptual system that is, on the one hand, free from immediate behavioral expression and the potential punishing consequences of such expressions—and, on the other hand, free to play and experiment mentally with possible choices of action before implementing an action. Fourth, worry may involve semantic satiation. Interviews of clients with GAD and introspective observations both suggest that worrying about a concern tends to be repetitive (i.e., mentally saying basically the same things over and over). Empirically, content analysis of stream-of-consciousness reports has shown that worry is characterized by significant decreases in topical shifts (Molina, Borkovec, Peasley, & Person, 1998). The cognitive psychology literature has demonstrated that the repetition of a word leads to a temporary weakening of the links to the rest of its associative network of meaning (e.g., Smith, 1984). By implication, if worrying contains the repetition of crucial, worry-related words, this repetition will result in lowered access to other elements of meaning (especially the affective and other response elements) contained within their network.

Finally, the combination of earlier-reviewed empirical features of GAD and worry also provides hints about other mechanisms that may interconnect some of those features. Clients with GAD are detecting threat frequently. Threat perception ordinarily (and evolutionarily, for the sake of survival) elicits fight-or-flight sympathetic activation to facilitate avoidance. There is rarely an overt behavioral avoidance response available to clients with GAD to remove the threat, and so they naturally turn to cognitive attempts to solve the problem. The problem, however, is frequently insoluble, because (1) the threat cues perceived exist solely in the mind; (2) those cues refer to possible bad events in the future, which do not actually exist in the present moment; and (3) the vast majority of bad events that are feared are not going to happen anyway (as we will document later). Under these circumstances (a fight-or-flight response with no place to go), sympathetic activation is not useful or adaptive and so is suppressed. Animal analogues exist wherein precisely these kinds of circumstances and effects occur. When some organisms are trapped in a threatening environment and escape is not possible, they freeze (increased muscle tone, reduced autonomic variability, and sympathetic inhibition).

Suppression of Affect in General

Consideration of the above-described findings about the nature of worry and GAD leads to the speculation that perhaps clients with GAD are less in tune with affective experience in general, and not merely with the somatic aspects of anxious responding. The only empirical evidence indirectly related to this possibility comes from studies finding that college students meeting criteria for GAD reported greater difficulty in identifying and describing their emotions on the Toronto Alexithymia Scale than did nonanxious controls (Abel, 1994; Yamas, Hazlett-Stevens, & Borkovec, 1997). Either persons with GAD may be actively avoiding emotion, or their constant focus of attention on thought activity may make them less aware of affective fluctuations throughout the day. Research focused on more valid assessments of general emotional experience in GAD is required to verify this speculation, but if it turns out to be correct, then future therapy developments for GAD could usefully incorporate measures to increase clients' processing of emotion in general.

Although worry has been demonstrated to suppress *immediate* somatic anxiety responses to threatening material and thus appears to serve as a negatively reinforced cognitive avoidance activity, it is also important to examine the evidence for our earlier logical conclusion that worry functions as an attempt to solve the problem of possible *future* bad environmental events and thus acts as an effort to avoid distal dangers as well.

Worrying to Avoid Future Bad Events

We have begun this chapter with the self-evident logic behind the proposition that worry functions to anticipate and avoid bad outcomes in the future. Empirical evidence indicates that people do at least believe that worry is an effective method of preventing disaster (see also Freeston, Rheaume, Letarte, Dugas, & Ladouceur, 1994, and Wells, Chapter 7, this volume, for a comprehensive discussion of both positive and negative beliefs about worry). Several years ago, Borkovec and his colleagues asked clients with GAD undergoing the Penn State treatment protocols (to be described later) what benefits they saw to worrying. Six common themes emerged. Worry was believed to be a way to (1) motivate oneself to get things done, (2) determine how to avoid or prevent bad events, (3) prepare for the worst, (4) problem-solve, (5) superstitiously lessen the likelihood of bad events, and (6) distract oneself from even more emotional topics. Each of these potential benefits of worrying functionally contains a negative reinforcement contingency (see Borkovec, Hazlett-Stevens, & Diaz, 1999, for a more detailed description of this for each belief). Results from a questionnaire constructed from these items and administered to college students who met or did not meet GAD criteria showed that all six reasons to worry were widely endorsed by both groups, with motivation, avoidance, and preparation being the most highly rated (Borkovec & Roemer, 1995). In addition, participants with GAD scored significantly higher on the item involving distraction from more emotional topics in two separate studies. Although most of the items reflect both psychodynamic and learning theory views of the neurotic paradox, this latter item, which distinguished GAD from nonanxious groups, is perhaps the quintessential example: Humans may create distress for themselves in order to preclude even greater subsequent pain.

It may be the case that merely believing that a negative reinforcement contingency exists is sufficient for an activity like worry actually to be maintained. However, some of the empirical research mentioned earlier and additional research described below provide evidence that a functional basis may indeed exist for some (perhaps all) of the positive beliefs about worry listed above. Negative reinforcement requires that a behavior be followed by the removal of a punishing state. The punishing state includes both the bad environmental events and the feelings of fear themselves. In Mowrer's (1947) terms, the rat's avoidance response terminates both the internal (conditioned response) fear cues and the possibility of being exposed to punishment (the aversive unconditioned stimulus). If we found evidence that worry is associated with either or both of these events, then we would have evidence consistent with the hypothesis that worry is potentially being negatively reinforced.

Given that worry immediately mitigates somatic reactions to phobic images (a direct demonstration of its ability to reduce feelings of fear and create Mowrer's "good" state), it may well provide sufficient historical experience to support a belief that worry does indeed prepare one for the worst. If, in addition, one has multiple experiences of worrying about potential bad events, and the worry process itself is associated with lessened somatic anxiety, then one might reasonably conclude that worry is an effective way to prepare oneself for catastrophe.

In terms of negative reinforcement from the avoidance of more temporally distant punishing environmental events (solving the problem presented by perceived threat), there is clear evidence that the vast majority of things about which people worry never happen (Borkovec et al., 1999). College students with and without GAD, as well as clients with GAD from our therapy protocols, have kept daily diaries over 2 or more weeks in which they noted every topic about which they worried and then rated the eventual environmental outcomes once they happened. The rating for each outcome was made on the basis of whether the outcome turned out as bad as feared or better or worse than feared. Seventy percent of the students' worries turned out better than they had feared. This was true regardless of GAD status, although the participants with GAD spent much more time worrying during a typical day. For the clients, 85% of their worries had positive outcomes. Because clients with GAD typically fear not being able to cope with negative events, the clients in this research also rated how well they coped with those bad outcomes that did happen. The results indicated better-than-expected coping in 79% of those cases. What these data importantly indicate is that worry is typically followed by the nonoccurrence of the feared event. This was especially the case for clients with GAD, and the nonoccurrences included both the feared environmental catastrophes and the feared inability to cope. Under these schedules of negative reinforcement, the chronic worry seen in GAD is both strengthened by frequent negative reinforcement and becomes resistant to extinction, due to the type of schedule of reinforcement that the world provides.

Given these contingencies, a direct functional basis for two of the positive beliefs about worry can be seen—namely, that worry can help one to find effective ways to avoid or prevent bad events, and that worry somehow superstitiously lessens the likelihood of such events. Although the possibility has not yet been empirically tested, it is likely that self-monitoring of outcomes related to two of the other beliefs (problem solving and motivation) would show similar results indicating superstitious reinforcement. Worry is necessary neither for engaging in problem solving (indeed, anxiety generally interferes with complex task performances) nor for motivating adaptive behavior (positive contingencies could be adaptively substituted to achieve the same goal). In either case, however, the outcomes are quite likely to turn out better than feared, regardless of whether the person chooses positive or aversive self-control strategies, and will thus similarly reflect the operation of a variable schedule of superstitious reinforcement.

Worrying to Avoid More Emotional Topics

No direct evidence exists as yet for the possibility that worry might function as a cognitive means of avoiding more emotional topics. If indeed such topics do exist, and if worry does in fact function to avoid exposure to them, however, then there are intriguing possibilities for what those more emotional topics might be. These possibilities come in two forms with regard to likely associative network organization.

Topic-Related Underlying Fears

In the vertical form of network organization, it may be that the conscious content of a worry typically involves only the most superficial elements of its worrisome fear structure and does not access deeper representations of the threat underlying those elements. Under this circumstance, superficial worrisome thoughts are distractions from, and therefore ways of avoiding, thoughts about the more anxiety-provoking levels of content. The use of decatastrophizing methods in cognitive therapy assumes that this is the case; such methods are used to access the clients' deeper underlying fears, reflected by the more distal anxious thoughts typically reported by clients initially. One study is potentially supportive of the possibility that worry is avoidant of deeper threat (Vasey & Borkovec, 1992). "Worriers" and "nonworriers" were asked to indicate what would be bad or fearful about each step in the process of catastrophizing their most worrisome topic. Worriers generated a significantly greater number of steps, and most importantly, they showed increasing levels of discomfort over the consecutive steps; nonworriers maintained low levels of discomfort throughout the catastrophizing sequence. Thus some of the conditions necessary to support the hypothesis that chronic worriers worry at a superficial level in order to avoid more anxiety-provoking material were present—namely, a rich associative network of worry-related steps, with increasing discomfort during the accessing of those steps.

In the horizontal form of network organization, worrying about a particular topic may function to distract a person from completely different content—content that is more anxiety-provoking in nature. What such content might be has not been empirically established, but research on

GAD has determined at least three domains in which significantly negative historical or current events may contribute to negative emotional experiences about which the person would rather not think.

Past Trauma

Theories of GAD have proposed that stressful life events play a causal role in two of the central characteristics of the disorder—namely, chronic anxious apprehension (Barlow, 2002) and excessive perceptions of the world as a dangerous place (Beck & Emery with Greenberg, 1985). Indeed, Beck and colleagues (1985) suggested that exposure to a single potentially traumatic life event might be sufficient for the development of GAD. Furthermore, traumatic life events occurring after the onset of GAD would reasonably contribute to its maintenance or exacerbation, given that such events would be likely to reinforce an individual's perceptions of the world as threatening and/or perceptions that he or she may not be able to cope. If past trauma is frequent among people suffering from GAD, then it may represent the "more emotional topic" from which their daily worry and its content are a distraction.

In both undergraduate and client samples, individuals meeting criteria for GAD have been found to report a significantly greater frequency of past traumatic events than participants without GAD (Roemer, Molina, Litz, & Borkovec, 1997). Similarly, a GAD diagnosis is associated with a higher frequency of at least one unexpected, major negative life stressor (Blazer, Hughes, & George, 1987). Of course, a reported history of trauma is common as well in persons with other psychiatric disorders, including other anxiety disorders (Fierman, Hunt, Pratt, & Warshaw, 1993; Herman, Perry, & van der Kolk, 1989; Jordan et al., 1991). Thus a history of trauma may simply make individuals more susceptible to psychopathology in general, as opposed to GAD in particular. Some empirical research offers hints of specificity, however. Zuellig, Newman, Alcaine, and Behar (1999) conducted childhood diagnostic interviews with three groups of college students: those who met criteria for adult GAD, those who met criteria for adult panic disorder without GAD, and those who met no adult diagnostic criteria. They found significantly higher rates of retrospectively reported childhood posttraumatic stress disorder in the group with GAD. Similarly, clients diagnosed with GAD have reported experiencing the death of a parent before the age of 16 significantly more often than clients with panic disorder (Torgersen, 1986). Although further comparisons with other anxiety disorder groups would be important, extant data do suggest that individuals with GAD may indeed have more traumatic histories than do individuals with at least one other anxiety disorder. Caution is advised in interpreting these data, given that retrospective reports can in general be unreliable; mood-congruent memory may play a role in selective recall and/or interpretation of past events by a client with GAD; only 50% of the group with GAD in the Roemer, Molina, Litz, and Borkovec (1997) study reported traumas (indicating the likelihood that other historical factors must be playing an etiological role); and no investigation to date has explored whether the reported traumatic experiences occurred prior to or after the onset of GAD.

If the past experiences of some people with GAD do indeed contain more traumatic events than is true for other individuals, then investigating the relationship between the content of their traumas and the content of their worry topics might reveal evidence about whether or not these individuals might be using worries about current concerns to avoid memories of those past experiences. In the Roemer, Molina, Litz, and Borkovec (1997) investigation, groups with GAD reported more frequent occurrences of such events as death, illness, injury, and assault. Importantly, however, these are precisely the topics about which people with GAD worry the least (Roemer, Molina, & Borkovec, 1997). So, although these individuals report having experienced these traumatic occurrences, they now fail to worry about those topics that are most directly relevant to the past traumas that they have experienced. This important discrepancy leads us to consider two possibilities: Either they have habituated to cognitive activity dealing with traumatic material about physical threats, or they are avoiding memories about these more emotionally distressing topics by worrying about other things.

Early Childhood Relationships

Extremely stressful or life-threatening events are of course not the only historical aversive experiences that people might wish to avoid in their daily recollections. Recent investigations into what individuals with GAD remember from childhood relationships with their primary caregivers provide another clue about what the avoided content of their "more emotional topics" might be. Bowlby (1982) hypothesized that insecure attachments in early childhood may lead to anxiety later in life. Attachment, he theorized, is a child's attempt to seek safety and comfort whenever threat is perceived in the environment. If the child repeatedly experiences the unavailability of an attachment figure, the child may come to perceive the world as a dangerous, frightening place. The result may be a tendency to overestimate the likelihood and severity of feared events, as well as to underestimate resources available to cope with those threats. Such perceptions are remarkably similar to those of adult clients with GAD.

Clients with GAD (Cassidy, 1995) as well as undergraduates meeting criteria for GAD (Cassidy, 1995; Schut et al., 1997), have completed the Inventory of Adult Attachment (Lichtenstein & Cassidy, 1991), a questionnaire designed to assess reports of attachment-related memories from childhood. In both investigations, the groups with GAD reported more role-reversed/enmeshed relationships: As children, they had to take care of their primary caregivers (instead of being taken care of). Thus they had to anticipate dangers not only for themselves but for those primary caregivers as well. This provides an understandable, early childhood basis for the view of the world in adulthood GAD—that is, as a potentially threatening place where the person's ability to cope is limited and threat must be constantly anticipated. Also in both studies, the groups with GAD indicated greater current levels of unresolved anger toward and vulnerability to their childhood primary caregivers.

Although the groups with GAD in the Cassidy (1995) and Schut and colleagues (1997) studies reported the existence of these role-reversed/enmeshed relationships with residual anger and vulnerability, they also reported having greater difficulty remembering their childhood relationships. Although alternative hypotheses exist (e.g., chronic, constant thought activity may simply make recall of distant past events more difficult), it is also possible that this report indicates an avoidance of negative attachment-related memories. As would be the case for the many other instances of negative emotional experience in the daily life of a client with GAD, worry may be avoidant by filling the mind with superficial conceptual activity when it might otherwise shift to thoughts of a distressing and anger-inducing childhood, while simultaneously inhibiting the imagery and somatic activation potentially accompanying those memories.

Current Interpersonal Relationships

Perhaps past trauma or negative childhoods are not the sources of difficulty that lead individuals with GAD to claim that their worrying distracts them from more emotional topics. It may be the case that the hypothetical horizontal distraction has to do with present life concerns that are simply too difficult to allow very frequently into awareness.

Although clients with GAD worry about a multitude of topics, interpersonal situations are particular causes of concern and anxiety for them. Social phobia is the most frequent comorbid diagnosis for GAD (Barlow, 1988; Brown & Barlow, 1992); trait worry correlates more highly with social fears than it does with nonsocial fears (Borkovec, Robinson, et al., 1983); and content analysis of worry topics reveals that interpersonal concerns are more frequent than any other topical area (Roemer, Molina, & Borkovec, 1997). More exciting has been the identification of specific types of current interpersonal concerns among clients with GAD (Pincus & Borkovec, 1994), as determined by the Inventory of Interpersonal Problems (Horowitz, Rosenberg, & Bartholomew, 1993). Not only did the group with GAD show greater levels of distress and rigidity in their interpersonal relationships than did nonanxious controls, but cluster analysis revealed that the largest grouping (62.1% of clients with GAD) involved an interpersonal style characterized by being "overly nurturant and intrusive" in their relationships (the other two, smaller clusters were "cold/vindictive" and "socially avoidant/nonassertive"). What is exciting about this outcome is that it connects conceptually so well with the childhood attachment findings. It appears that the majority of the clients with GAD learned in childhood to take care of others in order to receive love and nurturance, and that they continue to do this in their adulthood relationships, possibly for the same reason. Worry may thus function as a method for anticipating the needs of significant others in an attempt to satisfy one's most important interpersonal needs and/or as a distraction from the realization that those needs are indeed not being met.

Although we have speculated earlier that people with GAD may experience lowered affect in general, they may, on the other hand, develop a particular sensitivity to other people's emotional experience. This would make sense, because role reversal in childhood as well as nurturant roles in current relationships would require that they learn to detect the feeling states of significant others in their lives. Indeed, participants meeting GAD criteria have been found to report significantly greater empathy with others, and especially greater ability to feel the pain of others, than nonanxious participants report (Peasley, Molina, & Borkovec, 1994).

IMPLICATIONS OF WORRY AS A NEGATIVELY REINFORCED COGNITIVE AVOIDANCE RESPONSE

The review above empirically documents several of the immediate consequences of worry. The worry process, however, has potentially broader implications, described below.

Emotional Processing

The most significant implication of worry as cognitive avoidance is, of course, the fact that it probably precludes emotional processing and thus maintains anxious meanings. In Foa and Kozak's (1986) model, the entire fear structure must be accessed if extinction is to take place. This structure contains stimulus, response, and meaning propositions (Lang, 1985). Failure to access any of these elements implies that extinction will be retarded or nonexistent during either *in vivo* or imaginal exposures to disorder-relevant stimuli, and regardless of whether these exposures are taking place in daily life or in systematic therapeutic applications. Overt behavioral avoidance obviously precludes exposure. Analogously, if worry is functioning to help a person escape or avoid each periodic occurrence of catastrophic images, it minimizes exposure to the imaginally represented stimulus elements that represent the threat. If worry suppresses somatic reactions to such feared material, it reduces exposure to crucial response elements (in Mowrer's terms, the conditioned fear responses) of its fear structure. If worry is superficial in either a horizontal or a vertical sense, it prevents exposure to the stimulus, response, and meaning elements of the underlying fear.

The research reviewed throughout this chapter supports the conclusion that worry does indeed have these characteristics and consequences. What is even more remarkable is that separate research has shown that worry can interfere with a dramatically different type of emotional processing. If one imagines an unconditioned stimulus (UCS) previously employed in an aversive conditioning task, this UCS rehearsal will enhance subsequent fear responses to a previously established conditioned stimulus (Jones & Davey, 1990). If one worries prior to the UCS rehearsal, however, no enhancement of fear occurs, whereas either prior neutral thinking or somatically anxious thinking does strengthen the conditioned response (Davey & Matchett, 1994). This is remarkable because it indicates that worry reduces extinction effects during repeated exposure tasks, but at the same time mitigates the strengthening of anxiety during UCS rehearsal tasks. Because these are diametrically opposite outcomes whose common ingredient is emotional processing, the impact of worry on both processes suggests that its pathway of effect is through interference with that processing.

A separate literature shows that worry after exposure to a stressor also mitigates adaptive emotional processing of the distressing material. Both Butler, Wells, and Dewick (1995) and Wells and Papageorgiou (1995) found that intrusive images during the 3 days subsequent to the viewing of a stressful film were greater among participants who had worried for 4 minutes about the just-seen film in comparison to control conditions. In the former study, worry also had an immediate effect on reducing subjective distress about the film. The fact that this effect was not replicated in the latter study suggests that worry sometimes does and sometimes does not produce some immediate relief from exposure to distressing material. When it does, another example of potential negative reinforcement of worry is provided.

Strengthening of Anxious Meanings

Worry may also have consequences beyond mere prevention of the otherwise naturally occurring extinction effects of repeated exposure. Worry may, by its process or content, actually increase anxious meanings as well. Although worry reduces some aspects of fear responding, it still generates aversive emotional states and includes periodic aversive images. In the process of worry, worrisome thinking is not only occurring in constant response to periodic aversive images, but is also followed by such images. In such a sequence, conditions exist for evaluative conditioning to take place, with anxiety-provoking images serving as UCSs. We already know that images can function as UCSs (Davey & Matchett, 1994; Jones & Davey, 1990). A more recent study has shown that even worry-related words can serve that function: Clients with GAD developed a conditioned orienting response to a neutral cue paired with threat words, whereas nonanxious control participants did not (Thayer, Friedman, Borkovec, Johnsen, & Molina, 2000). This finding also describes one possible mechanism for the growth of hypervigilance in GAD. Moreover, only the clients with GAD showed cardiovascular accelerations to the threat word presentations. This finding suggests the possibility of motivated inattention (cognitive avoidance) (Jennings, 1986) and provides psychophysiological evidence for Mathews's (1990) view that worry sequentially involves ongoing selective vigilance to threat followed by evasion of that threat. Finally, the very act of avoiding something (overtly or covertly) may, from the James–Lange perspective on the nature of emotion (see Fehr & Stern, 1970), strengthens the anxious meanings associated with stimuli so avoided ("If I am worrying about it, the topic must contain danger"). An analogous process has been shown in the thought suppression literature, wherein suppression even of a neutral thought leads to an increase in the anxiety-provoking value of that suppressed thought (Roemer & Borkovec, 1994).

Relevance to Other Anxiety Disorders

Based on early age of onset, chronicity, and lack of treatment responsiveness, Brown, Barlow, and Liebowitz (1994) have argued that GAD may be the basic anxiety disorder out of which other anxiety and mood disorders emerge. Furthermore, although worry is the central defining feature of GAD, it is also pervasive in these other disorders (Barlow, 1988), and GAD is one of their most frequent comorbid conditions (Brown & Barlow, 1992). Given these observations, it follows that everything we know about the nature and functions of worry becomes potentially relevant to the understanding and treatment of any disorder of the emotions. If worry precludes emotional processing, and if other emotional disturbances require such processing for their amelioration, then worry may be a factor in their maintenance and/or therapeutic attempts to reduce them. Surprisingly, however, little systematic research on the role of worry in other disorders has yet been conducted; such research remains as a potentially crucial area for further empirical pursuit. One investigation that underscores the potential importance of this domain discovered that successful treatment of principal GAD eliminates nearly all comorbid conditions by follow-up assessment (Borkovec, Abel, & Newman, 1995).

Relevance to Physical Health

The habitual, rigid nature of the cognitive, physiological, and interpersonal systems found to exist in GAD may well have health implications beyond psychological dysfunction. This appears to be particularly likely because of their distinctive psychophysiologies, characterized by parasympathetic deficiency. Evidence strongly suggests that reduced physiological variability (especially in the cardiovascular system) is implicated in numerous physical pathologies, such as sudden cardiac death, hypertension, ventricular fibrillation, and coronary atherosclerosis (Goldberger, 1992). It is not surprising, then, that a 20-year longitudinal study found that worry predicts an increased incidence of coronary heart disease (Kubzansky et al., 1997); that worry affects the immune response to phobic stimuli (Segerstrom, Glover, Craske, & Fahey, 1999); and that GAD is associated with significant utilization of family doctors and other (nonpsychiatric) medical specialists (Greenberg et al., 1999), as well as with significant social and occupational impairment (Roy-Byrne, 1996).

Absence of Present-Moment Focus of Attention

The most poignant feature of a life spent lost in one's thoughts, especially thoughts that constantly create negative experiences based upon the illusion of nonexistent futures, is that such a way of being disconnects the person from present-moment experiences—which are, in the final analysis, the only reality that is available to us. It is simply a matter of attentional resources: The more attention is allocated to an illusory inner world, the less attention can be devoted to what is right in front of us. Primary emotional experiences (as opposed to secondary or instrumental emotions; see Greenberg & Safran, 1987) in response to immediately available events, the information contained in the world from which we can learn and grow, connection to the people in our lives—these things that give us aliveness and adaptiveness are compromised in their positive influence if they are not attended to and processed. Perhaps this is the characteristic of GAD that is most in need of change.

THE SEARCH FOR EFFECTIVE THERAPIES FOR WORRY AND GAD

The Traditional Cognitive-Behavioral Approach to GAD

As mentioned before, GAD did not lend itself well to the exposure models and techniques of early behavior therapy, given its diffuse nature, lack of identifiable and circumscribed anxiety elicitors, and consequential absence of clear avoidance behaviors. The growing use of cognitive therapy with anxiety disorders, and a shift to coping-oriented rather than mastery-oriented therapeutic approaches, provided at least a beginning point for the development of psychological interventions for this previously neglected disorder. By the early 1980s, a package of cognitive-behavioral therapy (CBT) techniques had been created and applied to the treatment of GAD (see Leahy, Chapter 11). These techniques typically involved three primary elements. First, the clients were taught relaxation methods as generalizable skills; emphasis was placed on deployment of relaxation strategies throughout the day and at any time when anxiety or worry might be noticed (e.g., Öst's [1987] applied relaxation method). Second, because GAD involves frequent detection and/or interpretation of threat, cognitive therapy, often based on Beck and colleagues' (1985) technique descriptions, was employed to help the clients generate alternative ways of perceiving and believing that were less anxiety-provoking. Third, some element of rehearsal of these relaxation and cognitive skills was often provided, in order to build up their habit strength and to make it more likely that clients would remember to make use of these coping strategies throughout their daily life and in response to stressors and stress (e.g., Suinn & Richardson's [1971] anxiety management training and Goldfried's [1971] self-control desensitization). In each instance, clients repeatedly imagined incipient anxiety or worry and their associated cues, and then imagined applying their newly learned coping responses within those situations. Although controlled clinical trials conducted on various versions of this CBT package have documented its efficacy, reviews of this literature (Borkovec & Ruscio, 2001; Borkovec & Whisman, 1996; Chambless & Gillis, 1993; see also Gould, Safren, Washington, & Otto, Chapter 10, this volume) have also indicated that only about half of the clients so treated achieve high end-state functioning at follow-up assessments. It is clear that further improvements in therapy for GAD are needed.

The Current CBT Approach at the Penn State GAD Project

Our current CBT approach being used in our GAD efficacy research at Penn State is grounded in the techniques described above, but we have modified or expanded those interventions based on our growing knowledge about the nature and functions of worry and GAD. Below we briefly describe some salient examples of these treatment developments.

Response Prevention

To confront their fears, people need to prevent their avoidance responses. But how to stop uncontrollable worry is precisely the problem that the client with GAD faces. Its uncontrollable nature is likely due to the fact that worry is a strongly reinforced habit, and as long as the perception of threat remains and no behavioral response provides a solution to the perceived threats, worry will continue. We have found one technique that holds some partial promise for reducing the amount of worrying that is taking place. Because people can worry at any time and in any place as long as the environment is not demanding their attention, worry as an operant activity becomes associated with, and thereby is triggered by, many times and places; it is under poor discriminative control. Although telling clients with GAD to stop worrying and be happy will not be effective, they can comply successfully with a request to gradually restrict the time and place in which their worrying is occurring in order to achieve some degree of stimulus control of the activity. In its empirically validated version (Borkovec, Wilkinson, Folensbee, & Lerman, 1983), this stimulus control program instructs people to establish a worry period at the same time and place each day; to monitor their worrying during the day and to learn to recognize its initiation; and to postpone the worrying upon detection to the worry period, reminding themselves that they will have the opportunity to devote their full energy to worrying and problem solving later, and that they can more adaptively focus their attention now on whatever task is at hand. A second version created by one of our therapists, Mary Boutselis, involves determining a daily time, place, or activity that will become a "worry-free zone," wherein any detected worrying is merely put off until the client is outside that zone. Over sessions, the client expands the zone to include more times, places, and activities.

Worry Outcome Monitoring

As we have described earlier, because many individuals with chronic worry or GAD believe that worrying serves some adaptive functions (e.g., prevention of bad events and preparation for the worst), we ask clients to (1) write down in a daily diary each worry that they notice during the day and its feared outcome; and (2) evaluate at the end of each day any outcomes relevant to a diary entry, what the actual outcome was, and how well they coped with it. This process results in their being frequently exposed to significant corrective experiences. They discover that most of the things that they worry about do not happen, and that they cope quite well with those that do. At the same time, they are building in memory a history of accurate evidence from which they can draw for making predictions in the future. All of this information contributes to a decline in their general tendency to perceive threat in their futures.

Present-Moment Focus of Attention

One of the ultimate goals for both relaxation techniques and cognitive therapy methods is to have clients learn to live more fully in the present

moment. Clients with GAD spend excessive time living in a largely negative world that does not exist. This illusion is created by their focus of attention on worrisome thoughts and images that refer to the past or to possible (though highly unlikely) futures. If they are to find relief from this
incessant world, they must usefully learn to shift their attention to what is
real, and the only reality that exists is in the present moment right before
their eyes. It is in this present moment that adaptive information, new
learning, growth, and development exist. Because anxiety is always antici-
patory, by definition there can be no anxiety in the present moment. So
our clients are encouraged to practice focusing their attention more and
more often on the present moment (e.g., the task at hand, the sensations
provided by the external world, or the information being offered by that
world). Relaxation practice and applied relaxation, with their inherent request to "let go" of everything (including thoughts) and to focus only on
the feelings of relaxation, provide initial experiences of pleasant present
moments. Over time, clients are increasingly asked to practice opening up
and attending to other present-moment experiences being offered by the
world from this relaxed and tranquil place. Cognitive therapy also proceeds in stages leading to the present moment. In the first stage, we help
our clients to recognize the frequent inaccuracy of their predictions about
the future and to replace these predictions, as soon as they are detected,
with alternative perspectives that are more accurate. In the second stage,
we encourage them to notice that no prediction about a future event is
ever completely accurate, and we invite them to begin to spend increasing
time living an "expectancy-free" life. Clients who have begun to recognize
through their self-monitoring that things usually turn out fine, and that
they are indeed quite successful in coping with whatever comes down the
road, can discover that living in the present without the need to think very
much about the future at all can be a very pleasant way to be. The goal is
to encourage them to let go of the felt need for certainty in an uncertain
world and to trust themselves in the face of that reality (see Dugas, Buhr,
& Ladouceur, Chapter 6, this volume, for other approaches to the intolerance of uncertainty). In the third stage, once clients are focused more on
the present, we can begin to work with them on ways of constructing the
meaning of that present moment. We now encourage our clients to focus
on the intrinsics of whatever present moment they face. Special emphasis
is placed on using perspectives that contain the clients' values and/or can
bring joy to the moment.

Throughout both relaxation training and cognitive therapy, we also
emphasize flexibility, in contrast to the rigidity that is typical both in our
clients' psychophysiology and in their patterns of thought. Specifically, we
teach our clients multiple methods of relaxing (progressive relaxation,
meditation, slowed and paced diaphragmatic breathing, and relaxing imagery), and we make sure in cognitive therapy applications that a client

and therapist generate multiple perspectives for any given event or situation. Underlying these approaches is the notion of playing and experimenting with multiple ways of being.

The Use of Imagery

Because of our clients' hypothetical escape and avoidance of negative images, we employ the typical self-control desensitization technique: Clients repeatedly imagine worrisome or other anxiety-provoking circumstances until negative emotions are being experienced, at which time they imagine relaxing themselves in the situation and shifting their perspectives to the more accurate ones developed during earlier cognitive therapy. Although this method provides some exposure to feared internal and external anxiety cues, its primary purpose is to rehearse the deployment of somatic and cognitive coping responses. Once an image is well rehearsed, we finish the imagery with the imagination of the most likely outcome, based on logic, history, and evidence. Most importantly, we ask our clients to shift to an image of the most likely outcome any time during the day when they detect a worrisome concern. In certain functional senses, imagery is reality: Images can generate the same physiological responses as real-life events do (Lang, 1985), and imagined events stored in memory can at times be confused with actual historical events (Garry, Manning, & Loftus, 1996). Such processes may be the basis for the familiar client comment that new, alternative perspectives do not initially feel as true or believable as their anxious perspectives feel. The frequent imagination of catastrophes has indeed established "evidence" in memory that such things have happened, even though they have not. Creation of a new history of evidence through imagining the most likely outcomes and verifying these outcomes in daily diaries would reasonably counteract these processes.

Identification and Targeting of Core Fears That Are Avoided

If we could identify specific circumstances that create anxiety for our clients, then therapy techniques to deal with these circumstances (including customarily powerful exposure methods) could be usefully employed. As we have seen, GAD is not obviously associated with circumscribed anxiety triggers. The possibility remains, however, that core fears do exist that underlie clients' numerous and constantly changing sources of worrisome concern. Earlier, we have reviewed research suggesting that GAD is often associated with traumatic histories, attachment-related problems in childhood, and current interpersonal problems that prevent clients from having their needs met. These may well represent the underlying source of the clients' view that the world is a dangerous place and that they may not be able to cope. Although we have periodically made use of such themes in standard CBT applications in our previous clinical trials, we have not done so in any systematic fashion. Furthermore, the focus of CBT in our trials has largely been on current concerns, and the scientific questions of those studies have revolved around changing intrapersonal processes and precluded attempts to change interpersonal behavior. But the quest to identify functionally important, underlying core fears is likely to promote greater understanding of the etiological and maintaining conditions of GAD, and the development of therapy methods specifically targeting those fears may well provide the needed ingredients for discovering a truly effective approach for this difficult-to-treat disorder.

Our current efforts to do so stem from findings concerning our clients' characteristic interpersonal problems, and from evidence that these problems predict poor short-term and long-term outcome among clients treated solely with CBT methods (Borkovec, 1995). If insecure attachment in childhood has led to generally muted affective experience and to rigid ways of establishing relationships with others in adulthood that preclude meeting one's most basic interpersonal needs, and if this sequence is the foundation for the origins and maintenance of GAD, then a therapy that not only provides cognitive and behavioral coping responses for anxious experience, but also accesses emotion and modifies interpersonal behavior in adaptive ways, may provide the most effective form of intervention for this disorder. We should know the answer to this question in another few years, when a clinical trial contrasting CBT with and without an interpersonal/emotional processing therapy has been completed (see Newman, Castonguay, Borkovec, & Molnar, Chapter 13, this volume).

SUMMARY

Evidence suggests that worry is predominantly thought activity that focuses on attempts to avoid the occurrence of future catastrophe, and that it thereby functions as a cognitive avoidance maneuver in response to perceived threats. The worry process appears to be negatively reinforced both by immediate suppression of sympathetic reactions to anxiety-provoking material and by the more long-term nonoccurrence of predicted feared events. Worry may also be superficial in its content, reflecting an avoidance of more distressing thoughts and emotions deriving from past traumas, negative childhood attachment experiences, or current interpersonal difficulties. As is the case for any type of avoidance response, worry precludes emotional processing and thus prevents extinction, and it may also strengthen the anxious meanings surrounding its topics and their content. In that case, worry is likely to be relevant to understanding and treating not only GAD, but any emotional disorder wherein emotional processing is important to the amelioration of the problem. Moreover, chronic worry has been associated with significant physical health problems, and its excessively negative valence and its detrimental impact on ability to live in and fully experience the present moment create an inflexible, maladaptive, and unhappy internal world. Although various forms of CBT have been shown to be effective for GAD, half of the clients so treated fail to achieve high end-state functioning. Ideally, new therapeutic developments based on the increasing knowledge of the nature and functions of worry will lead to more effective interventions in the future. Promising examples of such developments include the monitoring of actual worry outcomes, learning increasingly to live in the present moment, imagery rehearsals of effective coping, replacing catastrophic images with images of likely outcomes, identification and therapeutic targeting of fears that potentially underlie superficial avoidant worries, and the targeting of current interpersonal difficulties.

ACKNOWLEDGMENTS

Preparation of this chapter was supported in part by National Institute of Mental Health Grant No. MH-58593 to Thomas D. Borkovec.

REFERENCES

Abel, J. L. (1994, November). *Alexithymia in an analogue sample of generalized anxiety disorder and non-anxious matched controls*. Paper presented at the annual meeting of the Association for Advancement of Behavior Therapy, San Diego, CA.

American Psychiatric Association (APA). (1980). *Diagnostic and statistical manual of mental disorders* (3rd ed.). Washington, DC: Author.

American Psychiatric Association (APA). (1987). *Diagnostic and statistical manual of mental disorders* (3rd ed., rev.). Washington, DC: Author.

American Psychiatric Association (APA). (1994). *Diagnostic and statistical manual of mental disorders* (4th ed.). Washington, DC: Author.

Bandura, A. (1969). *Principles of behavior modification*. New York: Holt, Rinehart & Winston.

Barlow, D. H. (1988). *Anxiety and its disorders: The nature and treatment of anxiety and panic*. New York: Guilford Press.

Barlow, D. H. (2002). *Anxiety and its disorders: The nature and treatment of anxiety and panic* (2nd ed.). New York: Guilford Press.

Beck, A. T., & Emery, G., with Greenberg, R. L. (1985). *Anxiety disorders and phobias: A cognitive perspective*. New York: Basic Books.

Blazer, D., Hughes, D., & George, L. K. (1987). Stressful life events and the onset of a generalized anxiety syndrome. *American Journal of Psychiatry, 144*, 1178–1183.

Borkovec, T. D. (1972). Effects of expectancy on the outcome of systematic desensitization and implosive treatments for analogue anxiety. *Behavior Therapy, 3*, 29–40.

Borkovec, T. D. (1974). Heart-rate process during systematic desensitization and implosive therapy for analogue anxiety. *Behavior Therapy, 5*, 636–641.

Borkovec, T. D. (1979). Extensions of two-factor theory: Cognitive avoidance and autonomic perception. In N. Birbaumer & H. D. Kimmel (Eds.), *Biofeedback and self-regulation* (pp. 139–148). Hillsdale, NJ: Erlbaum.

Borkovec, T. D. (1985). Worry: A potentially useful construct. *Behaviour Research and Therapy, 23,* 481–482.

Borkovec, T. D. (1995, July). *Implication of basic research for treatment developments in generalized anxiety disorder.* Paper presented at the World Congress of Behavioural and Cognitive Therapies, Copenhagen.

Borkovec, T. D., Abel, J. L., & Newman, H. (1995). The effects of therapy on comorbid conditions in generalized anxiety disorder. *Journal of Consulting and Clinical Psychology, 63,* 479–483.

Borkovec, T. D., Hazlett-Stevens, H., & Diaz, M. L. (1999). The role of positive beliefs about worry in generalized anxiety disorder and its treatment. *Clinical Psychology and Psychotherapy, 6,* 126–138.

Borkovec, T. D., & Hu, S. (1990). The effect of worry on cardiovascular response to phobic imagery. *Behaviour Research and Therapy, 28,* 69–73.

Borkovec, T. D., & Inz, J. (1990). The nature of worry in generalized anxiety disorder: A predominance of thought activity. *Behaviour Research and Therapy, 28,* 153–158.

Borkovec, T. D., Lyonfields, J. D., Wiser, S. L., & Diehl, L. (1993). The role of worrisome thinking in the suppression of cardiovascular response to phobic imagery. *Behaviour Research and Therapy, 31,* 321–324.

Borkovec, T. D., Ray, W. J., & Stöber, J. (1998). Worry: A cognitive phenomenon intimately linked to affective, physiological, and interpersonal behavioral processes. *Cognitive Therapy and Research, 22,* 561–576.

Borkovec, T. D., Robinson, E., Pruzinsky, T., & DePree, J. A. (1983). Preliminary exploration of worry: Some characteristics and processes. *Behaviour Research and Therapy, 21,* 9–16.

Borkovec, T. D., & Roemer, L. (1995). Perceived functions of worry among generalized anxiety disorder subjects: Distraction from more emotional topics? *Journal of Behavior Therapy and Experimental Psychiatry, 26,* 25–30.

Borkovec, T. D., & Ruscio, A. (2001). Psychotherapy for generalized anxiety disorder. *Journal of Clinical Psychiatry, 62,* 37–45.

Borkovec, T. D., & Whisman, M. A. (1996). Psychological treatment for generalized anxiety disorder. In M. R. Mavissakalian & R. F. Prien (Eds.), *Long-term treatments of anxiety disorders* (pp. 171–199). Washington, DC: American Psychiatric Press.

Borkovec, T. D., Wilkinson, L., Folensbee, R., & Lerman, C. (1983). Stimulus control applications to the treatment of worry. *Behaviour Research and Therapy, 21,* 247–251.

Bowlby, J. (1982). *Attachment and loss: Vol. 1. Attachment* (2nd ed.). New York: Basic Books.

Brown, T. A., & Barlow, D. H. (1992). Comorbidity among anxiety disorders: Implications for treatment and DSM-IV. *Journal of Consulting and Clinical Psychology, 60,* 835–844.

Brown, T. A., Barlow, D. H., & Liebowitz, M. R. (1994). The empirical basis of generalized anxiety disorder. *American Journal of Psychiatry, 151,* 1272–1280.

Butler, G., Wells, A., & Dewick, H. (1995). Differential effects of worry and imagery after exposure to a stressful stimulus: A pilot study. *Behavioural and Cognitive Psychotherapy, 23,* 45–56.

Carter, W., Johnson, M., & Borkovec, T. D. (1986). Worry: An electrocortical analysis. *Advances in Behaviour Research and Therapy, 8,* 193–204.

Cassidy, J. (1995). Attachment and generalized anxiety disorder. In D. Cicchetti & S. Toth (Eds.), *Rochester Symposium on Developmental Psychopathology : Vol. 6. Emotion, cognition and representation* (pp. 343–370). Rochester, NY: University of Rochester Press.

Chambless, D. L., & Gillis, M. M. (1993). Cognitive therapy of anxiety disorders. *Journal of Consulting and Clinical Psychology, 61,* 248–260.

Davey, G. C. L., & Matchett, G. (1994). Unconditioned stimulus rehearsal and the retention and enhancement of differential "fear" conditioning: Effects of trait and state anxiety. *Journal of Abnormal Psychology, 103,* 708–718.

Deffenbacher, J. L. (1980). Worry and emotionality in test anxiety. In I. G. Sarason (Ed.), *Test anxiety: Theory, research and application* (pp. 111–128). Hillside, NJ: Erlbaum.

Fehr, F. S., & Stern, J. A. (1970). Peripheral physiological variables and emotion: The James–Lange theory revisited. *Psychological Bulletin, 74,* 411–424.

Fierman, E. J., Hunt, M. F., Pratt, L. A., & Warshaw, M. G. (1993). Trauma and post-traumatic stress disorder in subjects with anxiety disorders. *American Journal of Psychiatry, 150,* 1872–1874.

Foa, E. B., & Kozak, M. J. (1986). Emotional processing of fear: Exposure to corrective information. *Psychological Bulletin, 99,* 20–35.

Freeston, M. H., Dugas, M. J., & Ladouceur, R. (1996). Thoughts, images, worry, and anxiety. *Cognitive Therapy and Research, 20,* 265–273.

Freeston, M. H., Rheaume, J., Letarte, H., Dugas, M. J., & Ladouceur, R. (1994). Why do people worry? *Personality and Individual Differences, 17,* 791–802.

Garry, M., Manning, C. G., & Loftus, E. F. (1996). Imagination inflation: Imagining a childhood event inflates confidence that it occurred. *Psychonomic Bulletin and Review, 3,* 208–214.

Goldberger, A. L. (1992). Applications of chaos to physiology and medicine. In J. H. Kim & J. Stringer (Eds.), *Applied chaos* (pp. 321–329). New York: Wiley.

Goldfried, M. R. (1971). Systematic desensitization as training in self-control. *Journal of Consulting and Clinical Psychology, 37,* 228–234.

Goldstein, A. J., & Chambless, D. L. (1978). A reanalysis of agoraphobia. *Behavior Therapy, 9,* 47–59.

Gray, J. A. (1982). Precis of "The neurophysiology of anxiety: An enquiry into the functions of the septo-hippocampal system. " *Behavioral and Brain Sciences, 5,* 469–534.

Grayson, J. B., & Borkovec, T. D. (1978). The effects of expectancy and imagined response to phobic stimuli on fear reduction. *Cognitive Therapy and Research, 2,* 11–24.

Grayson, J. B., Foa, E. B., & Steketee, G. (1982). Habituation during exposure treatment: Distraction vs. attention-focusing. *Behaviour Research and Therapy, 20,* 323–328.

Greenberg, L. S., & Safran, J. D. (1987). *Emotion in psychotherapy.* New York: Guilford Press.

Greenberg, P. E., Sisitsky, T., Kessler, R. C., Finklestein, S. N., Berndt, E. R., Davidson, J. R. T., Ballenger, J. C., & Fyer, A. J. (1999). The economic burden of anxiety disorders in the 1990s. *Journal of Clinical Psychiatry, 60,* 427–435.

Grossman, P., Stemmler, G., & Meinhardt, E. (1990). Paced respiratory sinus arrythmia as an index of cadiac parasympathetic tone during varying behavioral tasks. *Psychophysiology, 27,* 404–416.

Grossman, P., & Svebak, S. (1987). Respiratory sinus arrhythmia as an index of parasympathetic cardiac control during active coping. *Psychophysiology, 24,* 228–235.

Hazlett-Stevens, H., & Borkovec, T. D. (2001). Effects of worry and progressive relaxation on the reduction of fear in speech phobia: An investigation of situational exposure. *Behavior Therapy, 32,* 503–517.

Heller, W., Nitschke, J., Etienne, M., & Miller, G. (1997). Patterns of regional brain activity differentiate types of anxiety. *Journal of Abnormal Psychology, 106,* 376–385.

Herman, J. L., Perry, J. C., & van der Kolk, B. A. (1989). Childhood trauma in borderline personality disorder. *American Journal of Psychiatry, 146,* 490–495.

Hoehn-Saric, R., & McLeod, D. R. (1988). The peripheral sympathetic nervous system: Its role in normal and pathological anxiety. *Psychiatric Clinics of North America, 11,* 375–386.

Hoehn-Saric, R., McLeod, D. R., & Zimmerli, W. D. (1989). Somatic manifestations in women with generalized anxiety disorder: Physiological responses to psychological stress. *Archives of General Psychiatry, 46,* 1113–1119.

Horowitz, L. M., Rosenberg, S. E., & Bartholomew, K. (1993). Interpersonal problems, attachment styles, and outcome in brief dynamic therapy. *Journal of Consulting and Clinical Psychology, 61,* 549–560.

Jennings, J. R. (1986). Bodily changes during attention. In M. Coles, E. Donchin, & S. W. Porges (Eds.), *Psychophysiology: Systems, processes, and applications* (pp. 268–290). New York: Guilford Press.

Jones, T., & Davey, G. C. (1990). The effects of cued UCS rehearsal on the retention of differential "fear" conditioning: An experimental analogue of the "worry" process. *Behaviour Research and Therapy, 28,* 159–164.

Jordan, R. K., Schlenger, W. E., Hough, R., Kulka, R. A., Weiss, D., Fairbank, J. A., & Marmar, C. R. (1991). Lifetime and current prevalence of specific psychiatric disorders among Vietnam veterans and controls. *Archives of General Psychiatry, 48,* 207–215.

Kosslyn, S. M. (1983). *Ghosts in the mind's machine: Creating and using images in the brain.* New York: Norton.

Kubzansky, L. D., Kawachi, I., Spiro, A., III, Weiss, S. T., Vokonas, P. S., & Sparrow, D. (1997). Is worrying bad for your heart?: A prospective study of worry and coronary heart disease in the Normative Aging Study. *Circulation, 95,* 818–824.

Lang, P. J. (1985). The cognitive psychophysiology of emotion: Fear and anxiety. In A. H. Tuma & J. D. Maser (Eds.), *Anxiety and the anxiety disorders* (pp. 131–170). Hillsdale, NJ: Erlbaum.

Lichtenstein, J., & Cassidy, J. (1991, March). *The Inventory of Adult Attachment: Validation of a new measure.* Paper presented at the biennial meeting of the Society for Research in Child Development, Seattle, WA.

Lyonfields, J. D., Borkovec, T. D., & Thayer, J. F. (1995). Vagal tone in generalized anxiety disorder and the effects of aversive imagery and worrisome thinking. *Behavior Therapy, 26,* 457–466.

Marten, P. A., Brown, T. A., Barlow, D. H., Borkovec, T. D., Shear, M. K., & Lydiard, R. B. (1993). Evaluation of the ratings comprising the associated symptom criterion of DSM-III-R generalized anxiety disorder. *Journal of Nervous and Mental Disease, 181,* 676–682.

Mathews, A. (1990). Why worry?: The cognitive function of anxiety. *Behaviour Research and Therapy, 28,* 455–468.

McGuire, W. J., & McGuire, C. V. (1991). The content, structure, and operation of thought systems. In R. S. Wyer & T. K. Srull (Eds.), *Advances in social cognition* (pp. 1–78). Hillside, NJ: Erlbaum.

Molina, S., Borkovec, T. D., Peasley, C., & Person, D. (1998). Content analysis of worrisome streams of consciousness in anxious and dysphoric participants. *Cognitive Therapy and Research, 22,* 109–123.

Mowrer, O. H. (1947). On the dual nature of learning: A re-interpretation of "conditioning" and "problem-solving. " *Harvard Educational Review, 17,* 102–148.

Öst, L. (1987). Applied relaxation: Description of a coping technique and review of controlled studies. *Behaviour Research and Therapy, 25,* 397–409.

Paivio, A. (1986). *Mental representations: A dual coding approach.* New York: Oxford University Press.

Paivio, A., & Marschark, M. (1991). Integrative processing of concrete and abstract sentences. In A. Paivio (Ed.), *Images in the mind: The evolution of a theory* (pp. 134–154). New York: Harvester Wheatsheaf.

Peasley, C. E., Molina, S., & Borkovec, T. D. (1994, November). *Empathy in generalized anxiety disorder.* Paper presented at the annual meeting of the Association for Advancement of Behavior Therapy, San Diego, CA.

Peasley-Miklus, C., & Vrana, S. R. (2000). Effect of worrisome and relaxing thinking on fearful emotional processing. *Behaviour Research and Therapy, 38,* 129–144.

Pincus, A. L., & Borkovec, T. D. (1994, June). *Interpersonal problems in generalized anxiety disorder: Preliminary clustering of patients' interpersonal dysfunction.* Paper presented at the annual meeting of the American Psychological Society, New York.

Porges, S. W. (1992). Autonomic regulation and attention. In B. A. Campbell, H. Hayne, & R. Richardson (Eds.), *Attention and information processing in infants and adults* (pp. 201–223). Hillside, NJ: Erbaum.

Pruzinsky, T., & Borkovec, T. D. (1990). Cognitive and personality characteristics of worriers. *Behaviour Research and Therapy, 28,* 507–512.

Roemer, L., & Borkovec, T. D. (1994). Effects of suppressing thoughts about emotional material. *Journal of Abnormal Psychology, 103,* 467–474.

Roemer, L., Molina, S., & Borkovec, T. D. (1997). An investigation of worry content among generally anxious individuals. *Journal of Nervous and Mental Disease, 185,* 314–319.

Roemer, L., Molina, S., Litz, B. T., & Borkovec, T. D. (1997). Preliminary investigation of the role of previous exposure to potentially traumatizing events in generalized anxiety disorder. *Depression and Anxiety, 4,* 134–138.

Roy-Byrne, P. P. (1996). Generalized anxiety and mixed anxiety–depression: Association with disability and health care utilization. *Journal of Clinical Psychiatry, 57,* 86–91.

Schut, A., Pincus, A., Castonguay, L. G., Bedics, J., Kline, M., Long, D., & Seals, K. (1997, November). *Perceptions of attachment and self-representations at best and worst states in generalized anxiety disorder.* Poster session presented at the annual meeting of the Association for Advancement of Behavior Therapy, Miami Beach, FL.

Segerstrom, S. C., Glover, D. A., Craske, M. G., & Fahey, J. L. (1999). Worry affects the immune response to phobic fear. *Brain, Behavior, and Immunity, 13,* 80–92.

Smith, L. C. (1984). Semantic satiation affects category membership decision time but not lexical priming. *Memory and Cognition, 12,* 483–488.

Stampfl, T. G., & Levis, D. J. (1967). Essentials of implosive therapy: A learning-theory-based psychodynamic behavioral therapy. *Journal of Abnormal Psychology, 72,* 496–530.

Stöber, J. (1998). Worry, problem elaboration and suppression of imagery: The role of concreteness. *Behaviour Research and Therapy, 36,* 751–756.

Stöber, J., Tepperwien, S., & Staak, M. (2000). Worrying leads to reduced concreteness of problem elaborations: Evidence for the avoidance theory of worry. *Anxiety, Stress, and Coping, 13,* 217–227.

Suinn, R. M., & Richardson, F. (1971). Anxiety management training: A nonspecific behavior therapy program for anxiety control. *Behavior Therapy, 2,* 498–510.

Thayer, J. F., Friedman, B. H., & Borkovec, T. D. (1996). Autonomic characteristics of generalized anxiety disorder and worry. *Biological Psychiatry, 39,* 255–266.

Thayer, J. F., Friedman, B. H., Borkovec, T. D., Johnsen, B. H., & Molina, S. (2000). Phasic heart period reactions to cued threat and non-threat stimuli in generalized anxiety disorder. *Psychophysiology, 37,* 361–368.

Torgersen, S. (1986). Childhood and family characteristics in panic and generalized anxiety disorders. *American Journal of Psychiatry, 143,* 630–632.

Tucker, D. M., Antes, J. R., Stenslie, C. E., & Barnhardt, T. M. (1978). Anxiety and lateral cerebral function. *Journal of Abnormal Psychology, 87,* 380–383.

Tucker, D. M., & Newman, J. P. (1981). Verbal versus imaginal cognitive strategies in the inhibition of emotional arousal. *Cognitive Therapy and Research, 5,* 197–202.

Tyler, S., & Tucker, D. (1982). Anxiety and perceptual structure: Individual differences in neuropsychological function. *Journal of Abnormal Psychology, 91,* 210–220.

Vasey, M. W., & Borkovec, T. D. (1992). A catastrophizing assessment of worrisome thoughts. *Cognitive Therapy and Research, 16,* 1–16.

Vrana, S. R., Cuthbert, B. N., & Lang, P. J. (1986). Fear imagery and text processing. *Psychophysiology, 23,* 247–253.

Wells, A., & Papageorgiou, C. (1995). Worry and the incubation of intrusive images following stress. *Behaviour Research and Therapy, 33,* 579–583.

Yamas, K., Hazlett-Stevens, H., & Borkovec, M. (1997, November). *Alexithymia in generalized anxiety disorder.* Paper presented at the annual meeting of the Association for Advancement of Behavior Therapy, Miami Beach, FL.

Zuellig, A. R., Newman, M. G., Alcaine, O. A., & Behar, E. S. (1999, November). *Childhood history of post-traumatic stress disorder in adults with generalized anxiety disorder, panic disorder, and non-disordered controls.* Poster presented at the annual meeting of the Association for Advancement of Behavior Therapy, Toronto.

CHAPTER 5

Information-Processing Approaches

Assessing the Selective Functioning of Attention, Interpretation, and Retrieval

COLIN MacLEOD
ELIZABETH RUTHERFORD

It is well established that patients with generalized anxiety disorder (GAD) report worrying with greater frequency and intensity than is the case for most individuals in the normal population (Beck, Stanley, & Zebb, 1996; Dugas et al., 1998). Worry is a mode of cognitive processing within which threatening thoughts are overrepresented (Borkovec, 1994; Borkovec & Inz, 1990; Borkovec & Lyonfields, 1993; Borkovec, Ray, & Stöber, 1998), and it tends to be accompanied by the concomitant experience of state anxiety, even when it is directly elicited by experimental instructions (Molina, Borkovec, Peasley, & Person, 1998). Accordingly, researchers have sought to identify the patterns of information processing that give rise to this type of cognitive experience, in order to address the possibility that the causal basis of GAD symptomatology might reside in the functioning of these underlying cognitive processes.

Though worry represents a characteristic feature of GAD, it is also common in nonpathological anxiety. Factor-analytic studies of state anxiety symptoms in the normal population consistently have revealed a major worry factor (Endler, Parker, Bagby, & Cox, 1991; Steptoe & Kearsley, 1990). The tendency to experience elevated state anxiety varies across the normal population as a function of trait anxiety (see Spielberger, 1972). Therefore, the tendency of patients with GAD to worry with disproportionate frequency and intensity is shared by those members of the nonclinical population who display high levels of trait anxiety (Eysenck & van Berkum, 1992). Further evidence of an association between high trait anxiety and GAD comes from the common finding that patients with GAD typically score very highly on measures of trait anxiety (Rapee, 1991) and from the observation that a heightened level of trait anxiety represents a risk factor for the development of GAD (Eysenck, 1992). Although the nature and content of worry in patients with GAD differs little from that observed in the nonclinical population (Borkovec, Shadick, & Hopkins, 1991), patients typically report having less ability to consciously control their worrying than do nonpatients who worry (Craske, Rapee, Jackel, & Barlow, 1989; Sanderson & Barlow, 1990). This clinical feature is captured in the fourth edition of the *Diagnostic and Statistical Manual of Mental Disorders* (DSM-IV; American Psychiatric Association, 1994), which explicitly requires that worry must be experienced as difficult to control before a diagnosis of GAD can be given. Thus, although patients with GAD and members of the nonclinical population with high trait anxiety share certain cognitive characteristics, they also display potentially important cognitive differences.

In this chapter, we provide an overview of research designed to illuminate the types of cognitive operations most often implicated in information-processing theories of GAD. The various experimental approaches that have been employed are critically evaluated. Reference is also made where appropriate to work that has examined patterns of selective information processing in populations with high trait anxiety, primarily to highlight similarities and potential discrepancies between the information-processing characteristics of GAD and high trait anxiety. We conclude the chapter by considering the likely causal role played by observed information biases in the mediation of anxiety symptomatology.

INFORMATION-PROCESSING ACCOUNTS OF GAD

Although cognitive models of anxiety vulnerability and anxiety disorders vary greatly in terms of their architecture, they share the common feature that susceptibility to anxiety and its associated disorders is attributed to the operation of selective processing biases within the cognitive system (see MacLeod, 1999). Most commonly, such accounts consider anxiety disorders such as GAD to result from the tendency to preferentially encode threatening information, to draw threatening inferences under conditions of ambiguity, and/or to preferentially retrieve threatening information from memory.

The influence exerted by the early theories of Aaron Beck (1976; Beck & Emery with Greenberg, 1985; Beck, Rush, Shaw, & Emery, 1979) and G. H. Bower (1981, 1983) in stimulating and directing research on the selective processing biases associated with anxiety cannot be overemphasized, as has been recognized elsewhere (see Mathews & MacLeod, 1994). Beck and his colleagues developed a schema model (see Graesser & Nakamura, 1982) to explain the genesis and maintenance of emotional disorders. They attributed GAD to the impact of maladaptive cognitive structures termed "danger schemata," which automatically facilitate the encoding and retrieval of threatening information, as well as the threatening interpretation of ambiguous information. In contrast, Bower proposed that anxiety is sustained and exacerbated by the automatic spread of activation from anxiety nodes within semantic memory, which serves to "prime" threat-related information, thereby rendering it disproportionately available to other cognitive processes. Although the models of Beck and Bower were developed from different theoretical perspectives, both predict that anxious individuals should display enhanced encoding and retrieval of threatening information, and should exhibit an elevated tendency to impose threatening interpretations upon ambiguous material. Furthermore, these biases should occur quite automatically, in the sense that they should not depend upon conscious mediation.

Although growing diversity has accompanied their proliferation, other cognitive models of anxiety tend to share these same characteristics. For example, in response to the constraints imposed by the emerging body of experimental findings, Williams, Watts, MacLeod, and Mathews (1988, 1997) have proposed an account of anxiety vulnerability within which particular emphasis is placed upon the degree to which different types of cognitive representations undergo what Graf and Mandler (1984) have termed "integrative processing." This automatic process involves the temporary strengthening of a mental representation's internal structure and serves to make that representation more accessible, in that it will come to mind more readily when only some of its features are processed. According to Williams and colleagues' model, vulnerability to anxiety is associated with a disproportionate tendency to carry out integrative processing upon threatening mental representations. The resulting enhanced accessibility of these representations causes threat-related stimuli to "pop out" of stimulus arrays in a manner that recruits selective attention and increases the ease with which threatening interpretations of ambiguity are apprehended. Williams et al. consider anxiety symptoms to result directly from this preferential automatic processing of threatening information, which they believe causally underpins the development of GAD.

Many other influential models place similar emphasis upon the role of selective information processing in the genesis of anxious symptomatology (see MacLeod, 1991, 1999; Mogg & Bradley, 1998). Öhman (1993,

1999), for example, has developed an account of anxiety that implicates an underlying bias in the preattentive processing of threatening information. Eysenck's (1997) unified theory of anxiety places principal importance upon hypervigilance for threat information and the tendency to impose unduly threatening interpretations upon ambiguity in explaining the development and maintenance of GAD. Mogg and Bradley (1998) have put forward a cognitive–motivational theory of anxiety, which also predicts that GAD should be associated with automatic attentional orientation toward minor threat cues. Mathews and Mackintosh (1998) have advanced a model of anxiety within which processing options appraised to be highly threatening automatically will recruit disproportionate processing resources in individuals with elevated levels of anxiety vulnerability, thereby eliciting the symptoms of anxiety. However, these authors also suggest that the degree to which such automatic processing biases influence emotional state may depend upon whether they can be overridden by controlled cognitive operations, which they propose is more likely for nonpatients with high trait anxiety than for patients with GAD. In a refinement of Beck's original model, Beck and Clark (1997) similarly identify a potential role for controlled processes to modify the automatic processing biases assumed to be associated with anxiety vulnerability. This refined model continues to propose that vulnerability is characterized by the rapid automatic detection of threat stimuli, but postulates that this is followed by more controlled semantic elaboration. Beck and Clark argue that this controlled elaboration stage can be employed adaptively to moderate the anxiety elicited during earlier stages of processing—for example, by engaging in "defensive" activity. However, in patients with GAD, they consider this controlled stage to involve sustained selective processing of threatening information, now with the accompanying elaboration that elicits the conscious experience of worry. Thus, despite their differences, these various cognitive models of anxiety—and many more besides (e.g., Rapee, 2001; Wells, 1995; Woody & Rachman, 1994)—have in common the central idea that automatic biases in the selective processing of threat-related information may make an important causal contribution to the development and maintenance of GAD.

Given that such a wide variety of cognitive models share the core premise that GAD symptomatology may result from selective processing biases operating automatically to favor threatening information during encoding, interpretation, and/or retrieval, it is not surprising that many researchers have now directly investigated the patterns of processing selectivity that patients with GAD display across these three classes of cognitive operation. The remainder of the chapter provides a review of the experimental literature designed to establish not only the processing biases that characterize patients with GAD, but also the degree to which these are similar to, or different from, those that characterize nonpatients with high trait anxiety. One possibility, highlighted within several models discussed earlier, is that GAD pathology may reflect the inability to employ controlled processing to modify biases that, for both patients and highly trait-anxious nonpatients, originate at an automatic level of cognition. To appraise the viability of this position, we contrast, whenever possible, the patterns of processing selectivity displayed by patients with GAD and participants with high trait anxiety across tasks that preclude or encourage the use of controlled processing.

ASSESSING BIASES IN THE ENCODING OF THREATENING INFORMATION

Researchers have adopted a wide array of experimental techniques to assess whether anxiety vulnerability is associated with biased patterns of selective processing during the encoding of emotional information. Often participants are directly instructed to ignore the emotional stimulus information, which is presented as a potential source of distraction while they carry out some central task. The encoding of this emotional information then is revealed by the degree to which its presence serves to disrupt, or interfere with, the execution of the principal task. Such interference approaches have provided a wealth of evidence to support the presence of an encoding advantage for threatening stimuli in patients with GAD.

In one early interference study, Mathews and MacLeod (1986) presented patients with GAD and nonanxious controls with either threatening or neutral stimulus words to one ear, which these participants were instructed to ignore. Simultaneously with the presentation of this emotional information, participants were required to monitor the display of a computer, which occasionally instructed them to press a response key as quickly as possible and recorded the speed with which their response was executed. It was reasoned that performance on this central task would be most efficient to the extent that participants were able to avoid the diversion of processing resources toward the distracting auditory information. For the nonanxious controls, response latencies on the central task were equivalent regardless of the emotional valence of the auditory distractors, suggesting that these individuals could equally well avoid encoding either neutral or threatening information. However, the patients with GAD displayed a significant slowing of responses on this central task in the presence of threatening compared to neutral distractors, suggesting that this anxiety disorder is indeed characterized by a tendency to preferentially encode threatening information, even under instructions to ignore this information.

This tendency for patients with GAD to demonstrate disproportionate performance disruption on a central task when trying to ignore threatening distractor information has now been confirmed repeatedly (see McNally, 1995, 1998). Probably the greatest wealth of evidence has come from an interference procedure that represents an adaptation of the classic Stroop color-naming task (Stroop, 1935), which has become known as the "emotional Stroop paradigm" (see Williams, Mathews, & MacLeod, 1996). This procedure involves presenting participants with threatening and neutral words in different ink colors, and instructing them to rapidly name the colors of these words while ignoring their semantic content. The tendency to selectively encode the content of threatening stimuli should be revealed by slowed color naming. Consistent with the hypothesis that patients with GAD preferentially encode threat-related information, Mathews and MacLeod (1985) demonstrated that, compared to nonanxious individuals, such patients did indeed display disproportionately slow color-naming latencies on threat words relative to neutral words. This tendency for patients with GAD to display exaggerated color-naming interference effects on threat words has since been replicated a great many times, across studies that have employed a wide variety of stimulus presentation formats (e.g., Azaies, Granger, & Debray, 1994; Bradley, Mogg, Millar, & White, 1995; Mogg, Bradley, Williams, & Mathews, 1993; Mogg, Mathews, & Weinman, 1989).

Delayed color naming of threatening words has also been observed in nonpatients with high trait anxiety (Fox, 1993; Mogg et al., 2000; Richards & Millwood, 1989). Like patients with GAD, highly trait-anxious persons also demonstrate threat interference effects across a wide variety of stimuli, spanning the full range of social and physical threat. Although the similar broad scopes of their attentional biases are consistent with the possibility that high trait anxiety and GAD may represent related conditions, it is also appropriate to note certain differences in the manifestation of these effects within each population. Unlike patients with GAD, who appear to display chronically heightened threat interference effects, individuals with high trait anxiety may not reliably display these effects unless they are exposed to a stressor. Thus, for example, we (MacLeod & Rutherford, 1992) observed no difference in the profiles of color-naming latencies shown by students high and low in trait anxiety on a computerized variant of the emotional Stroop task when these participants were tested at a time of low stress. However, as the proximity of important examinations increased, the high-anxiety students became slower to color-name threat words relative to neutral words, whereas the low-anxiety students developed the reverse tendency. This has led to the conclusion that high levels of trait anxiety are characterized not by the constant presence of a selective attentional bias toward threatening information, as is the case for patients with GAD, but rather by the tendency to develop such a biased pattern of information processing in response to stress (Mathews, 1993; Mogg & Bradley, 1998). Of course, if such a pattern of attentional selectivity does contribute to the development of GAD, then this may explain why individuals with high trait anxiety are particularly susceptible to developing GAD, especially when exposed to extended periods of environmental stress.

Although patterns of performance on interference tasks have lent considerable support to the idea that patients with GAD selectively attend to threatening information, this methodological approach inevitably has also attracted its share of criticism. One reason for concern is that such patients might show performance decrements in the presence of threatening information for reasons that have nothing to do with the selective processing of this information. For example, it has been suggested that patients and controls may afford the same processing to threatening information, but that such information may provoke a more intense anxiety response among patients (MacLeod & Mathews, 1991). Disruptions of task performance, then, may reflect only the general cognitive impairment associated with high levels of state anxiety (see Eysenck, 1982), rather than being caused by an underlying pattern of selective processing. A second concern is that slowed color naming of threat words may result from a tendency to display attentional avoidance of threatening information, rather than attentional vigilance for such information (de Ruiter & Brusschot, 1994). For example, patients with GAD could be slow to color-name threat words because they allocate attention away from such stimuli altogether, thereby impairing the registration of other attributes such as color. The viability of such an account is reinforced by Lavy and van den Hout's (1994) demonstration that instructing participants to attentionally avoid certain classes of words during performance of a color-naming task leads to a slowing rather than to a speeding of color naming for these stimuli.

If exaggerated threat interference effects truly reflect the enhanced encoding of threatening stimuli, then it should be possible to create circumstances under which heightened anxiety vulnerability is associated with superior task performance in the presence of threatening stimuli. All this requires is the construction of tasks within which performance would be facilitated by the enhanced encoding of threatening information. A number of such tasks have been developed, and the resulting patterns of performance provide converging support for the hypothesis that anxiety vulnerability is associated with an encoding advantage for threatening information.

For example, researchers have employed the lexical decision task (Forbach, Stanners, & Hochhaus, 1974) to assess whether patients with GAD encode threat-related words with disproportionate ease. In this experimental procedure, participants are presented with letter strings and must quickly press either of two response buttons to indicate whether or not each string represents a legitimate word. The rapidity with which they can accurately classify the lexical status of genuine words reflects the speed with which they can encode these stimuli. MacLeod and Mathews

(1991) found no evidence that patients with GAD, when presented with the task of classifying the lexical status of single letter strings, displayed disproportionately fast lexical decision latencies on threat words. However, when these researchers employed a double-string variant of the lexical decision task (which required participants to assign priorities to the processing of alternative stimulus options), then they did indeed find that patients with GAD, unlike nonanxious controls, displayed speeded lexical decisions on threat words. Similar findings have been reported by Mogg, Mathews, Eysenck, and May (1991). This pattern of facilitated performance suggests that GAD is associated not with an increased ability to encode threatening stimuli, but rather with a tendency to assign a disproportionately high priority to the encoding of threatening stimuli, under circumstances that present alternative processing options.

More direct measures of attentional allocation have yielded further evidence that patients with GAD direct processing resources toward threatening information. For example, MacLeod, Mathews, and Tata (1986) briefly presented patients with GAD and nonanxious controls with pairs of words, separated on the vertical axis of a computer screen. On critical trials, one member of this pair was a threatening word, and the other was a neutral word. Following the termination of each such display, a small dot probe could appear on the screen within the spatial location previously occupied by either of these two words. Participants were required to press a key whenever a probe was detected, and their response latencies were recorded. It was reasoned that if attention was drawn selectively toward the more threatening words within each stimulus pair, then probes presented to this same spatial area should be detected more rapidly than those presented to the other screen location. MacLeod and colleagues observed that patients with GAD displayed speeded detection responses for probes that appeared in the same locations as the threatening stimulus words, suggesting that GAD is associated with the selective allocation of attention toward the source of threatening information. Interestingly, the nonanxious controls tended to display the reverse pattern of detection latencies, suggesting that these individuals may have systematically diverted their attentional resources away from the locus of the threatening stimuli.

Numerous variants of this attentional probe paradigm have now served to reinforce this conclusion. Most have employed verbal stimuli similar to those presented by MacLeod and colleagues (1986) and have confirmed that patients with GAD, but not nonanxious controls, reliably demonstrate speeded processing of visual probes presented in the spatial vicinity of threatening stimulus words (e.g., Mogg, Bradley, & Williams, 1995; Mogg, Mathews, & Eysenck, 1992). Other versions of the attentional probe task have employed pictorial stimuli, such as angry and neutral faces, and have demonstrated that patients with GAD also show more rapid responses to probes appearing in the vicinity of threatening rather than neutral pictures (Bradley, Mogg, White, Groom, & de Bono, 1999).

Attentional probe studies have also yielded compelling evidence to indicate that attentional orientation toward threatening stimuli may be characteristic of elevated trait anxiety in the nonclinical population. Some of these studies have shown that participants with high trait anxiety display a relative speeding to process probes presented in the spatial vicinity of threatening verbal stimuli (Mogg, Bradley, & Hallowell, 1994), while others have demonstrated similar effects with pictorial stimuli (Bradley, Mogg, & Millar, 2000). As has been the case in emotional Stroop studies of nonpatients with high trait anxiety, evidence from some attentional probe studies suggests that this tendency to orient attention toward threatening information can remain latent in such nonpatients until evoked by stressors that elevate state anxiety (Broadbent & Broadbent, 1988; MacLeod & Mathews, 1988). For example, MacLeod and Mathews (1988) found students high and low in trait anxiety not to differ in their patterns of probe detection latencies at a time of low stress. However, as these students approached the week of an important examination, those who reported high levels of trait anxiety came to display speeded detection of probes in the vicinity of threat words, suggesting the development of attentional orientation toward such stimuli. In contrast, for students with low trait anxiety, the advent of this stressor was associated with the emergence of disproportionately slow detection latencies for probes presented in the vicinity of threat words, suggesting that these individuals came to orient attention away from such threat stimuli in response to this stressor. Once again, therefore, it would appear that high levels of trait anxiety in the nonclinical population may be associated with the latent tendency to develop the same pattern of attentional bias as the one displayed by patients with GAD, but that this tendency becomes manifest only in response to environmental stress. This style of attentional response to stress may help explain why individuals high in trait anxiety are at increased risk of developing GAD.

The range of experimental methodologies that have been adopted to investigate the patterns of selective attention shown by patients with GAD continues to expand. For example, in a study cited by Mogg and Bradley (1998), Mogg, Bradley, and Millar employed eye movement measures to demonstrate that patients with GAD showed a greater probability than nonanxious controls of shifting their gaze toward images of faces that display threatening expressions. Furthermore, the patients were also found to orient their gaze toward such stimuli with disproportionate speed. Despite the great variation in the methodologies that have been utilized, the findings yielded by this diverse range of experimental paradigms converge reassuringly upon the same conclusion: Together, these findings represent very strong evidence that GAD is characterized by a disproportionate tendency to selectively encode a broad range of threatening information. Thus the evidence is quite consistent with the possibility that selective encoding of threatening information may indeed contribute to the development and maintenance of this clinical disorder.

ASSESSING BIASES IN THE INTERPRETATION OF AMBIGUOUS INFORMATION

People's everyday environments frequently present them with ambiguous information permitting, but not requiring, interpretations that could evoke anxiety. The offhand comment of an acquaintance, a friend's ambivalent expression, the unexpected interest of a stranger, or newly developed somatic sensations could all be accommodated by either threatening or nonthreatening interpretations. A tendency to systematically impose more threatening interpretations on such ambiguity would give people increased grounds for worry, and would be likely to elicit elevated levels of anxiety. The possibility that interpretative biases may underpin the symptomatology of GAD has led a number of investigators to examine directly whether patients with GAD display an elevated likelihood of interpreting ambiguity in a threatening manner.

In order to avoid the methodological limitations associated with self-report studies, investigators have developed various paradigms that use task performance measures to reveal the interpretations that patients with GAD actually do make when required to process ambiguous information. One such approach has involved giving participants a small battery of psychometric tests, within which is included a simple spelling test that requires participants to write down words presented on audiotape. Embedded among a substantial number of unambiguous words are critical homophones that each permit a threat-related and a neutral meaning, such as "pain"/"pane" or "die"/"dye." The spellings participants use when they write down these words yield a measure of the interpretations they impose on this ambiguous information. Consistent with the hypothesis that patients with GAD interpret ambiguity in a disproportionately threatening manner, these individuals display a greater tendency than controls to write down the more negative interpretations when presented with such homophones (Mathews, Richards, & Eysenck, 1989; Mogg, Bradley, Miller, & Potts, 1994).

Many researchers have reported that the tendency to display a pattern of biased spelling of homophones is also associated with high trait anxiety in the nonclinical population. Repeatedly, participants high in trait anxiety have shown a greater tendency than individuals low in trait anxiety to provide the more threatening spelling for these homophones (Byrne & Eysenck, 1993; Richards, Reynolds, & French, 1993; Russo, Patterson, Roberson, & Stevenson, 1996). This suggests the possibility that the selective imposition of threatening spelling shown by patients with GAD might reflect their elevated trait anxiety levels. Indeed, in a study reported by Eysenck, MacLeod, and Mathews (1987), which compared patients with GAD and nonclinical controls, the degree to which threatening spellings were given for homophones was found to reflect trait anxiety level more directly than clinical status.

However, some investigators have drawn attention to the possibility that the patterns of spelling commonly produced by patients with GAD on this task may reflect the operation of a response bias rather than a genuine bias in interpretative processing (see Mathews & MacLeod, 1994). Specifically, it has been pointed out that on some trials, participants may access both meanings of a homophone and so must select which of the two possible responses to provide on the spelling task. If patients with GAD show a greater tendency to favor the more threatening response option on these occasions, then the observed effect would be obtained. Thus, in the homophone task, a bias in response selection could be mistaken for a bias in interpretation. Nevertheless, converging support for the conclusion that patients with GAD demonstrate disproportionately threatening interpretations of ambiguity has come from other studies using different performance measures, many of which are less susceptible to response bias explanations.

One such approach has involved the use of recognition memory measures. Eysenck, Mogg, May, Richards, and Mathews (1991) presented patients with GAD and nonanxious controls with an assortment of sentences in an initial encoding task. Included were a number of ambiguous sentences, each permitting a threatening and a nonthreatening interpretation (e.g., "The two men discussed the best way to blow up the boat"). After a delay, participants were given a recognition memory test, within which they were shown a number of sentences and asked to indicate which of these had been presented earlier. The sentences employed in this recognition memory test included disambiguated versions of the original ambiguous items, now constrained to either their threatening meaning (e.g., "The men talked about how they should destroy the boat") or to their nonthreatening meaning (e.g., "The men talked about how they should inflate the boat"). As predicted by the hypothesis that GAD is associated with a negative interpretative bias, the patients with GAD claimed to recognize disproportionately more of the threatening disambiguations. In a second study, Eysenck and his colleagues replicated this finding. Furthermore, by including emotionally valenced foils in the recognition test, they were also able to exclude the possibility that the effect was due to a response bias impelling the patients to endorse any threatening candidate sentences in the recognition task. The patients were found only to display elevated endorsement rates for threatening candidates that represented possible interpretations of originally presented ambiguous sentences. The investigators concluded that their patients with GAD did indeed selectively impose the more threatening interpretations on these ambiguous sentences.

Some critics of the recognition memory approach to the assessment of interpretation have argued that although the obtained patterns of effects clearly cannot be attributed to an anxiety-linked response bias, it remains possible that these effects might reflect the operation of an anxiety-related memory bias rather than an interpretative bias (MacLeod & Cohen, 1993). That is, patients with GAD and controls may impose threatening and nonthreatening interpretations upon the original ambiguous sentences with equal frequency, but the patients may subsequently better remember those sentences that they interpret in a threatening manner. Although such a possibility cannot be excluded, it is reassuring to observe that experimental techniques developed to provide online measures of interpretation, which are susceptible to the influence of neither response bias nor memory bias, continue to provide compelling evidence for an anxiety-linked bias in interpretation. These techniques commonly make use of semantic priming effects to determine the meanings that participants impose on ambiguous information.

It has long been appreciated that the processing of a target stimulus, such as a word, is facilitated when it is preceded by a semantically related prime stimulus (see Neely, 1991). It has also been demonstrated that if such a prime is ambiguous, and only one of its possible meanings is semantically related to the target, then facilitated processing of this target normally will occur only when this particular meaning has been imposed on the prime (Marcel, 1980). Therefore, it follows that the relative degree to which an ambiguous prime stimulus facilitates the processing of target stimuli related to either of its possible meanings can serve to reveal participants' preferred interpretations of this ambiguous prime. Given its methodological advantages, it is somewhat surprising to find that no research has yet capitalized upon this priming approach to assess the patterns of interpretation shown by patients with GAD. However, findings from such priming methodologies strongly suggest that elevated levels of trait anxiety are associated with an increased tendency to interpret ambiguity in a threatening manner.

This conclusion has sometimes been drawn from studies that have employed single ambiguous words as prime stimuli. For example, a series of three experiments by Richards and French (1992) examined the degree to which the prior presentation of homographs, each permitting a threatening and a nonthreatening interpretations, served to reduce lexical decision latencies on subsequently presented target words related to either of these meanings. They found that for participants high in trait anxiety, such priming effects were disproportionately pronounced on targets related to the threatening interpretations of the primes, suggesting that these individuals were particularly inclined to impose the more negative meanings on the ambiguous stimuli. Equivalent findings have been obtained in studies that, instead of using single-word homographs, have employed ambiguous sentences or passages as primes (Calvo, Eysenck, & Estevaz, 1994; Hirsch & Mathews, 1997). Furthermore, the results have been replicated when target word-naming latencies, rather than lexical decision latencies, have been used to compute priming effects (Calvo & Castillo, 1997; Calvo & Eysenck, 2000). Indeed, in some naturalistic variants of such priming paradigms, participants have been required simply to read short passages at a self-paced rate, and silent reading time has been recorded. It has been found that, following the presentation of an ambiguous sentence within such passages, individuals with high (but not those with low) trait anxiety are disproportionately quick to read subsequent text that is consistent with its more threatening rather than its less threatening interpretation (Calvo, Eysenck, & Castillo, 1997; MacLeod & Cohen, 1993). Overall, these findings represent convincing evidence that high levels of trait anxiety are associated with an increased tendency to interpret ambiguous information in a threatening manner.

It remains for future research to determine whether these kinds of priming methodologies will also support the presence of an interpretative bias in GAD. However, the experimental literature reviewed in this section provides good grounds for expecting this to be the case. Across a diverse range of studies, employing a wide variety of different methodologies, the findings consistently have indicated that patients with GAD do indeed display an elevated tendency to interpret ambiguity in its more threatening manner. Although each type of experimental paradigm has been subject to particular criticisms, the wealth of evidence converges on the conclusion that GAD is characterized by an interpretative bias that favors threatening resolutions of ambiguity. Because a similar pattern of biased interpretation is also evident in nonpatients with high trait anxiety, it seems possible that this cognitive characteristic of GAD may be related to the high levels of trait anxiety associated with the disorder. Nevertheless, it is quite possible that this bias in interpretation may play a causal role in the development and maintenance of GAD, and this possibility is discussed in more detail later in this chapter.

ASSESSING BIASES IN THE RETRIEVAL OF THREATENING INFORMATION

In contrast to the compelling evidence that patients with GAD display both an attentional bias favoring the encoding of threatening stimuli and an interpretative bias favoring threatening resolutions of ambiguity, experimental researchers have obtained less support for the hypothesis that these patients show enhanced memory for threatening information.

Burke and Mathews (1992) obtained some empirical support for this possibility when they examined cued recall from autobiographical memory. Patients with GAD judged their retrieved memories to be more negative than was the case for control subjects, recalled more negative memories than the control subjects, and accessed negative autobiographical memories with disproportionate speed. However, it seems likely that such group differences in the cued recall of autobiographical memories may not reflect biases in the retrieval process at all; rather, patients with GAD actually may have experienced a disproportionate number of negative events in their pasts.

To exclude the possible influence of different encoding experiences, researchers have investigated the ease with which patients with GAD and controls can recollect from memory emotional stimuli encoded earlier in the experimental session. Such studies have typically yielded no evidence that these patients demonstrate a superior ability to recollect more threatening stimuli, regardless of whether they have assessed cued recall (Mathews, Mogg, May, & Eysenck, 1989), free recall (Becker, Roth, Andrich, & Margraf, 1999; Bradley, Mogg, & Williams, 1995), or recognition memory (Mogg, Gardiner, Stavrou, & Golombok, 1992). Indeed, when Mogg, Mathews, and Weinman (1987) employed signal detection analysis to separate genuine memory sensitivity from response bias effects, patients with GAD actually were found to display selectively impaired memory sensitivity for anxiety-related stimuli.

Even when memory for emotional information has been assessed following encoding tasks on which patients with GAD have displayed attentional biases toward the more threatening stimuli, these patients typically show no superior ability to recollect such materials. For example, after having found that their patients with GAD, relative to their control subjects, displayed disproportionately slow color naming of threatening words, both Mathews and MacLeod (1985) and Mogg, Mathews, and Weinman (1989) then asked participants to freely recall the words presented in this color-naming task. The recall performance of the patients did not differ from that displayed by the control subjects, providing no evidence to suggest that GAD was associated with enhanced recall of the more threatening words. Using a recognition memory test, MacLeod and McLaughlin (1995) similarly failed to find any evidence that patients with GAD displayed a heightened capacity to recognize threat stimuli initially presented in an emotional Stroop task. Of course, it remains possible that under certain conditions these patients might display facilitated recall or recognition of threatening information, and more recently Friedman, Thayer, and Borkovec (2000) have reported results suggesting that prolonged exposure to stimuli during encoding may elicit a subsequent recall advantage for threatening words in such patients. However, an explicit memory advantage for threat certainly does not appear to be a particularly robust characteristic of patients with GAD.

The same appears to be true of members of the nonclinical population with high trait anxiety, as numerous researchers have reported failures to observe either recall or recognition memory advantages for threatening information in high-anxiety relative to low-anxiety individuals (Bradley, Mogg, & Williams, 1994; Dalgleish, 1994; Nugent & Mineka, 1994). On those few occasions when participants high in trait anxiety have been found to display enhanced recall or recognition memory for emotionally negative information, experimenters either have reported difficulty distinguishing whether these effects are related to trait anxiety or to depression (Eysenck & Byrne, 1994), or else have statistically demonstrated them to be a function of depression rather than trait anxiety (Reidy & Richards, 1997). As with patients who have GAD, therefore, there would appear to be little basis for concluding that individuals who report high levels of trait anxiety are characterized by a robust tendency to display enhanced explicit memory for threatening information.

More support for the existence of a selective memory advantage for threatening information in patients with GAD has been forthcoming when implicit, rather than explicit, memory has been examined. On implicit memory tasks, the memorial impact of previously presented information is assessed not on the basis of participants' recollective experience (as is the case on explicit memory tasks), but rather by observing the degree to which such memory traces affect other aspects of performance (see Roediger, Guynn, & Jones, 1994). Several studies have found that patients with GAD display enhanced implicit memory for threatening words, even though these individuals show no evidence of superior explicit memory for these same stimulus materials. Such an implicit memory bias was first demonstrated in patients with GAD by Mathews, Mogg, May, and Eysenck (1989). After an encoding task that involved exposing participants to threatening and neutral words, Mathews and colleagues then gave these participants incomplete word stems and directed them simply to complete each stem to make the first word that came to mind. Implicit memory was revealed by the finding that the prior presentation of a word made it more likely that participants would complete word stems to produce this same word. The degree to which this implicit memory effect occurred was found to be disproportionately great for threatening words in participants with GAD, but not in controls. Using a rather different experimental paradigm, MacLeod and McLaughlin (1995) also obtained evidence of an implicit memory advantage for threatening words in patients with GAD. In this experiment, following an encoding task that required the processing of threatening and neutral words, participants were instructed to identify single words presented very briefly on a computer display. Implicit memory for the originally presented words was revealed by the finding that these previously exposed words could be more readily identified on this subsequent perceptual task than could new words. Once again, in patients with GAD compared to nonanxious controls, this implicit memory effect was disproportionately large for the threatening words. Several investigators also have reported finding that high trait anxiety in the nonclinical population is associated with enhanced implicit memory for threatening words, as revealed by performance on word stem completion tasks (Eysenck & Byrne, 1994; Richards & French, 1992).

This implicit memory advantage for threatening information has not always replicated consistently, either in studies of patients with GAD (Bradley, Mogg, & Williams, 1995; Mathew, Mogg, Kentish, & Eysenck, 1995) or in studies of nonpatients with high trait anxiety (Nugent & Mineka, 1994; Russo, Fox, & Bowles, 1999). Therefore, although research findings suggests that both GAD and high trait anxiety may be more strongly associated with an implicit than with an explicit memory advantage for threatening information, Coles and Heimberg (2002) correctly note that there is a need for further research designed to examine the potential influence of encoding tasks, retrieval tasks, and stimulus materials, before firm conclusions can be drawn concerning the association between anxiety and selective memory. For the moment, it is perhaps most appropriate to conclude that the evidence for a memory bias favoring threatening information in GAD is less compelling than is the evidence that patients with GAD selectively encode threatening information and selectively impose threatening interpretations upon ambiguity.

ASSESSING AUTOMATIC AND CONTROLLED ASPECTS OF SELECTIVE INFORMATION PROCESSING: SIMILARITIES AND DIFFERENCES BETWEEN GAD AND HIGH TRAIT ANXIETY

It will be recalled from the beginning of this chapter that the DSM-IV diagnostic criteria for GAD make direct reference to the apparent lack of control such patients seem to have over the central cognitive activity that defines this disorder. It will also be recalled that the major information-processing theories of GAD, which attribute this cognitive symptomatology to underlying patterns of selective information processing, also typically place emphasis upon the supposed automaticity of these processing biases. When considering, in the light of these observations, how to explain the similarities and differences between patients with GAD and members of the nonclinical population with high trait anxiety, we have identified one possibility that implicates the balance between automatic and controlled aspects of their selective processing biases. We have suggested that GAD pathology may reflect an inability to employ controlled processing to modify biases that, for both patients and highly anxious nonpatients, originate at an automatic level of cognition. The plausibility of this account is now evaluated against the relevant evidence from studies capable of dissociating automatic and controlled aspects of the information-processing biases shown by patients with GAD and by individuals with high trait anxiety.

In general, there is agreement among theorists that automatic cognitive processing commonly is initiated without intentional volition, tends to take place rapidly, and can proceed without the need for conscious awareness. In contrast, controlled cognitive processing typically is initiated intentionally, proceeds more slowly, and can be carried out only on information that is represented within conscious awareness (see McNally, 1995, 1996). As McNally has pointed out, it is not always the case that a given process necessarily meets all or none of the criteria associated with either classification. Therefore, when one is considering whether any instance of selective cognition represents an automatic or a controlled processing bias, it is appropriate to make explicit the criteria being used to guide this classification. Two issues are addressed in this section concerning the degree to which observed patterns of processing selectivity meet these various criteria. First, it is considered whether the evidence supports the view that the selective processing advantages for threatening information shown by both patients with GAD and nonpatients with high trait anxiety are indeed initiated automatically within the cognitive system. Second, the evidence is examined to determine whether support can be found for the idea that the patients lack the ability, which nevertheless is shown by the nonpatients, to moderate these cognitive biases through the use of controlled processing.

Across both patients with GAD and nonpatients with high trait anxiety, the greatest evidence of a memory advantage for threatening information has come from task variants that seem likely to be particularly sensitive to automatic processes. Implicit memory tasks appraise the impact of remembered information without the volitional engagement of effortful retrieval, and previous research has established that implicit memory effects continue to be shown even when individuals have no conscious awareness that the relevant memory traces even exist (see Rugg, 1995). Therefore, it is tempting to suggest that the biased implicit memory occasionally observed in patients with GAD by researchers such as Mathews, Mogg, May, and Eysenck (1989), and in nonpatients with high trait anxiety by investigators such as Richards and French (1992), might be taken as evidence that this enhanced memory for threat originates at an automatic level of processing in both these populations.

Interpretative biases favoring threatening resolutions of ambiguity have been shown to be a reliable characteristics of both GAD and elevated trait anxiety, but the experimental paradigms employed to assess this effect typically do not permit discrimination of the contributions made by automatic and controlled processing. In virtually all cases, the ambiguous stimulus materials can be consciously apprehended by participants; the tasks permit the engagement of intentional interpretative strategies; and sufficient processing time is provided to permit the execution of such effortful cognitive activity. Because the methodologies permit both automatic and controlled processing to influence the interpretations that are imposed, it is impossible to know which class of processing represents the locus of the biased interpretation that is observed.

Some researchers have suggested that priming approaches to the assessment of interpretation may permit this issue to be resolved, by manipulating the stimulus onset asynchrony (SOA) of the prime and target in order to reveal the relative speeds with which alternative meanings of ambiguous prime stimuli are accessed. For example, in the homograph priming study conducted on students high and low in trait anxiety by Richards and French (1992), the prime–target SOAs were either 500 milliseconds, 750 milliseconds, or 1,250 milliseconds. The exaggerated priming effects shown by the students high in trait anxiety on targets related to the threatening meanings of the homograph primes were evident only on the two longer SOAs, leading these investigators to suggest that trait anxiety may not have been associated with an automatic bias in the interpretation of the ambiguous stimuli. However, at the 500-millisecond SOA, large and equivalent priming effects already had fully developed for targets related to both meanings of the ambiguous primes (and differential priming effects then emerged at longer SOAs because of the differing rates at which each of these priming effects then dropped off). Therefore, even shorter SOAs would have been required to reveal whether the participants with high trait anxiety did indeed access the threatening meanings of the ambiguous prime stimuli with disproportionate speed, as would be expected to result from an automatic interpretative bias. On the basis of convincing experimental evidence, Neely (1977) advises that prime–target SOAs below 250 milliseconds are required to clearly identify those priming effects that result from the automatic processing of prime stimuli.

When we turn to consider those tasks that have been employed to assess patterns of biased attention, it becomes easier to draw conclusions about the automaticity of the cognitive operations that mediate the observed effects. Given that the elevated threat interference effects shown by both patients with GAD and individuals high in trait anxiety (see Williams et al., 1996) occur despite participants' active efforts to ignore the emotional distractor information, it would seem reasonable to argue that such biases are automatic, at least in the sense that they represent involuntary attentional effects. However, even better evidence for the automaticity of these interference effects has come from studies that have examined subjective awareness of this distractor information. For example, in the study of dichotic listening interference in patients with GAD by Mathews and MacLeod (1986), participants were unable to report the identity of the unattended emotional distractor stimuli, could not accurately identify these stimuli on a recognition test, and even failed to perform above chance levels when forced to guess whether these distractors were threatening or neutral in content. Yet, despite this apparent lack of awareness for these distractors, these patients evidenced disproportionate interference on the central reaction time task in the presence of threatening rather than neutral distractor stimuli. The implication that this bias operated upon information that was not represented within conscious awareness invites the conclusion that it reflected automatic processing selectivity.

Interference studies that have more rigorously manipulated conscious awareness of distracting emotional stimuli, by presenting them for only a few milliseconds and using backward masking procedures (see Turvey, 1973), have provided converging support for the conclusion that the attentional bias displayed by patients with GAD is not dependent upon conscious awareness of the emotional information being processed. Despite an inability to report the presence of distractor words under such exposure conditions, such patients continue to display disproportionately long color-naming latencies in the presence of threatening items (Bradley, Mogg, Millar, & White, 1995; Mogg et al., 1993). Parallel findings have been reported when patients with GAD and nonanxious controls have performed variants of the attentional probe task, within which the use of brief exposures and backward masking has eliminated their ability to report the content of the presented word pairs. For example, Mogg, Bradley, and Williams (1995) found that, despite being unable to consciously apprehend these stimuli, patients continued to show speeded detection of probes presented in the vicinity of the more threatening words, suggesting that they selectively oriented attention toward the locus of threatening information that was not consciously represented. Clearly, such findings demand the conclusion that the tendency of patients with GAD to attend selectively toward threatening information does indeed originate as an automatic processing bias within the cognitive system.

The performance of participants with high trait anxiety on similar masked versions of these tasks requires the same conclusion. Across a range of studies that have exposed individuals high and low in trait anxiety to briefly presented backward-masked words that they are unable to report, the high-anxiety participants have reliably displayed disproportionately slow color-naming latencies in the presence of threatening rather than neutral stimuli (MacLeod & Hagan, 1992; MacLeod & Rutherford, 1992; Mogg, Bradley, & Hallowell, 1994; van den Hout, Tenney, Huygens, Merckelbach, & Kindt, 1995). On variants of the attentional probe task, too, individuals with high trait anxiety have been found to display speeded processing of probes presented in the vicinity of briefly presented masked threatening stimuli, despite demonstrating an inability to report their content (Mogg & Bradley, 1999). Such results strongly suggest that the attentional bias to threat shown by nonpatients with high trait anxiety, like that observed in patients with GAD, originates at an automatic level of processing.

It does indeed appear to be the case, therefore, that patients with GAD and nonpatients with high trait anxiety do share an automatic cognitive bias that operates to favor the processing of threatening information. Potentially, this may help to explain the similarities between members of these two populations, who also have in common the tendency to experience unusually pronounced elevations in their levels of state anxiety. Yet clearly the two populations differ in important ways, not least in terms of the degrees to which their elevated levels of anxiety tend to become extreme, prolonged, and disabling. Is there evidence to support the possibility that these differences in symptomatology may reflect differing abilities to employ controlled processing in a manner that moderates the impact of these automatic patterns of selectivity? Actually, there are rather good grounds for believing that this may be the case.

When patients with GAD have been exposed to different versions of cognitive experimental tasks, designed either to permit or to preclude the influence of controlled information processing, these patients typically have demonstrated equivalent evidence of biased cognitive functioning under both conditions. Consider, for example, how such patients perform on the masked and unmasked versions of the emotional Stroop task. The masked version of this assessment paradigm presents stimuli in a manner that precludes the influence of controlled cognitive operations, and the fact that patients display increased interference from threatening materials on this task indicates a biased pattern of selectivity in their automatic processing. In contrast, the unmasked, more conventional version of the emotional Stroop task does permit some opportunity to employ controlled cognitive operations in a manner that influences the processing of the emotional information. However, patients with GAD continue to demonstrate exaggerated threat interference under this condition also, indicating that this opportunity to modify the expression of their automatically initiated patterns of processing selectivity is not exploited by these patients. Interestingly, though, the situation has often appeared quite different when individuals with high trait anxiety, but without a diagnosis of GAD, have been exposed to these same two presentation conditions. A number of researchers have reported that under such circumstances, elevated levels of trait anxiety are associated with exaggerated threat interference effects in the masked exposure condition, which prevents the influence of controlled processing, but not in the unmasked exposure condition, which permits the influence of such controlled processing (MacLeod & Hagan, 1992; van den Hout et al., 1995). Such findings are entirely consistent with the possibility that individuals with high trait anxiety, unlike patients with GAD, do indeed engage controlled processing to counter the expression of their automatically initiated processing bias favoring threatening information.

For example, we (MacLeod & Rutherford, 1992) employed a modified version of the emotional Stroop task that presented trials in both masked and unmasked exposure conditions, to assess processing selectivity in students high and low in trait anxiety who were approaching an important examination. Under the masked exposure condition, as the exam stressor approached, the high-anxiety individuals displayed increasing threat interference across all threat words, suggesting the facilitated automatic processing of threatening information by these individuals. For the low-anxiety individuals under this same masked exposure condition, the approach of the exam stressor instead was associated with the reduction of threat interference, suggesting the inhibited automatic processing of threat information by these participants. Under the unmasked exposure condition, however, the approach of the exam stressor was associated in both groups of participants with the reduction of threat interference effects, especially on those threat words most closely associated with exam-related concerns. The conclusion drawn was that, in response to the impending stressor, the participants high in trait anxiety employed controlled processing to override and reverse a developing automatic tendency to selectively process threatening information, and that this controlled inhibition was focused most directly on the processing of threat information most relevant to the source of their anxiety.

A parallel study (Locke, 1991, reported by MacLeod & Rutherford, 1998) employed a rather different priming methodology to assess selective attention in students high and low in trait anxiety approaching an examination; it also manipulated prime–target SOAs to dissociate the influence of automatic and controlled processing. The results were fully consistent with our conclusions (MacLeod & Rutherford, 1992). At the short SOA (250 milliseconds), which permitted the least influence from controlled processing, high-anxiety individuals responded to the impending examinations by selectively activating the threatening prime stimuli, whereas low-anxiety individuals responded by selectively inhibiting the processing of these threatening primes. However, at the long SOA (2,000 milliseconds), which permitted a considerably greater opportunity for controlled processing, the high-anxiety students now shared the low-anxiety students' tendency to inhibit the processing of threat primes as the examination approached, and did so principally on those threatening primes most strongly associated with exam-related concerns. Once again, this pattern of findings represents good evidence that individuals high in trait anxiety can engage controlled cognitive operations to negate, or even to reverse, their automatic tendency to selectively favor the processing of threat information.

It would be incorrect to imply that members of the normal population with high trait anxiety never appear to selectively process threatening information under circumstances that might permit the engagement of controlled cognitive operations. For example, using an unmasked version of the emotional Stroop task, Mogg and colleagues (2000) recently obtained evidence of elevated threat interference effects in a nonclinical sample of individuals with high trait anxiety. However, it does appear to be the case that such individuals are capable of exercising controlled processing to negate such patterns of cognitive selectivity. Furthermore, the fact that they seem particularly disposed to do so when exposed to stressful situations suggests that they may employ this ability adaptively, to ameliorate the likely emotional consequences that would result from selectively processing threatening information under such circumstances. In contrast, patients with GAD demonstrate no such ability to employ controlled processing in this manner, and the lack of this ability may reduce their capacity to adaptively regulate their emotional reactions to situational stressors. For an appropriate test of this intriguing possibility, it will be necessary to execute future experiments that directly compare patients with GAD, high-anxiety nonpatients, and low-anxiety nonpatients, on paradigms capable of dissociating automatic and controlled patterns of processing selectivity—ideally, when all these participants are exposed to situational stressors. However, it is acknowledged that the chronically elevated levels of state anxiety in patients with GAD may render it difficult to identify specific situations that are sufficiently stress-inducing for all participants. Clearly, however, the present proposal that the emotional similarities and differences between GAD and high trait anxiety may result from underlying similarities and differences in their patterns of selective cognition presupposes that such processing biases can play a causal role in the mediation of anxiety vulnerability. The final section of this chapter considers the degree to which the experimental evidence is consistent with the premise that selective information processing may causally contribute to anxiety vulnerability.

ASSESSING THE CAUSAL ROLE OF SELECTIVE PROCESSING BIASES IN THE MEDIATION OF ANXIETY VULNERABILITY

As the preceding review has demonstrated, a substantial body of empirical evidence has now accumulated to support the central tenet that underpins information-processing accounts of GAD. Consistent with such theories, patients suffering from this disorder are indeed characterized by the operation of cognitive biases that selectively favor the processing of information related to threat. These biases are most evident on tasks that assess selective encoding and interpretation, and have also been observed on implicit memory tasks. There are reasonable grounds for concluding that such selectivity has its origins in automatic cognitive operations. When only automatic processing has been permitted, the patterns of bias displayed by patients with GAD seem to be equivalent to those shown by nonclinical individuals whose high levels of trait anxiety suggest the disposition to develop GAD. However, in contrast to these nonpatients, the patients show no evidence of any capacity to override or negate these automatically initiated biases, when task conditions permit the strategic use of controlled information processing. Overall, then, the empirical findings are consistent with the hypothesis that the presence of selective processing biases, leading to the overrepresentation of threatening information within the cognitive system, may play a causal role in precipitating and sustaining the clinical symptomatology of GAD.

Undoubtedly, it is this particular causal interpretation of the observed association between selective cognition and GAD that lends such findings their greatest clinical relevance. From a theoretical perspective, such a causal account offers the richest potential to advance understanding of the mechanisms that mediate the development of this disorder. Furthermore, when causality is construed in this manner, then very direct applied implications also follow. Specifically, according to this position, the measurement and manipulation of these selective processing biases should serve to predict and to modify, respectively, the manifestation of GAD symptomatology. Given these exciting possibilities, many researchers have been tempted to entertain this type of causal interpretation when discussing their own experimental findings.

Of course, the demonstration of a mere association between selective information processing and anxiety vulnerability cannot permit the conclusion that the former plays a causal role in the development of the latter. Quite the reverse causal relationship could equally well underpin such an association, with cognitive selectivity developing only in response to anxiety symptomatogy, once this has become established. However, studies that have taken a developmental approach to the investigation of anxiety-linked processing biases provide no support for this alternative causal interpretation. In general, it has been found that even in young children, anxiety pathology is associated with the manifestation of a processing advantage for threatening information, and the degree to which such biases are demonstrated appears unrelated either to age or to the preceding duration of the anxiety symtomatology (see Vasey & MacLeod, 2001).

Furthermore, some adult studies now have yielded direct evidence that the selective processing of threatening information can precede, and can predict the development of, anxious symptomatology. For example,

MacLeod and Hagan (1992) used an emotional Stroop task, containing both masked and unmasked trials, to assess individual differences in attentional selectivity within a population of women who were undergoing a cervical examination. Several weeks later, they followed up those women who later received a diagnosis of cervical pathology, to assess individual differences in the emotional impact of this subsequent stressful event. The degree to which women initially displayed an automatic attentional bias to threat, as evidenced by slowed color naming on masked threat trials relative to masked neutral trials in the emotional Stroop task, most powerfully predicted the degree to which these women later experienced intensely negative emotional reactions to the subsequent stress of diagnosis. Indeed, this measure of automatic attentional bias to threat predicted these later emotional reactions to the subsequent stressor considerably better than did any questionnaire measure of emotional vulnerability, and it retained this predictive capacity even when the influence of such questionnaire measures was statistically removed. This demonstration that a bias in selective processing can precede and predict the development of emotional symptoms, which other studies since have replicated with different types of stressors (see MacLeod & Rutherford, 1998), is clearly consistent with the view that cognitive bias may play a causal role in the mediation of emotional symptomatology.

Additional evidence to support this causal hypothesis has been provided by studies that have examined the emotional consequences of manipulating cognitive variables. When conventional cognitive therapies have been employed to treat patients with GAD, it has commonly been observed that reduction of their anxiety symptoms is associated with reduction in their tendency to selectively process threatening information. Mathews and colleagues (1995), for example, found that the degree to which cognitive therapy served to ameliorate such patients' anxiety symptoms depended upon the degree to which it reduced the threat interference effects the patients displayed on an emotional Stroop task. Mogg, Bradley, Millar, and White (1995) also report finding that cognitive therapy reduced anxiety symptomatology to the greatest degree in those patients with GAD who displayed the greatest reduction in their threat interference effects. A similar reduction in interpretative bias has also been associated with clinical recovery in such patients (Eysenck et al., 1991; Mathews, Richards, & Eysenck, 1989). Although such findings once again are clearly consistent with the proposal that cognitive bias may play a causal role in GAD, it could perhaps be argued that the reduction of cognitive bias observed in these treatment studies might be a direct consequence of symptom improvement, rather than representing a mechanism that functionally mediates the efficacy of cognitive therapy. However, it does not appear to be the case that the successful elimination of GAD symptoms through the use of benzodiazepines is associated with any similar reduction of the selective processing preference these patients display for threatening information (Golombok, Stavrou, Bonn, & Mogg, 1991). The fact that changes in the selective processing of threat predicts the therapeutic efficacy only of those GAD treatments that plausibly represent direct manipulations of cognitive biases lends further weight to the view that biased cognition has causal status in its relationship with anxiety vulnerability.

The most direct evidence to support this conclusion comes from those studies that have employed the most direct manipulations of processing selectivity (see Mathews & MacLeod, 2002). Across a series of experiments, Mathews and his colleagues have recently developed training variants of tasks previously employed only to assess interpretative bias; the variants are designed instead to experimentally induce the tendency to impose either more or less threatening interpretations of ambiguity (Grey & Mathews, 2000; Mathews & Mackintosh, 2000). For example, in one such training task, participants were required to read a large number of short ambiguous sentences and, in each case, to supply the final word by completing a word fragment that appeared at the end of the sentence. For every ambiguous sentence, two possible word fragments were constructed; one permitted only a completion consistent with its threatening interpretation, and the other permitted only a completion consistent with its nonthreatening interpretation. For one group of participants, all the word fragments given in the training task were of the former type, and so success on this version of the task required these individuals to consistently access the more threatening meanings of the ambiguous text. It was expected that extended performance on this task variant would train participants to selectively impose threatening interpretations on ambiguous information. For the other group, all the word fragments given in the training task were consistent with the nonthreatening meanings of the ambiguous sentences, and it was expected that extended performance on this version of the task would train these individuals to selectively impose nonthreatening interpretations on ambiguous information. Mathews and his coworkers delivered these and similar training tasks to volunteers whose trait anxiety levels fell within the normal range, and were able to confirm their efficacy in inducing the target interpretative biases by assessing participants' interpretations of subsequently presented ambiguous materials. Furthermore, Mathews and Mackintosh (2000) were able to demonstrate that the induction of these differential styles of interpretative bias did indeed directly affect participants' anxiety. Specifically, those individuals trained to interpret ambiguity in its more threatening manner came to display greater levels of anxious symptomatology than did those individuals trained to impose the less threatening interpretations upon ambiguity.

In a parallel program of research, we (MacLeod, Campbell, &

Rutherford, 1997) have developed cognitive experimental procedures designed to induce selective patterns of attentional response to threatening information. Once again, these tasks represent variants of methodologies previously used only to assess patterns of selective attention, but now incorporating contingencies that directly encourage the development of attentional bias in nonclinical participants. For example, in two experiments, we (MacLeod, Rutherford, Campbell, Ebsworthy, & Holker, 2002) gave a training variant of the attentional probe task to two groups of participants drawn from the midrange of trait anxiety levels. For one group, across hundreds of trials, virtually all the probes appeared in the vicinity of the more threatening stimulus words, and it was intended that this training would induce the development of an attentional bias toward threatening information. In contrast, for the other group of participants, nearly every probe appeared in the opposite screen location from that in which the threatening stimulus had appeared, and it was anticipated that this training condition would induce the development of an attentional bias away from threat. The efficacy of the training procedure in inducing the target attentional biases was confirmed by the patterns of performance that participants came to display on critical test trials, which violated this training contingency. Of greatest importance for present considerations, assessment of participants' emotional reactions to a subsequent anagram stress task also confirmed the prediction that this direct manipulation of attentional bias would serve to modify anxiety vulnerability. Although participants exposed to each of the two training conditions did not report experiencing differing mood states at the end of the training procedure, those in the group that had acquired an attentional bias toward threat displayed a disproportionately intense negative emotional reaction to this subsequent stressor. Furthermore, across all participants, the degree to which the training procedure served to modify the intensity of the state anxiety responses shown on this stress task was found to be a direct function of the degree to which it served to induce the target pattern of attentional bias.

Therefore, despite the difficulties associated with the determination of causality, it would be fair to say that a substantial amount of evidence now bears upon the hypothesis that selective patterns of information processing may exert a causal influence over the development and maintenance of dysfunctional anxiety. Individual differences in the manifestations of such biases have been shown to precede and predict variations in the emotional responses individuals display to stressful life events. It has been found that cognitive therapies for GAD serve to modify such patterns of processing selectivity, and that the degree to which patients with GAD exposed to such therapies display an improvement in their clinical symptoms is directly associated with the degree to which they demonstrate reductions in their selective processing of threatening information.

Cognitive experimental procedures designed to directly manipulate patterns of selective attention or selective interpretation have also been shown to modify vulnerability to anxiety. Taken together, this evidence represents impressive converging support for the proposal that the attentional and interpretative biases now known to be associated with GAD may indeed play a causal role in the mediation of the anxiety symptomatology displayed by individuals who suffer from this disorder.

SUMMARY AND CONCLUSIONS

As increasing clinical emphasis has been placed upon cognitive aspects of GAD over the past 20 or so years, so too have theoreticians become increasingly disposed to implicate cognitive variables in their conceptual explanations of this condition. Although they vary considerably in their details, many models of GAD now share the core premise that the cognitive symptomatology of this disorder stems from a pattern of selective processing that operates quite automatically to favor threatening information. The idea has been put forward that patients with GAD, in contrast to nonpatients with high trait anxiety, may lack the ability to negate or reverse such automatic patterns of selectivity using controlled cognitive processes.

Compelling converging evidence has accumulated to demonstrate that patients with GAD do indeed selectively attend to threatening stimuli during the encoding of information and also selectively impose threatening interpretations on ambiguous information. These patients, and nonpatients with elevated levels of trait anxiety, display similar patterns of processing biases on tasks that minimize the potential influence of cognitive strategies, suggesting that such selectivity originates at an automatic level of cognition. However, the patients and nonpatients have often been found to differ when the task format makes it possible for controlled processing to influence expression of their automatic patterns of selectivity. The nonpatients commonly seem to capitalize upon this opportunity, by displaying patterns of controlled processing selectivity that negate or reverse their automatic preference for threatening information. In contrast, the patients demonstrate no such ability to use controlled processing in this adaptive manner. Such observations suggest that an automatic tendency to preferentially process threatening information may give rise to the heightened anxiety vulnerability evident in both nonpatients with high trait anxiety and patients with GAD. However, the ability to negate or reverse this pattern of selectivity, using controlled cognitive processes, may protect the nonpatients from the disabling emotional consequences suffered by the patients, who lack the capacity to employ controlled processing for this purpose.

The possibility that patterns of biased cognition, selectively favoring the processing of threatening information, may play a causal role in the mediation of GAD symptomatology has been supported by a number of empirical observations. Such patterns of processing selectivity have been found to precede and predict the development of negative emotional reactions to stressful life events. Furthermore, the manipulation of these selective processing biases has been shown to directly modify the patterns of anxiety symptomatology associated with GAD.

On the basis of such findings, it would appear reasonable to conclude that the theoretical rationale underpinning cognitive approaches to the treatment of GAD is based upon solid empirical foundations. As we move forward to enhance our capacity to treat this common and disabling disorder, it seems likely that the research partnership between clinical and cognitive experimental psychologists will continue to be a productive one. Across the past decade or more, this partnership has done much to illuminate the information-processing characteristics of GAD, in ways that have greatly advanced our theoretical understanding of this disorder. Perhaps it is not unreasonable to hope that as it extends across the coming decade, this same partnership will also facilitate the development and evaluation of new therapeutic techniques, designed to alleviate this clinical condition by modifying the patterns of selective information that seem likely to causally underpin the disorder.

REFERENCES

American Psychiatric Association. (1994). *Diagnostic and statistical manual of mental disorders* (4th ed.). Washington, DC: Author.

Azaies, F., Granger, B., & Debray, Q. (1994). Interférence sémantique et pathologie anxieuse: Approche experimentale dans l'anxiété generalisée. *Annales Médico-Psychologiques, 152,* 458–461.

Beck, A. T. (1976). *Cognitive therapy and the emotional disorders.* New York: International Universities Press.

Beck, A. T., & Clark, D. A. (1997). An information processing model of anxiety: Automatic and strategic processes. *Behaviour Research and Therapy, 35,* 49–58.

Beck, A. T., & Emery, G., with Greenberg, R. C. (1985). *Anxiety disorders and phobias: A cognitive perspective.* New York: Basic Books.

Beck, A. T., Rush, A., Shaw, B., & Emery, G. (1979). *Cognitive therapy of depression.* New York: Guilford Press.

Beck, J. G., Stanley, M., & Zebb, B. (1996). Characteristics of generalized anxiety disorder in older adults: A descriptive study. *Behaviour Research and Therapy, 34,* 225–234.

Becker, E. S., Roth, W. T., Andrich, M., & Margraf, J. (1999). Explicit memory in anxiety disorders. *Journal of Abnormal Psychology, 108,* 153–163.

Borkovec, T. D. (1994). The nature, function and origin of worry. In G. C. L. Davey & F. Tallis (Eds.), *Worrying: Perspectives on theory, prevention and treatment* (pp. 467–484). Chichester, UK: Wiley.

Borkovec, T. D., & Inz, J. (1990). The nature of worry in generalized anxiety disorder: A predominance of thought activity. *Behaviour Research and Therapy, 28,* 153–158.

Borkovec, T. D., & Lyonfields, J. (1993). Thought suppression of emotional processing. In H. W. Krohne (Ed.), *Attention and avoidance: Strategies in coping with aversiveness.* Göttingen, Germany: Hogrefe & Huber.

Borkovec, T. D., Ray, W. J., & Stöeber, J. (1998). Worry: A cognitive phenomenon intimately linked to affective, physiological and interpersonal behavioral processes. *Cognitive Therapy and Research, 22,* 561–576.

Borkovec, T. D., Shadick, R. N., & Hopkins, M. (1991). The nature of normal and pathological worry. In R. M. Rapee & D. H. Barlow (Eds.), *Chronic anxiety: Generalized anxiety disorder and mixed anxiety–depression* (pp. 29–51). New York: Guilford Press.

Bower, G. H. (1981). Mood and memory. *American Psychologist, 36,* 129–148.

Bower, G. H. (1983). Affect and cognition. *Philosophical Transactions of the Royal Society of London, B302,* 387–402.

Bradley, B. P., Mogg, K., & Millar, N. H. (2000). Covert and overt orienting of attention to emotional faces in anxiety. *Cognition and Emotion, 14,* 789–808.

Bradley, B. P., Mogg, K., Millar, N., & White, J. (1995). Selective processing of negative information: Effects of clinical anxiety, concurrent depression, and awareness. *Journal of Abnormal Psychology, 104,* 532–536.

Bradley, B. P., Mogg, K., White, J., Groom, C., & de Bono, J. (1999). Attentional bias for emotional faces in generalized anxiety disorder. *British Journal of Clinical Psychology, 38,* 267–278.

Bradley, B. P., Mogg, K., & Williams, R. (1994). Implicit and explicit memory for emotional information in non-clinical subjects. *Behaviour Research and Therapy, 32,* 65–78.

Bradley, B. P., Mogg, K., & Williams, R. (1995). Implicit and explicit memory for emotion-congruent information in clinical depression and anxiety. *Behaviour Research and Therapy, 33,* 755–770.

Broadbent, D. E., & Broadbent, M. (1988). Anxiety and attentional bias: State and trait. *Cognition and Emotion, 2,* 165–183.

Burke, M., & Mathews, A. (1992). Autobiographical memory and clinical anxiety. *Cognition and Emotion, 6,* 23–35.

Byrne, A., & Eysenck, M. W. (1993). Individual differences in positive and negative interpretive biases. *Personality and Individual Differences, 14,* 849–851.

Calvo, M. G., & Castillo, D. (1997). Mood-congruent bias in interpretation of ambiguity: Strategic processes and temporary activation. *Quarterly Journal of Experimental Psychology: Human Experimental Psychology, 50,* 163–182.

Calvo, M. G., & Eysenck, M. W. (2000). Early vigilance and late avoidance of threat processing: Repressive coping versus low/high anxiety. *Cognition and Emotion, 14,* 763–787.

Calvo, M. G., Eysenck, M. W., & Castillo, M. D. (1997). Interpretative bias in test anxiety: The time course of predictive inference. *Cognition and Emotion, 11,* 43–63.

Calvo, M. G., Eysenck, M. W., & Estevaz, A. (1994). Ego-threat interpretative bias in test anxiety: On-line inferences. *Cognition and Emotion, 2,* 127–146.

Coles, M. E., & Heimberg, R. G. (2002). Memory biases in the anxiety disorders: Current status. *Clinical Psychology Review, 22,* 587–627.

Craske, M. G., Rapee, R. M., Jackel, L., & Barlow, D. H. (1989). Qualitative dimensions of worry in DSM-III-R generalized anxiety disorder subjects and nonanxious controls. *Behaviour Research and Therapy, 27,* 397–402.

Dalgleish, T. (1994). The relationship between anxiety and memory biases for material that has been selectively processed in a prior task. *Behaviour Research and Therapy, 32*, 227–231.

de Ruiter, C., & Brosschot, J. F. (1994). The emotional Stroop interference effect in anxiety: Attentional bias or cognitive avoidance? *Behaviour Research and Therapy, 32*, 315–319.

Dugas, M. J., Freeston, M. H., Ladouceur, R., Rheaume, J., Provencher, M., & Boisvert, J.-M. (1998). Worry themes in primary GAD, secondary GAD, and other anxiety disorders. *Journal of Anxiety Disorders, 12*, 253–261.

Endler, N. S., Parker, J. D., Bagby, M. R., & Cox, B. J. (1991). Multidimensionality of state and trait anxiety: Factor structure of the Endler Multidimensional Anxiety Scales. *Journal of Personality and Social Psychology, 60*, 919–926.

Eysenck, M. W. (1982). *Attention and arousal, cognition and performance.* Berlin: Springer-Verlag.

Eysenck, M. W. (1992). *Anxiety: The cognitive perspective.* Hove, UK: Erlbaum.

Eysenck, M. W. (1997). *Anxiety: A unified theory.* Hove, UK: Erlbaum.

Eysenck, M. W., & Byrne, A. (1994). Implicit memory bias, explicit memory bias, and anxiety. *Cognition and Emotion, 8*, 415–431.

Eysenck, M. W., MacLeod, C., & Mathews, A. (1987). Cognitive functioning in anxiety. *Psychological Research, 49*, 189–195.

Eysenck, M. W., Mogg, K., May, J., Richards, A., & Mathews, A. (1991). Bias in the interpretation of ambiguous sentences related to threat in anxiety. *Journal of Abnormal Psychology, 100*, 144–150.

Eysenck, M. W., & van Berkum, J. (1992). Trait anxiety, defensiveness, and the structure of worry. *Personality and Individual Differences, 13*, 1285–1290.

Forbach, G. B., Stanners, R. F., & Hochhaus, L. (1974). Repetition and practice effects in a lexical decision task. *Memory and Cognition, 2*, 337–339.

Fox, E. (1993). Attentional bias in anxiety: Selective or not? *Behaviour Research and Therapy, 31*, 487–493.

Friedman, B. H., Thayer, J. F., & Borkovec, T. D. (2000). Explicit memory bias for threat words in generalized anxiety disorder. *Behavior Therapy, 31*, 745–756.

Golombok, S., Stavrou, A., Bonn, J., & Mogg, K. (1991). The effects of diazepam on anxiety-related cognitions. *Cognitive Therapy and Research, 15*, 459–467.

Graesser, A. C., & Nakamura, G. V. (1982). The impact of a schema on comprehension and memory. *Psychology of Learning and Motivation, 16*, 59–109.

Graf, P., & Mandler, G. (1984). Activation makes words more accessible but not necessarily more retrievable. *Journal of Verbal Learning and Verbal Behavior, 23*, 553–568.

Grey, S., & Mathews, A. (2000). Effects of training on interpretation of emotional ambiguity. *Quarterly Journal of Experimental Psychology: Human Experimental Psychology, 53*, 1143–1162.

Hirsch, C., & Mathews, A. (1997). Interpretive inferences when reading about emotional events. *Behaviour Research and Therapy, 35*, 1123–1132.

Lavy, E. H., & van den Hout, M. A. (1994). Cognitive avoidance and attentional bias: Causal relationships. *Cognitive Therapy and Research, 18*, 179–191.

MacLeod, C. (1993). Cognition in clinical psychology: Measures, methods or models? *Behaviour Change, 10*, 169–195.

MacLeod, C. (1999). Anxiety and anxiety disorders. In T. Dalgleish & M. Power (Eds.), *Handbook of cognition and emotion* (pp. 447–477). Chichester, UK: Wiley.

MacLeod, C., & Cohen, I. L. (1993). Anxiety and the interpretation of ambiguity: A text comprehension study. *Journal of Abnormal Psychology, 102*, 238–247.

MacLeod, C., & Hagan, R. (1992). Individual differences in the selective processing of threatening information, and emotional responses to a stressful life event. *Behaviour Research and Therapy, 30,* 151–161.

MacLeod, C., & Mathews, A. (1988). Anxiety and the allocation of attention to threat. *Quarterly Journal of Experimental Psychology: Human Experimental Psychology, 40,* 653–670.

MacLeod, C., & Mathews, A. (1991). Cognitive-experimental approaches to the emotional disorders. In P. R. Martin (Ed.), *Handbook of behavior therapy and psychological science: An integrative approach* (pp. 116–150). New York: Pergamon Press.

MacLeod, C., Mathews, A., & Tata, P. (1986). Attentional bias in emotional disorders. *Journal of Abnormal Psychology, 95,* 15–20.

MacLeod, C., & McLaughlin, K. (1995). Implicit and explicit memory bias in anxiety: A conceptual replication. *Behaviour Research and Therapy, 33,* 1–14.

MacLeod, C., & Rutherford, E. M. (1992). Anxiety and the selective processing of emotional information: Mediating roles of awareness, trait and state variables, and personal relevance of stimulus materials. *Behaviour Research and Therapy, 30,* 479–491.

MacLeod, C., & Rutherford, E. M. (1998). Automatic and strategic cognitive biases in anxiety and depression. In K. S. C. Kirsner (Ed.), *Implicit and explicit mental processes* (pp. 233–254). Mahwah, NJ: Erlbaum.

MacLeod, C., Campbell, L., & Rutherford, E. M. (1997, July). *Modification of anxiety vulnerability through direct manipulation of selective processing bias.* Paper presented at the 2nd Australian Anxiety Disorders Conference, Port Douglas, Queensland.

MacLeod, C., Rutherford, E., Campbell, L., Ebsworthy, G., & Holker, L. (2002). Selective attention and emotional vulnerability: Assessing the causal basis of their association through the experimental induction of attentional bias. *Journal of Abnormal Psychology, 111,* 107–123.

Marcel, A. J. (1980). Conscious and preconscious recognition of polysemous words: Locating the selective effects of prior verbal context. In R. S. Nickerson (Ed.), *Attention and performance* (Vol. 12, pp. 17–28). Hillsdale, NJ: Erlbaum.

Mathews, A. (1993). Attention and memory for threat in anxiety. In H. W. Krohne (Ed.), *Attention and avoidance: Strategies in coping with aversiveness* (pp. 119–135). Göttingen, Germany: Hogrefe & Huber.

Mathews, A., & Mackintosh, B. (1998). A cognitive model of selective processing in anxiety. *Cognitive Therapy and Research, 22,* 539–560.

Mathews, A., & Mackintosh, B. (2000). Induced emotional interpretation bias and anxiety. *Journal of Abnormal Psychology, 109,* 602–615.

Mathews, A., & MacLeod, C. (1985). Selective processing of threat cues in anxiety states. *Behaviour Research and Therapy, 23,* 563–569.

Mathews, A., & MacLeod, C. (1986). Discrimination of threat cues without awareness in anxiety states. *Journal of Abnormal Psychology, 95,* 131–138.

Mathews, A., & MacLeod, C. (1994). Cognitive approaches to emotion. *Annual Review of Psychology, 45,* 25–50.

Mathews, A., & MacLeod, C. (2002). Induced processing biases have causal effects on anxiety. *Cognition and Emotion, 16,* 301–315.

Mathews, A., Mogg, K., Kentish, J., & Eysenck, M. (1995). Effect of psychological treatment on cognitive bias in generalized anxiety disorder. *Behaviour Research and Therapy, 33,* 293–303.

Mathews, A., Mogg, K., May, J., & Eysenck, M. (1989). Implicit and explicit memory bias in anxiety. *Journal of Abnormal Psychology, 98,* 236–240.

Mathews, A., Richards, A., & Eysenck, M. (1989). Interpretation of homophones related to threat in anxiety states. *Journal of Abnormal Psychology, 98,* 31–34.

McNally, R. J. (1995). Automaticity and the anxiety disorders. *Behaviour Research and Therapy, 33,* 747–754.

McNally, R. J. (1996). Cognitive bias in the anxiety disorders. In D. A. Hope (Ed.), *Nebraska Symposium on Motivation: Vol. 43. Perspectives on anxiety, panic, and fear* (pp. 118–131). Lincoln: University of Nebraska Press.

McNally, R. J. (1998). Information-processing abnormalities in anxiety disorders: Implications for cognitive neuroscience. *Cognition and Emotion, 12,* 479–495.

Mogg, K., & Bradley, B. P. (1998). A cognitive–motivational analysis of anxiety. *Behaviour Research and Therapy, 36,* 809–848.

Mogg, K., & Bradley, B. P. (1999). Orienting of attention to threatening facial expressions presented under conditions of restricted awareness. *Cognition and Emotion, 13,* 713–740.

Mogg, K., Bradley, B. P., Dixon, C., Fisher, S., Twelftree, H., & McWilliams, A. (2000). Trait anxiety, defensiveness and selective processing of threat: An investigation using two measures of attentional bias. *Personality and Individual Differences, 28,* 1063–1077.

Mogg, K., Bradley, B. P., & Hallowell, N. (1994). Attentional bias to threat: Roles of trait anxiety, stressful events, and awareness. *Quarterly Journal of Experimental Psychology: Human Experimental Psychology, 47,* 841–864.

Mogg, K., Bradley, B. P., Millar, N., & White, J. (1995). Cognitive bias in generalized anxiety disorder: A follow-up study. *Behaviour Research and Therapy, 33,* 927–935.

Mogg, K., Bradley, B. P., Miller, T., & Potts, H. (1994). Interpretation of homophones related to threat: Anxiety or response bias effects? *Cognitive Therapy and Research, 18,* 461–477.

Mogg, K., Bradley, B. P., & Williams, R. (1995). Attentional bias in anxiety and depression: The role of awareness. *British Journal of Clinical Psychology, 34,* 17–36.

Mogg, K., Bradley, B. P., Williams, R., & Mathews, A. (1993). Subliminal processing of emotional information in anxiety and depression. *Journal of Abnormal Psychology, 102,* 304–311.

Mogg, K., Gardiner, J. M., Stavrou, A., & Golombok, S. (1992). Recollective experience and recognition memory for threat in clinical anxiety states. *Bulletin of the Psychonomic Society, 30,* 109–112.

Mogg, K., Mathews, A., & Eysenck, M. (1992). Attentional bias to threat in clinical anxiety states. *Cognition and Emotion, 6,* 149–159.

Mogg, K., Mathews, A., Eysenck, M., & May, J. (1991). Biased cognitive operations in anxiety: Artefact, processing priorities or attentional search? *Behaviour Research and Therapy, 29,* 459–467.

Mogg, K., Mathews, A., & Weinman, J. (1987). Memory bias in clinical anxiety. *Journal of Abnormal Psychology, 96,* 94–98.

Mogg, K., Mathews, A., & Weinman, J. (1989). Selective processing of threat cues in anxiety states: A replication. *Behaviour Research and Therapy, 27,* 317–323.

Molina, S., Borkovec, T. D., Peasley, C., & Person, D. (1998). Content analysis of worrisome streams of consciousness in anxious and dysphoric participants. *Cognitive Therapy and Research, 22,* 109–123.

Neely, J. H. (1977). Semantic priming and retrieval from lexical memory: Roles of inhibitionless spreading activation and limited capacity attention. *Journal of Experimental Psychology: General, 106,* 226–254.

Neely, J. H. (1991). Semantic priming effects in visual word recognition: A selective review of current findings and theories. In D. Besner & G. W. Humphreys (Eds.), *Basic processes in reading: Visual word recognition*. Hillsdale, NJ: Erlbaum.

Nugent, K., & Mineka, S. (1994). The effect of high and low trait anxiety on implicit and explicit memory tasks. *Cognition and Emotion, 8,* 147–163.

Öhman, A. (1993). Fear and anxiety as emotional phenomena. In M. Lewis & J. M. Haviland (Eds.), *Handbook of emotions* (511–536). New York: Guilford Press.

Öhman, A. (1999). Unconscious emotional processing. In T. Dalgleish & M. Power (Eds.), *Handbook of cognition and emotion* (pp. 321–352). Chichester, UK: Wiley.

Rapee, R. M. (1991). Generalized anxiety disorder: A review of clinical features and theoretical concepts. *Clinical Psychology Review, 11,* 419–440.

Rapee, R. M. (2001). The development of generalized anxiety. In M. W. Vasey & M. R. Dadds (Eds.), *The developmental psychopathology of anxiety* (pp. 481–503). New York: Oxford University Press.

Reidy, J. R., & Richards, A. (1997). Anxiety and memory: A recall bias for threatening words in high anxiety. *Behaviour Research and Therapy, 35,* 531–542.

Richards, A., & French, C. C. (1992). An anxiety-related bias in semantic activation when processing threat/neutral homographs. *Quarterly Journal of Experimental Psychology, 45,* 503–525.

Richards, A., & Millwood, B. (1989). Colour-identification of differentially valenced words in anxiety. *Cognition and Emotion, 3,* 171–176.

Richards, A., Reynolds, A., & French, C. C. (1993). Anxiety and the spelling and use in sentences of threat/neutral homophones. *Current Psychology: Research and Reviews, 12,* 18–25.

Roediger, H. L., Guynn, M. J., & Jones, T. C. (1994). Implicit memory: A tutorial review. In G. d'Ydewalle & P. Eelen (Eds.), *International perspectives on psychological science: Vol. 2. The state of the art* (pp. 67–94). Hove, UK: Erlbaum.

Rugg, M. (1995). Memory and consciousness: A selective review of issues and data. *Neuropsychologia, 33,* 1131–1141.

Russo, R., Fox, E., & Bowles, R. J. (1999). On the status of implicit memory bias in anxiety. *Cognition and Emotion, 13,* 435–456.

Russo, R., Patterson, N., Roberson, D., & Stevenson, N. (1996). Emotional value of information and its relevance in the interpretation of homophones in anxiety. *Cognition and Emotion, 10,* 213–220.

Sanderson, W. C., & Barlow, D. H. (1990). A description of patients diagnosed with DSM-III-R generalized anxiety disorder. *Journal of Nervous and Mental Disease, 178,* 588–591.

Spielberger, C. D. (1972). Anxiety as an emotional state. In C. D. Spielberger (Ed.), *Anxiety: Current trends in theory and research* (pp. 73–88). New York: Wiley.

Steptoe, A., & Kearsley, N. (1990). Cognitive and somatic anxiety. *Behaviour Research and Therapy, 28,* 75–81.

Stroop, J. R. (1935). Studies of interference in serial verbal reactions. *Journal of Experimental Psychology, 18,* 643–662.

Turvey, M. (1973). On peripheral and central processes in vision: Inferences from an information-processing analysis of masking with patterned stimuli. *Psychological Review, 80,* 1–52.

van den Hout, M., Tenney, N., Huygens, K., Merckelbach, H., & Kindt, M. (1995). Responding to subliminal threat cues is related to trait anxiety and emotional vulnerability: A successful replication of MacLeod and Hagan (1992). *Behaviour Research and Therapy, 33,* 451–454.

Vasey, M. W., & MacLeod, C. (2001). Information-processing factors in childhood anxiety: A review and developmental perspective. In M. W. Vasey & M. R. Dadds (Eds.), *The developmental psychopathology of anxiety* (pp. 253–277). New York: Oxford University Press.

Wells, A. (1995). Meta-cognition and worry: A cognitive model of generalized anxiety disorder. *Behavioural and Cognitive Psychotherapy, 23,* 301–320.

Williams, M., G., Mathews, A., & MacLeod, C. (1996). The emotional Stroop task and psychopathology. *Psychological Bulletin, 120,* 3–24.

Williams, J. M. G., Watts, F. N., MacLeod, C., & Mathews, A. (1988). *Cognitive psychology and the emotional disorders.* Chichester, UK: Wiley.

Williams, J. M. G., Watts, F. N., MacLeod, C., & Mathews, A. (1997). *Cognitive psychology and the emotional disorders* (2nd ed.). Chichester, UK: Wiley.

Woody, S., & Rachman, S. (1994). Generalized anxiety disorder (GAD) as an unsuccessful search for safety. *Clinical Psychology Review, 14,* 743–753.

CHAPTER 6

The Role of Intolerance of Uncertainty in Etiology and Maintenance

MICHEL J. DUGAS
KRISTIN BUHR
ROBERT LADOUCEUR

By the late 1980s, effective cognitive-behavioral interventions for many anxiety disorders had been developed and validated. Panic disorder with agoraphobia, social phobia, specific phobia, and even obsessive–compulsive disorder were being treated with relative efficacy via specific cognitive-behavioral approaches (see Barlow, Craske, Cerny, & Klosko, 1989; Foa, Steketee, & Ozarow, 1985; Heimberg et al., 1990; Rachman, 1990). Generalized anxiety disorder (GAD), however, was often treated with general anxiety reduction techniques that did not specifically target its main feature—excessive and uncontrollable worry. Although these treatments were effective to some extent, residual worry and anxiety as well as high relapse rates were common (Dugas & Ladouceur, 1998). Given these considerations, many researchers set out to identify the specific cognitive and behavioral processes that might be involved in GAD.

Based on clinical experience, our research group postulated that "intolerance of uncertainty" might represent an important cognitive process involved in worry and GAD. Intolerance of uncertainty can be defined as the tendency to react negatively on an emotional, cognitive, and behavioral level to uncertain situations and events. More specifically, individuals who are intolerant of uncertainty find ambiguity stressful and upsetting, and have difficulty functioning in uncertain situations. Moreover, they believe that uncertainty is negative and should be avoided, and that being uncertain is unfair. As everyday life is filled with uncertainty, a person who is intolerant of uncertainty can easily find numerous "reasons" to worry. In fact, many patients with GAD report that "even if everything is going well now, I worry that things will change." This statement captures the essence of intolerance of uncertainty.

A number of clinical observations led us to make a connection between intolerance of uncertainty and GAD. First, we noticed that standard cognitive correction techniques did not necessarily decrease worry and anxiety about feared outcomes for many patients with GAD. Although cognitive correction helped these patients arrive at more "realistic" estimates of the probability and consequences of a feared outcome, they often could not help worrying because there was a chance that "it could still happen." Second, many of our patients with GAD were not able to solve relatively simple problems. Once they had identified the most appropriate course of action, they frequently did not implement the solution because there was a chance that it might not lead to the desired outcome. Even if they had successfully identified the "best" solution, our patients often did not apply it because they appeared to be looking for the "perfect" solution (i.e., one that was "guaranteed" to work). Stated differently, many patients with GAD seemed to be immobilized by even small amounts of uncertainty, which are an unavoidable part of both a problem situation and the problem-solving process.

Our third clinical observation that suggested the importance of intolerance of uncertainty to GAD was the most striking. Contrary to what might be expected, some of our patients with GAD actually reported that they would prefer a problem to have a negative outcome than an uncertain one. For example, one patient reported that she had begun to experience problems in her relationship with her husband. Although her difficulties appeared to be relatively minor and transient, she stated that she would prefer it if her husband would "leave me now rather than [my] not knowing what might come of our relationship." It seemed that this patient favored a negative outcome (separation from her husband) over an uncertain one (not knowing how things would be resolved). Another patient reported something even more remarkable: He stated that he would prefer to know that he would pass away at the age of 55, rather than knowing that he would die at some unspecified age between 60 and 70. For this patient, not knowing exactly when he would die was intolerable; like the first patient mentioned, he preferred a negative outcome (dying sooner) to an uncertain one (not knowing when he would die). Clinical observations such as these appeared to corroborate our hypothesis that intolerance of uncertainty plays a key role in high levels of worry and GAD. Consequently, we used empirical means to investigate the relationship between intolerance of uncertainty and worry.

This chapter describes the course of our research on intolerance of uncertainty, beginning with the development and validation of the Intolerance of Uncertainty Scale. Following this, our research on the relationship between intolerance of uncertainty and worry in both nonclinical and clinical populations is reviewed. The nature of the relationship between intolerance of uncertainty and GAD, and the role of intolerance of uncertainty in the etiology and maintenance of GAD, are then discussed. Finally, the potential developmental origins of intolerance of uncertainty are explored.

DEVELOPMENT AND VALIDATION OF THE INTOLERANCE OF UNCERTAINTY SCALE

In an attempt to better understand intolerance of uncertainty and its relationship to worry, our research group developed a questionnaire to assess intolerance of uncertainty. The Intolerance of Uncertainty Scale (IUS; Freeston et al., 1994) was devised from a pool of 74 items corresponding to various aspects of intolerance of uncertainty. These include the consequences of being uncertain, the way uncertainty reflects on a person's character, expectations about the predictability of the future, attempts to control the future, frustration related to uncertainty, and all-or-nothing responses to uncertainty. Items that were deemed irrelevant or redundant were eliminated, and the remaining 44 items were administered to a group of 110 university students. The students were divided into three groups, based on whether they met GAD diagnostic criteria according to the Generalized Anxiety Disorder Questionnaire—Modified version (GADQ-M; Roemer, Posa, & Borkovec, 1991). The three groups of participants were defined as follows: (1) meeting cognitive and somatic criteria for GAD; (2) meeting somatic criteria only; and (3) meeting neither cognitive nor somatic criteria for GAD. Statistical procedures were used to determine which items distinguished the first two groups from the third group. We found that 23 items met this requirement, and an additional 4 items were kept because of their high correlation with the Penn State Worry Questionnaire (PSWQ; Meyer, Miller, Metzger, & Borkovec, 1990), a measure of the tendency to worry.

The final 27 items of the IUS are related to the idea that uncertainty is unacceptable, reflects badly on a person, leads to frustration and stress, and makes a person unable to take action. Examples of items include "Being uncertain means that a person is disorganized," "I can't stand being undecided about my future," and "One should always look ahead so as to avoid surprises." Items are rated on a 5-point Likert-type scale ranging from "not at all characteristic of me" to "entirely characteristic of me." The IUS, in its entirety, is presented in Appendix 6.1.

The psychometric properties of the IUS were assessed, and the scale showed excellent internal consistency (alpha = .91; Freeston et al., 1994), and good test–retest reliability over a 5-week period (r = .78; Dugas, Freeston, & Ladouceur, 1997). In terms of its factor structure, a five-factor solution was identified. Nine of the items loaded on the first factor, representing the belief that uncertainty is unacceptable and should be avoided. The second factor consisted of nine items concerning the idea that being uncertain reflects badly on a person. The four items that loaded on the third factor express the view that uncertainty results in frustration. The fourth factor had four items suggesting that uncertainty leads to stress, and the fifth factor included three items representing the idea that uncertainty prevents action. All factors were correlated with each other, with the overall IUS score, and with worry. Although the five factors of the IUS allow researchers to tap different aspects of an individual's intolerance of uncertainty, the overlap of the factors suggests that the total IUS score should be used. Overall, findings from the original validation study (i.e., Freeston et al., 1994) suggest that the IUS is a sound instrument for measuring intolerance of uncertainty.

ARE INTOLERANCE OF UNCERTAINTY AND WORRY DISTINCT CONSTRUCTS?

Given the strong correlations found between intolerance of uncertainty and worry, the possibility that they are not truly distinct constructs must be considered. "Worry" has been defined as concern about negative future events in which there is uncertainty about the outcome and where the individual experiences feelings of anxiety (MacLeod, Williams, & Bekerian, 1991). Although this definition of worry includes the notion of uncertainty, it essentially describes a *mental act* in response to a negative future event that may or may not actually occur. The definition of intolerance of uncertainty, on the other hand, emphasizes a low threshold of tolerance for the possibility that a negative event may occur at some time in the future (Dugas et al., 2001). Although both intolerance of uncertainty and worry refer to future negative events, there is an important distinction: Intolerance of uncertainty is defined as a *cognitive schema* or filter through which the individual views his or her environment, whereas worry can be seen as a cognitive reaction to potential negative events (i.e., worrying as a mental act). Consequently, worry might best be seen as a product of intolerance for uncertainty.

One way to investigate differences between worry and intolerance of uncertainty is to examine how measures of worry and intolerance of uncertainty relate to other constructs. The IUS appears to be a sound measure of intolerance of uncertainty. There are, of course, well-established instruments for assessing worry. For example, the PSWQ is recognized as a valid and reliable measure of the propensity for pathological worry (see Meyer et al., 1990). Accordingly, we (Ladouceur, Talbot, & Dugas, 1997) examined the relationships among the IUS, the PSWQ, and a series of behavioral tasks. Although intolerance of uncertainty as measured by the IUS and worry as measured by the PSWQ were related, they showed different patterns of correlations with specific behavioral tasks. In this study, participants were assessed on three experimental tasks that varied on level of uncertainty and difficulty. For example, a moderately uncertain task required participants to draw marbles from an opaque bag that contained either 85 black and 15 white marbles or 85 white and 15 black marbles. Participants were allowed to take as many marbles as they wanted before making a decision as to which bag they had been given. Worry was not correlated with performance on this task, but intolerance of uncertainty was. Specifically, individuals who scored high on intolerance of uncertainty drew a greater number of marbles before making a decision about which bag of marbles they had been given. However, high worry scores on the PSWQ were unrelated to performance on all tasks, regardless of the amount of uncertainty or level of difficulty.

Examination of gender differences on the IUS and the PSWQ also supports the notion that intolerance of uncertainty and worry are distinct constructs. Research has repeatedly shown that women report a greater tendency to worry than men. Recent data from our laboratory show that although women report a greater tendency to worry than men, women and men report similar levels of intolerance of uncertainty (Robichaud, Dugas, & Conway, 2003). Furthermore, this pattern of results (i.e., women reporting more worry than men, but similar levels of intolerance of uncertainty) was recently replicated in an adolescent sample (Laugesen, Dugas, & Bukowski, 2003). If intolerance of uncertainty and worry were essentially the same construct, we would expect women to report more intolerance of uncertainty than men. These findings corroborate the idea that although intolerance of uncertainty and worry are related, they are in fact different constructs.

Intolerance of Uncertainty and Nonclinical Worry

Worry is a common phenomenon in the general population; research suggests that as many as 38% of individuals in nonclinical samples worry at least once a day (Tallis, Davey, & Capuzzo, 1994). Research also suggests that similar processes are involved in both nonclinical and clinical worry (see Dugas & Ladouceur, 1998, for a review). Because of this, the study of nonclinical worry offers a unique opportunity to enhance our understanding of worry in both nonclinical and clinical populations. Although one cannot assume that findings obtained in nonclinical samples will always generalize to clinical worry, prior research into both clinical and nonclinical worry have often produced similar results.

Research in nonclinical samples has identified a strong relationship between intolerance of uncertainty and worry (Lachance, Ladouceur, & Dugas, 1999). Intolerance of uncertainty also appears to distinguish nonclinical subjects who meet GAD criteria by questionnaire from those who do not (Buhr & Dugas, 2002). Furthermore, although anxious and depressive symptoms are related to levels of worry in nonclinical populations, intolerance of uncertainty has emerged as a better predictor of worry in adolescents (Laugesen et al., 2003), adults (Dugas et al., 1997) and older adults (Doucet, Ladouceur, Freeston, & Dugas, 1998). Given the strength of the relationship among worry, anxiety, and depression, these findings suggest that intolerance of uncertainty represents a very important construct for the understanding of worry. In another study assessing differences in worry between adult men and women, intolerance of uncertainty was the best predictor of level of worry for both genders (Robichaud et al., 2003). These findings suggest that the relationship between intolerance of uncertainty and worry remains strong at different developmental stages as well as across gender, and lend further support to the proposal that it is a key worry process in nonclinical samples.

Given that intolerance of uncertainty is highly sensitive to worry, (e.g., people who are intolerant of uncertainty have high levels of worry and vice versa), it is important to assess the specificity of the relationship between intolerance of uncertainty and worry. In other words, is intolerance of uncertainty more highly related to worry than to other manifestations of anxiety and depression? In nonclinical samples, the answer to this question appears to be "yes." A study recently carried out by our research team showed that intolerance of uncertainty was highly related to worry, moderately related to obsessions/compulsions, and weakly related to panic sensations in a sample of undergraduate students (Dugas, Gosselin, & Ladouceur, 2001). Furthermore, the relationship between intolerance of uncertainty and worry remained strong after variance shared with other study variables was removed. A subsequent nonclinical study showed that intolerance of uncertainty was more highly related to worry than to depression, and that it predicted worry above and beyond symptoms of depression and social anxiety (Schwartz, Dugas, & Francis, 2000). Overall, these findings suggest that in the nonclinical adult population, intolerance of uncertainty is both sensitive and specific to worry. As such, the predictive capacity of intolerance of uncertainty to worry in clinical samples becomes an important question—particularly in the case of GAD, where the main feature is excessive and uncontrollable worry.

INTOLERANCE OF UNCERTAINTY AND GAD

The relationship between intolerance of uncertainty and GAD has now been examined in a number of studies. For example, in one study we assessed intolerance of uncertainty in patients with GAD and nonclinical controls, and found that the patients were significantly more intolerant of uncertainty than the control subjects (Dugas, Gagnon, Ladouceur, & Freeston, 1998). In fact, a discriminant function derived from the study variables was very effective in classifying GAD patients and nonclinical controls into their respective groups, as 82% of subjects were correctly classified. Furthermore, as expected, intolerance of uncertainty made the largest contribution to the discriminant function. A related study (Ladouceur, Blais, Freeston, & Dugas, 1998) assessed intolerance of uncertainty in patients with GAD, nonclinical analogues (subjects meeting GAD diagnostic criteria by questionnaire), and nonclinical participants with moderate worry levels. The patients with GAD and the analogue subjects had similar levels of intolerance of uncertainty, and both these groups were more intolerant of uncertainty than the group with moderate worry. Intolerance of uncertainty, therefore, appears to be more highly related to the presence of GAD symptoms than to clinical status.

Given these findings, some important research questions arise. For instance, how specific is intolerance of uncertainty to GAD? Is intolerance of uncertainty unique to GAD, or is it a cognitive process involved in other emotional disorders as well? One way to assess the uniqueness of intolerance of uncertainty is to determine whether it can successfully differentiate patients with GAD from patients with other anxiety disorders. In one study, the specificity of intolerance of uncertainty relative to GAD was assessed by examining intolerance of uncertainty in four subject groups: patients with primary GAD, patients with secondary GAD, patients with other anxiety disorders (primarily obsessive–compulsive disorder), and nonclinical controls (Ladouceur et al., 1999). In this study, the primary disorder was the most severe disorder as assessed by a standardized clinician rating. The patients with primary and secondary GAD had the highest levels of intolerance of uncertainty, followed by the patients with other anxiety disorders, followed by the nonclinical controls. These findings indicate that while intolerance of uncertainty may be a factor in other anxiety disorders, it appears to be relatively specific to GAD.

If, as this research suggests, intolerance of uncertainty is specific to GAD, an interesting issue becomes why patients with GAD seem to be more intolerant of uncertainty than patients with other anxiety disorders. Research has yet to be conducted on this question, but our clinical experience does support the notion that patients with other anxiety disorders can be intolerant of uncertainty. For example, patients with obsessive–

compulsive disorder sometimes report being intolerant of uncertainty (e.g., "Have I washed my hands thoroughly enough to be safe?"). Although we can only speculate at this time, patients with GAD may report being more intolerant of uncertainty because they have a low threshold of tolerance for the uncertainty in a wide variety of situations. In contrast to other anxiety disorders, where the focus of the threat is often specific, GAD is defined as worry and anxiety about a number of events or activities. Patients with GAD may be intolerant of the uncertainty involved in their relationships, their work performance, their health, and many other areas of their lives. In other words, for these patients, intolerance of uncertainty may be more of a generalized cognitive filter than it is for patients with other anxiety disorders.

WHAT IS THE NATURE OF THE RELATIONSHIP BETWEEN INTOLERANCE OF UNCERTAINTY AND GAD?

As evidenced by the findings presented above, it is clear that intolerance of uncertainty and worry are highly related. However, the exact nature of the relationship between intolerance of uncertainty and worry remains unclear: for example, is intolerance of uncertainty a causal risk factor for worry? According to Kraemer and colleagues (1997), a number of conditions must be met before one can conclude that a variable (in this case, intolerance of uncertainty) represents a causal risk factor for a second variable (in this case, worry). They suggest that the first step is to determine whether the variables are related; research has clearly established that intolerance of uncertainty and worry are in fact highly related (Dugas et al., 1997; Ladouceur et al., 1999). Second, Kraemer and colleagues state that changes in the "causal" variable must always precede changes in the other variable. Research has begun to assess whether changes in intolerance of uncertainty precede changes in worry. In a single-case study of a cognitive-behavioral treatment for GAD, time series analyses were used to assess the temporal relationship of changes in intolerance of uncertainty and changes in time spent worrying over the course of treatment. Changes in intolerance of uncertainty preceded changes in time spent worrying for three of the four study participants, whereas changes in time spent worrying never preceded changes in intolerance of uncertainty (Dugas & Ladouceur, 2000). In a larger study of the same cognitive-behavioral treatment for GAD, time series analyses revealed that 11 of 16 participants experienced changes in intolerance of uncertainty followed by changes in time spent worrying, and only 1 participant experienced changes in worry that preceded changes in intolerance of uncertainty (Dugas, Langlois, Rhéaume, & Ladouceur, 1998). Although these studies do not show that intolerance of uncertainty preceded the onset of GAD, they do show that changes in intolerance of uncertainty preceded changes in level of worry during treatment. Therefore, data from clinical trials suggest not only that intolerance of uncertainty is an important GAD treatment target, but that it may also represent a risk factor in the development of GAD worry.

Kraemer and colleagues (1997) propose a third condition necessary to ascertain whether a variable represents a causal risk factor by determining whether the variable can be changed or manipulated. Variables that cannot be changed are considered "fixed markers," whereas variables that can be manipulated are termed "causal risk factors." If a variable can be manipulated, it is only considered a causal risk factor when manipulation of that variable leads to changes in the second variable. In the case of intolerance of uncertainty, the question becomes whether intolerance of uncertainty can be manipulated, and, if so, whether this manipulation leads to changes in worry.

Whether intolerance of uncertainty can be considered a causal risk factor for worry was assessed in a study requiring subjects to participate in a roulette game, where the chances of winning were the same in all the conditions—that is, one out of three (Ladouceur, Gosselin, & Dugas, 2000). However, we manipulated the participants' level of intolerance of uncertainty by telling them that their chances of winning were either acceptable or unacceptable (when compared to the chances of winning in previous studies). Specifically, the participants were divided into two groups, and those in the first group were told that their chance of winning was less than in previous studies; therefore, this group's level of intolerance of uncertainty was *increased*. Those in the other group were told that their chance of winning was greater than in previous studies; therefore, this group's level of intolerance of uncertainty was *decreased*. Thus intolerance of uncertainty was being manipulated to allow us to assess the effect of this manipulation on worry. A manipulation check showed that the experimental procedure was successful: Participants who were told that their chances of winning were unacceptable (Group 1) reported being more intolerant of uncertainty than those who were told that their chances of winning were acceptable (Group 2). Participants in Group 1 (increased intolerance of uncertainty) reported more worries about the consequences of not winning than did participants in Group 2. These findings suggest that there may be a causal relationship between intolerance of uncertainty and worry: Changes in level of intolerance of uncertainty resulted in the predicted changes in level of worry. This result, combined with previous findings showing that changes in intolerance of uncertainty generally precede changes in worry over the course of treatment (Dugas & Ladouceur, 2000; Dugas, Langlois, et al., 1998), suggests that intolerance of uncertainty may be a *causal* risk factor for worry and GAD.

HOW MIGHT INTOLERANCE OF UNCERTAINTY LEAD TO GAD?

Intolerance of uncertainty may lead to worry both directly and indirectly. The direct link between intolerance of uncertainty and worry in GAD can be understood in terms of a patient's tendency to focus on potential negative outcomes, to overestimate the probability of the occurrence of these outcomes, and to exaggerate the negative consequences of these outcomes. Furthermore, when probability estimates and consequences are reevaluated (and made more realistic), the patient with GAD may still feel that the absence of a *guarantee* that the event will not occur is unacceptable. Intolerance of uncertainty, therefore, may directly lead to worry in many ways.

A number of studies support the direct links between intolerance of uncertainty and worry. For example, MacLeod and colleagues (1991) showed that individuals with high worry levels are more inclined to generate negative outcomes when faced with uncertain situations, and that they have an increased availability of explanations for why a negative event would be likely to occur. Since these individuals have a greater ability to formulate explanations for why negative events will occur, it is not surprising that they overestimate the probability that they will experience a negative outcome. Furthermore, such individuals are more likely than control subjects to overestimate their personal risk for threatening events (Vasey & Borkovec, 1992). In other words, those with high levels of worry believe that there is a greater chance of bad things happening to them and are more likely to conclude that the consequences of these events will be extremely costly. These findings are consistent with the idea that patients with GAD have adverse reactions to uncertain situations, and that intolerance of uncertainty may be the filter or schema through which these individuals interpret their environment. Stated differently, being intolerant of uncertainty may cause patients with GAD to focus on potential negative outcomes and to overestimate both the likelihood and personal cost of these events. This in turn could result in the development of worry concerning future negative outcomes. Furthermore, GAD may be resistant to change because intolerance of uncertainty may persist and lead to worry even when probability estimates and consequences are reevaluated, because the feared event "might still occur" (Dugas & Ladouceur, 1998). In these ways, intolerance of uncertainty may contribute directly to the development and maintenance of worry.

Conversely, the indirect link between intolerance of uncertainty and worry may operate quite differently and involve a separate set of processes. Our research team has proposed a model of worry that includes three process variables in addition to intolerance of uncertainty: positive beliefs about worry, negative problem orientation, and cognitive avoidance (Dugas, Gagnon, et al., 1998). The relationship between intolerance of uncertainty and each one of these processes may serve to clarify the in-direct effects of intolerance of uncertainty on worry.

Intolerance of Uncertainty and Positive Beliefs about Worry

Despite the fact that high levels of worry are associated with a loss of men-tal control and increased anxiety, patients with GAD hold a number of positive beliefs about worry (Wells, 1999; see also Wells, Chapter 7, this volume). In fact, such patients believe that worrying is more useful than do nonpatients with moderate levels of worry (Ladouceur et al., 1998). Our research team has identified five specific positive beliefs about worry that are related to excessive and uncontrollable worry (Francis & Dugas, 1999; Holowka, Dugas, Francis, & Laugesen, 2000). Interestingly, it has been shown that the successful treatment of GAD leads to a reduction in these positive beliefs about worry, and that the degree of change in posi-tive beliefs about worry predicts the extent of change in GAD symptoms (Laberge, Dugas, & Ladouceur, 2000).

The first type of positive belief about worry proposes that worrying helps an individual find better solutions to problems. These beliefs con-cern the usefulness of worrying in the problem-solving process, as well as in increasing vigilance and preparedness. The second type of belief about worry involves the idea that worrying motivates one to get things done. Stated differently, these beliefs imply that a decrease in worry would lead to complacency and inaction. The third set of beliefs about worry inti-mate that worrying offers protection from negative emotions. These in-clude beliefs that being worried in "advance" of some event offers protec-tion against surprise, sadness, or guilt, for example. The fourth belief about worry proposes that worrying, in and of itself, can prevent negative outcomes. This belief involves a type of magical thinking where worrying, on its own, can have an effect on the outcome of events. The fifth belief about worry proposes that worrying represents a positive personality trait. In this case, worrying is often confused with caring; worry is seen as a sign that the individual is conscientious and responsible—a person who "takes care of things."

Intolerance of uncertainty may well contribute to the formation of positive beliefs about worry. For example, a person who is intolerant of uncertainty may develop the belief that worrying will help him or her find better solutions to problems because the person has difficulty dealing with the uncertainty of the problem-solving process. This belief in the use-fulness of worrying could in turn reinforce the tendency to worry, and ul-timately sustain intolerance of uncertainty. As an example, an individual's belief in the usefulness of worrying will be positively reinforced when his or her worry coincides with the successful resolution of a problem. More-over, the individual may feel that he or she has "avoided" the uncertainty of the problem-solving process by worrying, as worrying makes the person feel as though he or she has considered every possible aspect of the problem. Thus, in this case, successful problem resolution will reinforce and maintain both the person's intolerance of uncertainty and his or her worry. As a second example, an individual who is intolerant of uncertainty may develop the belief that worrying protects him or her from negative emotions because, by imagining all possible negative outcomes, the person has eliminated the element of surprise or uncertainty related to these outcomes. If this individual worries about a loved one dying, the worry may make him or her feel more prepared and believe that the uncertainty of the situation has been reduced. However, this attempt to eliminate all uncertainty through worry prevents the individual from coming to terms with uncertainty and accepting a certain amount of uncertainty as a normal and inevitable part of life. Again, uncertainty will have been avoided, and intolerance of uncertainty will be sustained. In summary, it appears that intolerance of uncertainty contributes to the development of positive beliefs about worry. Moreover, these positive beliefs often lead to the perceived avoidance of uncertainty, which in turn reinforces both worry and intolerance of uncertainty.

Intolerance of Uncertainty and Negative Problem Orientation

Intolerance of uncertainty may lead to negative problem orientation by affecting both the individual's appraisal of the problem and his or her problem-solving ability. This negative problem orientation could then contribute to the development and maintenance of worry. Problem orientation reflects the awareness and appraisal of problems, and the assessment of one's problem-solving skills. All problems, by definition, contain some elements of uncertainty, as there is no way to be certain of how the situation will ultimately be resolved. A person who is intolerant of uncertainty may be more likely to focus on uncertain aspects of a problem and to interpret these aspects as threatening (Dugas et al., 1997), which in turn would interfere with the problem-solving process.

Intolerance of uncertainty may also affect an individual's appraisal of his or her own problem-solving ability. Because intolerance of uncertainty may lead to stress, anxiety, and frustration in problem situations, it may also reduce the cognitive and emotional resources needed for problem solving. Furthermore, high levels of negative emotions may lead to biased perceptions of one's problem-solving skills. In fact, research has demonstrated that patients with GAD have poorer problem-solving confidence than patients with panic disorder (Dugas, Marchand, & Ladouceur, 1999) or nonclinical controls (Dugas, Gagnon, et al., 1998). Research also shows that changes in problem-solving confidence can have a causal effect on catastrophic worrying (Davey, Jubb, & Cameron, 1996). In summary, intolerance of uncertainty may contribute to negative problem orientation by leading to biased appraisals of the problem and of problem-solving ability. Given that a negative problem orientation interferes with problem solving, it is clear how ineffective problem solving would lead to increased worry and anxiety.

Intolerance of Uncertainty and Cognitive Avoidance

Research shows that worry consists primarily of verbal/linguistic thought (i.e., an internal monologue) rather than mental images (Borkovec & Inz, 1990; Freeston, Dugas, & Ladouceur, 1996). Compared to verbal/linguistic thought, mental images of feared outcomes are often experienced as more subjectively unpleasant and are associated with greater physiological responding. In fact, mental images of feared outcomes may represent "core fears" that essentially drive an individual's worry. Some research suggests that worry, due to its verbal/linguistic nature, allows the individual to avoid the images and the unpleasant somatic activation they produce (Borkovec, Shadick, & Hopkins, 1991). Thus the individual who avoids a disturbing mental image by worrying is not only reinforcing his or her tendency to worry, but also rendering the image even more disturbing through avoidance. Paradoxically, therefore, avoidance of the threatening image prevents the individual from confronting and processing his or her fear, thereby maintaining the cycle of excessive worry. Some research does in fact suggest that avoidance of somatic activation may interfere with the emotional processing of core fears (see Foa & Kozak, 1986, for a review), and that it ultimately results in the maintenance of worry (Butler, Wells, & Dewick, 1995; Wells & Papageorgiou, 1995). Stated differently, when people who worry avoid threatening mental images, they may in fact be maintaining their worry in the same way that avoidance of a threatening stimulus slows down the process of extinction (Mathews, 1990).

Intolerance of uncertainty may contribute to the cognitive avoidance of threatening mental images, in the sense that images of potential ominous events will be difficult to tolerate. Consequently, the person may struggle not to think about the possible negative outcome and try to avoid any negative mental images associated with it. Rather than fully experiencing the negative mental images, the individual will attempt to avoid them, which will make the images even more threatening. Therefore, a person who is intolerant of uncertainty will use worry to anticipate negative outcomes and at the same time avoid threatening images, both of which may reinforce his or her worrying.

The following example illustrates how intolerance of uncertainty might ultimately lead to worry and anxiety. Imagine that Yvonne, a hypothetical person with GAD, is planning to take a trip during the holidays.

After booking her flight, she may begin to worry about the possibility that her airplane will crash. As her departure date approaches, she may increasingly overestimate the chances of her airplane crashing. Two weeks before Yvonne's scheduled departure, she may have reached a point where she believes that her airplane has a 50-50 chance of crashing. At this juncture, Yvonne may begin to feel that if she worries about her plane crashing, it will "magically" protect her from being in a plane crash. Although the function of this belief about the usefulness of worrying is to decrease the uncertainty of what might happen, Yvonne is now caught in a situation where she must worry until her departure. She may also want to obtain information about the crash record of the airplane model she will be taking. If Yvonne is intolerant of uncertainty, however, she may not call the airline because she is not certain of being able to obtain accurate information. In fact, she is unsure about where she should call to get this information, so that in the end she does not make the inquiry at all. Finally, because of her intolerance of uncertainty, Yvonne may avoid vivid and concrete mental images of what she fears (i.e., the plane crashing). This avoidance of mental images leads to a decrease in physiological arousal, which in turn interferes with the emotional processing of her fear. By now Yvonne is extremely worried about what might happen, and believes that she must keep worrying in order to protect herself; furthermore, she is paralyzed in her problem-solving attempts, and is not emotionally processing her fear. In this way, intolerance of uncertainty indirectly contributes to Yvonne's worries about her plane crashing. Let us now assume that Yvonne is given information about the actual probability of her plane crashing, which is extremely low. If she is intolerant of uncertainty, she will find it unacceptable that there is no guarantee that the plane will not crash (although the probability of such an event is extremely small). Therefore, if Yvonne remains intolerant of uncertainty, a simple reevaluation of the probability of a plane crash will be insufficient. As can be seen from this example, intolerance of uncertainty may lead to the development and maintenance of worry in a number of different ways.

INTOLERANCE OF UNCERTAINTY AND THE TREATMENT OF GAD

Recent investigations of intolerance of uncertainty suggest distinct intervention considerations—specifically, that patients with GAD should be encouraged to recognize and cope with a certain level of uncertainty in their environment. Our research group has developed a cognitive-behavioral treatment for GAD that helps patients recognize, accept, and develop strategies for dealing with uncertainty in their environment. This treatment targets intolerance of uncertainty by teaching these patients to distinguish between two types of worries (i.e., those about current problems and those about potential problems), and to apply a different strategy to each type of worry. Essentially, once patients have reevaluated their beliefs about the usefulness of worrying, they learn how to use sound problem-solving principles for worries about current problems and cognitive exposure for worries about potential problems. Each treatment component also aims to make patients with GAD more tolerant of uncertainty. For example, a component involving the reevaluation of the usefulness of worrying helps patients increase their tolerance of uncertainty, because they learn to deal with the uncertainty of future events rather than trying to control the events by worrying. The problem-solving training component helps patients to proceed with the problem-solving process even if they are unsure of its outcome, which targets their intolerance of uncertainty. Finally, cognitive exposure also helps patients increase their tolerance for uncertainty by modifying the catastrophic meaning they ascribe to threatening future events.

Thus far, our treatment for GAD has been assessed in two randomized controlled trials, both using wait-list control conditions. In the first trial, the cognitive-behavioral treatment was offered individually to 26 patients with GAD (Ladouceur, Dugas, et al., 2000). Results show that the treatment condition was statistically superior to wait-list on all study measures. Pre- to posttreatment effect sizes (Cohen's d') for primary outcome variables were $d' = 3.2$ for the standardized clinician rating of GAD symptoms, and $d' = 2.4$ for the self-report measure of pathological worry. Furthermore, 20 out of 26 participants (77%) no longer met GAD diagnostic criteria following treatment and these numbers were unchanged at 1-year follow-up. Interestingly, treatment outcome was related to change in intolerance of uncertainty. For example, every one of the 17 participants who had intolerance of uncertainty scores in the nonclinical range following treatment also had worry scores in the nonclinical range after treatment (Dugas, Langlois, et al., 1998). In the second trial, the treatment was offered in groups of 5–6 participants to 52 patients with GAD (Dugas et al., 2003). Again, the treatment condition was statistically superior to the wait-list condition on all study measures. Pre- to posttreatment effect sizes were $d' = 1.8$ for the standardized clinician rating of GAD symptoms, and $d' = 1.6$ for the self-report measure of pathological worry. Moreover, the treatment led to full remission in 60% of patients at posttest and this number increased to 95% at 2-year follow-up. Furthermore, intolerance of uncertainty scores significantly decreased during the follow-up phase of the study, which may help explain why many participants continued to improve after treatment had terminated. Taken together, these findings suggest that changes in intolerance of uncertainty are associated with changes in worry over the course of treatment and afterward, and underscore the importance of targeting intolerance of uncertainty in the treatment of GAD.

WHAT ARE THE ORIGINS OF INTOLERANCE OF UNCERTAINTY?

At present, we can only speculate about the origins of intolerance of uncertainty. Although the biological underpinnings of intolerance of uncertainty have yet to be examined, research into developmental factors associated with GAD has provided some interesting possibilities. In particular, early interactions between young children and their caregivers may play an important role in the later development of GAD through their effect on intolerance of uncertainty. Although research into early childhood interactions and GAD is just beginning, preliminary data suggest that specific types of attachment style can set the stage for the development of GAD. For example, Schut and colleagues (1997) found that individuals with GAD reported more insecure attachments to their primary caregivers than did healthy controls. In a related study, Cassidy (1995) found that the childhood experiences of individuals with GAD were characterized by more enmeshment than those of individuals without GAD. In this context, an "enmeshed" relationship is one in which the child attends to the needs of the caregiver, without necessarily having his or her own needs met. In other words, the parent–child relationship is marked by role reversal, with the child "taking care" of the parent.

Although no definite conclusions can be drawn from available data, it may be that an insecure attachment and an enmeshed relationship with a primary caregiver contribute to the development of intolerance of uncertainty. For example, if a child believes that the primary caregiver is weak and fragile, the child may constantly monitor the caregiver and the environment in an attempt to provide help if needed. Uncertainty would easily be construed as threatening, if the child views the caregiver as unable to deal with any problems that might arise. Furthermore, in addition to the caregiver having difficulties dealing with problems, the child may have limited resources to draw on if a real threat emerges, making uncertainty even more of a threat. This is especially true if one considers that the fragile caregiver may not be able to effectively model or teach the child how to deal with uncertainty. Given that intolerance of uncertainty seems to represent a relatively stable trait (Dugas et al., 1997), children who do not learn to deal successfully with uncertainty may be at risk for developing GAD later in life. Interestingly, Peasley, Molina, and Borkovec (1994) have shown that adults with GAD report more compassion and concern for the negative experiences of other people, as well as more anxiety and discomfort as a result of observing their negative experiences. It may be that the same enmeshed relationship that fosters intolerance of uncertainty also leads to overempathetic reactions to others later in life. In other words, it is conceivable that a child who learns at a very young age to tune into a parent's emotional states later becomes an adult who is very much attuned to the feelings of others.

In summary, early childhood interactions with a primary caregiver may contribute to the development of intolerance of uncertainty. Given that intolerance of uncertainty appears to be a stable cognitive characteristic, it may act as a cognitive diathesis that places an individual at risk for developing GAD at a later time. Intolerance of uncertainty may then interact with stressful life circumstances and lead to the development of GAD. It should be noted, however, that the stressful life circumstances ultimately leading to the development of GAD may be chronic stressors that do not necessarily involve traumatic experiences. In fact, most of the patients with GAD participating in our clinical trials reported that a gradual increase of responsibility at work and at home preceded the onset of their GAD. Thus an individual who is intolerant of uncertainty may be at considerable risk for developing GAD, because a gradual increase in responsibility and stress, which is quite common for adolescents and young adults, can trigger the onset of GAD. Once worry becomes excessive, other cognitive factors—such as positive beliefs about worry, negative problem orientation, and cognitive avoidance—may contribute to the maintenance of GAD.

Although the body of research on intolerance of uncertainty continues to grow, we are just beginning to understand its role in the etiology and maintenance of GAD. On the one hand, it is now well established that intolerance of uncertainty is highly and, for the most part, specifically related to worry and GAD. On the other hand, more research is needed to elucidate the nature of the relationship between intolerance of uncertainty and GAD. Using experimental manipulations and longitudinal designs, our research group has begun to address this issue. Given previous findings relating to intolerance of uncertainty, worry, and GAD, this line of research certainly seems promising.

REFERENCES

Barlow, D. H., Craske, M. G., Cerny, J. A., & Klosko, J. S. (1989). Behavioral treatment of panic disorder. *Behavior Therapy, 20,* 261–282.

Borkovec, T. D., & Inz, J. (1990). The nature of worry in generalized anxiety disorder: A predominance of thought activity. *Behaviour Research and Therapy, 28,* 153–158.

Borkovec, T. D., Shadick, R. N., & Hopkins, M. B. (1991). The nature of pathological and normal worry. In R. Rapee & D. Barlow (Eds.), *Chronic anxiety: Generalized anxiety disorder and mixed anxiety-depression* (pp. 29–51). New York: Guilford Press.

Buhr, K., & Dugas, M. J. (2002). The Intolerance of Uncertainty Scale: Psychometric properties of the English version. *Behaviour Research and Therapy, 40,* 931–945.

Butler, G., Wells, A., & Dewick, H. (1995). Differential effects of worry and imagery after exposure to a stressful stimulus: A pilot study. *Behavioural and Cognitive Psychotherapy, 23,* 45–56.

Cassidy, J. (1995). Attachment and generalized anxiety disorder. In D. Cicchetti & S. Toth (Eds.), *Rochester Symposium on Developmental Psychopathology: Vol. 6. Emotion, cognition, and representation* (pp. 343–370). Rochester, NY: University of Rochester Press.

Davey, G. C. L., Jubb, M., & Cameron, C. (1996). Catastrophic worrying as a function of changes in problem-solving confidence. *Cognitive Therapy and Research, 20,* 333–344.

Doucet, C., Ladouceur, R., Freeston, M. H., & Dugas, M. J. (1998). Thèmes d'inquiétudes et tendance à s'inquiéter chez les aînés. *Revue Canadienne du Vieillissement, 17,* 361–371.

Dugas, M. J., Freeston, M. H., & Ladouceur, R. (1997). Intolerance of uncertainty and problem orientation in worry. *Cognitive Therapy and Research, 21,* 593–606.

Dugas, M. J., Gagnon, F., Ladouceur, R., & Freeston, M. H. (1998). Generalized anxiety disorder: A preliminary test of a conceptual model. *Behaviour Research and Therapy, 36,* 215–226.

Dugas, M. J., Gosselin, P., & Ladouceur, R. (2001). Intolerance of uncertainty and worry: Investigating specificity in a nonclinical sample. *Cognitive Therapy and Research, 25,* 551–558.

Dugas, M. J., & Ladouceur, R. (1998). Analysis and treatment of generalized anxiety disorder. In V. E. Caballo (Ed.), *International handbook of cognitive-behavioural treatments of psychological disorders* (pp. 197–225). Oxford: Pergamon Press.

Dugas, M. J., & Ladouceur, R. (2000). Treatment of GAD: Targeting intolerance of uncertainty in two types of worry. *Behavior Modification, 24,* 635–657.

Dugas, M. J., Ladouceur, R., Léger, E., Freeston, M. H., Langlois, F., Provencher, M. D., & Boisvert, J.-M. (2003). Group cognitive-behavioral therapy for generalized anxiety disorder: Treatment outcome and long-term follow-up. *Journal of Consulting and Clinical Psychology, 71,* 821–825.

Dugas, M. J., Langlois, F., Rhéaume, J., & Ladouceur, R. (1998, November). Intolerance of uncertainty and worry: Investigating causality. In J. Stöber (Chair), *Worry: New findings in applied and clinical research.* Symposium presented at the annual meeting of the Association for Advancement of Behavior Therapy, Washington, DC.

Dugas, M. J., Marchand, A., & Ladouceur, R. (1999, November). *Problem solving in generalized anxiety disorder and panic disorder with agoraphobia.* Poster session presented at the annual meeting of the Association for Advancement of Behavior Therapy, Toronto.

Foa, E. B., & Kozak, M. J. (1986). Emotional processing of fear: Exposure to corrective information. *Psychological Bulletin, 99,* 20–35.

Foa, E. B., Steketee, G. S., & Ozarow, B. J. (1985). Behavior therapy with obsessive compulsives. In M. Mavissakalian, S. M. Turner, & L. Michelson (Eds.), *Obsessive–compulsive disorder* (pp. 49–129). New York: Plenum Press.

Francis, K., & Dugas, M. J. (1999, October). *Beliefs about the positive consequences of worrying: A specific relationship to excessive worry.* Poster session presented at the annual meeting of the Societé Québecoise pour la Recherche en Psychologie, Québec.

Freeston, M. H., Dugas, M. J., & Ladouceur, R. (1996). Thoughts, images, worry, and anxiety. *Cognitive Therapy and Research, 20,* 265–273.

Freeston, M. H., Rhéaume, J., Letarte, H., Dugas, M. J., & Ladouceur, R. (1994). Why do people worry? *Personality and Individual Differences, 17,* 791–802.

Heimberg, R. G., Dodge, D. A., Hope, D. A., Kennedy, C. R., Zollo, L., & Becker, R. E. (1990). Cognitive-behavior treatment for social phobia: Comparison with a credible placebo control. *Cognitive Therapy and Research, 14,* 1–23.

Holowka, D. W., Dugas, M. J., Francis, K., & Laugesen, N. (2000, November). *Measuring beliefs about worry: A psychometric evaluation of the Why Worry-II questionnaire.* Poster session presented at the annual meeting of the Association for Advancement of Behavior Therapy, New Orleans, LA.

Kraemer, H. C., Kazdin, A. E., Offord, D. R., Kessler, R. C., Jensen, P. S., & Kupfer, D. J. (1997). Coming to terms with the terms of risk. *Archives of General Psychiatry, 54,* 337–343.

Laberge, M., Dugas, M. J., & Ladouceur, R. (2000). Modification des croyances relatives aux inquiétudes après traitement du trouble d'anxiété généralisée. *Revue Canadienne des Sciences du Comportement, 32,* 91–96.

Lachance, S., Ladouceur, R., & Dugas, M. J. (1999). Éléments d'explication de la tendance à s'inquiéter. *Applied Psychology: An International Review, 48,* 187–196.

Ladouceur, R., Blais, F., Freeston, M. H., & Dugas, M. J. (1998). Problem solving and problem orientation in generalized anxiety disorder. *Journal of Anxiety Disorders, 12,* 139–152.

Ladouceur, R., Dugas, M. J., Freeston, M. H., Léger, E., Gagnon, F., & Thibodeau, N. (2000). Efficacy of a cognitive-behavioral treatment for generalized anxiety disorder: Evaluation in a controlled clinical trial. *Journal of Consulting and Clinical Psychology, 68,* 957–964.

Ladouceur, R., Dugas, M. J., Freeston, M. H., Rhéaume, J., Blais, F., Boisvert, J. M., Gagnon, F., & Thibodeau, N. (1999). Specificity of generalized anxiety disorder symptoms and processes. *Behavior Therapy, 30,* 191–207.

Ladouceur, R., Gosselin, P., & Dugas, M. J. (2000). Experimental manipulation of intolerance of uncertainty: A study of a theoretical model of worry. *Behaviour Research and Therapy, 38,* 933–941.

Ladouceur, R., Talbot, F., & Dugas, M. J. (1997). Behavioral expressions of intolerance of uncertainty in worry. *Behavior Modification, 21,* 355–371.

Laugesen, N., Dugas, M. J., & Bukowski, W. M. (2003). Understanding adolescent worry: The application of a cognitive model. *Journal of Abnormal Child Psychology, 31,* 55–64.

MacLeod, A. K., Williams, M. G., & Bekerian, D. A. (1991). Worry is reasonable: The role of explanations in pessimism about future personal events. *Journal of Abnormal Psychology, 100,* 478–486.

Mathews, A. (1990). Why worry?: The cognitive function of anxiety. *Behaviour Research and Therapy, 28,* 455–468.

Meyer, T. J., Miller, M. L., Metzger, R. L., & Borkovec, T. D. (1990). Development and validation of the Penn State Worry Questionnaire. *Behaviour Research and Therapy, 28,* 487–495.

Peasley, C. E., Molina, S., & Borkovec, T. D. (1994, November). *Empathy in generalized anxiety disorder.* Poster session presented at the annual meeting of the Association for Advancement of Behavior Therapy, San Diego, CA.

Rachman, S. (1990). The determinants and treatment of simple phobias. *Advances in Behaviour Research and Therapy, 12,* 1–30.

Robichaud, M., Dugas, M. J., & Conway, M. (2003). Gender differences in worry and associated cognitive-behavioral variables. *Journal of Anxiety Disorders, 17*, 501–516.

Roemer, L., Posa, S., & Borkovec, T. D. (1991, November). *A self-report measure of generalized anxiety disorder.* Poster session presented at the annual meeting of the Association for Advancement of Behavior Therapy, New York.

Schut, A. J., Pincus, A. L., Castonguay, L. G., Bedics, J., Kline, M., Long, D., & Seals, K. (1997, November). *Perceptions of attachment and self-representations at best and worst states in generalized anxiety disorder.* Poster session presented at the annual meeting of the Association for Advancement of Behavior Therapy, Miami Beach, FL.

Schwartz, A., Dugas, M. J., & Francis, K. (2000, November). *Intolerance of uncertainty and worry: Specificity with regards to social anxiety and depression.* Poster session presented at the annual meeting of the Association for Advancement of Behavior Therapy, New Orleans, LA.

Tallis, F., Davey, G. C. L., & Capuzzo, N. (1994). The phenomenology of non-pathological worry: A preliminary investigation. In G. C. L. Davey & F. Tallis (Eds.), *Worrying: Perspectives on theory, assessment and treatment* (pp. 61–89). New York: Wiley.

Vasey, M. W., & Borkovec, T. D. (1992). A catastrophising assessment of worrisome thoughts. *Cognitive Therapy and Research, 16*, 505–520.

Wells, A. (1999). A cognitive model of generalized anxiety disorder. *Behavior Modification, 23*, 526–555.

Wells, A., & Papageorgiou, C. (1995). Worry and the incubation of intrusive images following stress. *Behaviour Research and Therapy, 33*, 579–583.

APPENDIX 6.1. Intolerance of Uncertainty Scale

You will find below a series of statements that describe how people may react to the uncertainties of life. Please use the scale below to describe to what extent each item is characteristic of you. Please circle a number (1 to 5) that describes you best.

	Not at all characteristic of me		Somewhat characteristic of me		Entirely characteristic of me
1. Uncertainty stops me from having a firm opinion.	1	2	3	4	5
2. Being uncertain means that a person is disorganized.	1	2	3	4	5
3. Uncertainty makes life intolerable.	1	2	3	4	5
4. It's unfair not having any guarantees in life.	1	2	3	4	5
5. My mind can't be relaxed if I don't know what will happen tomorrow.	1	2	3	4	5
6. Uncertainty makes me uneasy, anxious, or stressed.	1	2	3	4	5
7. Unforeseen events upset me greatly.	1	2	3	4	5
8. It frustrates me not having all the information I need.	1	2	3	4	5
9. Uncertainty keeps me from living a full life.	1	2	3	4	5
10. One should always look ahead so as to avoid surprises.	1	2	3	4	5
11. A small unforeseen event can spoil everything, even with the best of planning.	1	2	3	4	5
12. When it's time to act, uncertainty paralyzes me.	1	2	3	4	5
13. Being uncertain means that I am not first-rate.	1	2	3	4	5
14. When I am uncertain, I can't go forward.	1	2	3	4	5
15. When I am uncertain I can't function very well.	1	2	3	4	5
16. Unlike me, others always seem to know where they are going with their lives.	1	2	3	4	5
17. Uncertainty makes me vulnerable, unhappy, or sad.	1	2	3	4	5
18. I always want to know what the future has in store for me.	1	2	3	4	5
19. I can't stand being taken by surprise.	1	2	3	4	5
20. The smallest doubt can stop me from acting.	1	2	3	4	5
21. I should be able to organize everything in advance.	1	2	3	4	5
22. Being uncertain means that I lack confidence.	1	2	3	4	5
23. I think it's unfair that other people seem sure about their future.	1	2	3	4	5
24. Uncertainty keeps me from sleeping soundly.	1	2	3	4	5
25. I must get away from all uncertain situations.	1	2	3	4	5
26. The ambiguities in life stress me.	1	2	3	4	5
27. I can't stand being undecided about my future.	1	2	3	4	5

Note. This is the first full-length publication of the "official" English translation of the IUS, which was originally prepared in French. A preliminary English translation appeared in Freeston, Rhéaume, Letarte, Dugas, and Ladouceur (1994). Copyright 1994 by Elsevier Science. Adapted by permission.

CHAPTER 7

A Cognitive Model of GAD

Metacognitions and Pathological Worry

ADRIAN WELLS

Generalized anxiety disorder (GAD) is a common and disabling condition that can persist for many years if untreated. It has been considered a "basic anxiety disorder" representing fundamental processes in all anxiety disorders (Barlow, 2002; Rapee, 1991), and Eysenck (1992) argues that there are important similarities between patients with GAD and non-patients who are high in trait anxiety. In view of the potential conceptual importance of GAD, it is surprising that there have been few attempts to construct models of the etiology and maintenance of the disorder. This state of affairs is reflected in studies that show relatively disappointing outcomes for psychological treatments of GAD, compared to the effectiveness of psychological interventions for other anxiety disorders (such as panic disorder or social phobia). Cognitive-behavioral treatments appear to be the most effective interventions, but only approximately 50% of patients achieve high end-state functioning or recovery (Durham & Allan, 1993; Fisher & Durham, 1999). In their reanalysis of data from six treatment trials, Fisher and Durham (1999) showed that approximately 60% of patients made some form of significant improvement following psychological therapy. Slightly less than 40% could be considered to be recovered in terms of scores on the Trait Anxiety subscale of the State–Trait Anxiety Inventory (Spielberger, Gorsuch, Lushene, Vagg, & Jacobs, 1983).

However, these overall figures tend to mask the considerable variability in outcome within and between studies. Overall, there is a predominance of relatively modest results, with few treatment conditions showing good outcomes (for further discussion, see Gould, Safren, Washington, & Otto, Chapter 10, this volume).

If treatments of GAD are to be improved, it will help to understand the mechanisms that contribute to and maintain excessive and uncontrollable worry, the predominant symptom of this disorder. This chapter describes a cognitive model of GAD (Wells, 1994a, 1997) that delineates particular mechanisms in the etiology and maintenance of pathological worry in GAD. The model is based on a synthesis of empirical work on the assessment of worry (Wells, 1994b) and clinical experience guided by a particular theoretical analysis of vulnerability to emotional disorders (Wells & Matthews, 1994).

Before I proceed with a description of the model, it is useful to briefly consider the characteristics of worry, since it appears to be distinct from other types of negative thinking. Armed with an idea of what worry is and its functional significance, we may begin to construct an understanding of the nature and regulation of negative thinking in GAD.

THE NATURE OF WORRY

Early conceptualizations of worry appeared in the literature on test anxiety (Sarason, 1972; Wine, 1971), where it was considered the cognitive component of anxiety responsible for performance decrements in anxiety-provoking evaluative situations. Subsequently, as a result of the pioneering work of Borkovec and colleagues (e.g., Borkovec, Robinson, Pruzinsky, & DePree, 1983), worry became more widely appreciated as an area of enquiry outside of the test anxiety arena. In this early work, Borkovec, Robinson, and colleagues (1983) defined worry as "a chain of thoughts and images negatively affect-laden and relatively uncontrollable" (p. 10). They considered worry a problem-solving activity closely related to fear processes. After exploring the nature of worry in clinical and nonclinical samples, Borkovec and colleagues suggested that worrying is predominantly a verbal rather than an imaginal process, and that it is an attempt to control future negative events and avoid current somatic arousal associated with imagery (Borkovec & Inz, 1990; Borkovec, Shadick, & Hopkins, 1991; Roemer & Borkovec, 1993). In a phenomenological study of nonclinical worrying, Tallis, Davey, and Bond (1994) described worry as a predominantly verbal thought process whose content is related to current concerns. However, the temporal focus of worry can also be on past or future issues. It appears that worry is predominantly ego-syntonic, and that it is perceived as serving an adaptive role in problem solving and motivation.

Differences appear to exist between worry and other varieties of negative thinking in emotional disorders, such as obsessions and depressive rumination. We (Wells & Morrison, 1994) demonstrated that nonclinical worries were more verbal, less involuntary, and more realistic than nonclinical obsessions, and were associated with a greater compulsion to act. Similar and additional differences were reported in a study by Clark and Claybourn (1997). In addition, they showed that worry was rated as focused more on the consequences of negative events. Studies of the cognitive variables that may relate uniquely to worry or obsessive–compulsive symptoms have found that different patterns of metacognitive beliefs predict these factors (Wells & Papageorgiou, 1998). Coles, Mennin, and Heimberg (2001) found that "thought–action fusion" (TAF; the tendency to appraise thoughts as causing external events) was significantly predictive of obsessive features when worry was controlled for; however, the association between TAF and worry was nonsignificant when obsessive features were controlled for. Studies have also examined the similarities and differences between worry and depressive rumination. In this context, we (Papageorgiou & Wells, 1999) demonstrated that worry and rumination differed significantly in 5 of 17 dimensions measured. Compared with rumination, worries consisted of greater verbal content and were associated with a greater compulsion to act, greater efforts to problem-solve, greater problem-solving confidence, and less of a past orientation.

In the cognitive model of GAD described in this chapter, two broad types of worry are separated for attention in conceptualizing pathological worry processes. The distinction is based on differences in the content and function that worry takes (Wells, 1995). "Type 1 worry" refers to worry about external events and internal noncognitive events (such as physical symptoms). "Type 2 worry," in contrast, consists of negative appraisal of and worry about one's own cognitive events and processes. This is essentially worry about worry—also known as "meta-worry," since it involves metacognitive processes of monitoring and appraising one's own thoughts. Examples of Type 1 worry include worrying about one's physical health or relationships, while meta-worry themes include appraisals of loss of control of thinking and of harm resulting from worry. The statistical independence of meta-worry from other worry domains (social and health worry) is reflected in the factorial structure of the Anxious Thoughts Inventory (Wells, 1994b).

To summarize, worry (1) consists of catastrophizing sequences of thoughts and is predominantly verbal; (2) is not merely a symptom of anxiety, but is in some forms a coping strategy; (3) can become excessive and seemingly uncontrollable (reflected in meta-worry appraisals); and (4) is distinguishable from other types of negative thoughts.

A COGNITIVE MODEL OF GAD

How can we account for the pervasive, excessive, and seemingly uncontrollable nature of worry in GAD? In this section, a cognitive model (Wells, 1994a, 1997) of the psychological mechanisms contributing to the development and maintenance of pathological worry in GAD is described. Figure 7.1 depicts these factors.

Metacognitive appraisals and beliefs are central to the development and maintenance of GAD in this model. "Metacognition" refers to the cognitive processes, strategies, and knowledge that are involved in the regulation and appraisal of thinking itself (Flavell, 1979; Wells, 2000). In GAD, worrying is used as a predominant means of coping with anticipated threat and is linked to the activation of positive metacognitive beliefs that guide the execution of worrying. These beliefs can be expressed verbally (e.g., "Worrying helps me cope," "If I worry I'll be prepared"). Although such beliefs are not exceptional, in people with GAD they are markers for implicit knowledge that supports the *active* use of worry as a coping strategy. As we shall see, however, the activation of negative beliefs about worry is central and more specific to the development of the problematic worrying found in GAD.

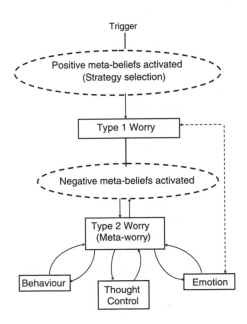

FIGURE 7.1. A cognitive model of GAD. From *Cognitive Therapy of Anxiety Disorders: A Practice Manual and Conceptual Guide* (p. 204) by A. Wells, 1997, Chichester, UK: Wiley. Copyright 1997 by John Wiley & Sons Ltd. Reproduced with permission.

In the model, a bout of worrying is triggered by an initial threatening experience of internal or external events. Such events can be sensations, emotions, cognitions, or external information. The initial interpretation often occurs in the form of "what if" questions with a catastrophic theme, such as "What if my children have meningitis?", "What if my partner is involved in an accident?", or "What if I get cancer?" These appraisals may also occur in the form of fleeting images of catastrophe, but patients with GAD shift to verbal-based worry processes in response to these triggers as a means of coping. Once a patient with GAD appraises a situation or event as potentially threatening, Type 1 worry is activated as a means of continued appraisal and coping. The Type 1 worry sequence is one in which answers to "what if" questions are contemplated and further "what if" questions are generated as a means of producing a range of coping strategies. Thus patients with GAD engage with their negative thoughts by activating Type 1 worry sequences in which they attempt to "work through" a negative thought or initial worry. This process of "working through" or Type 1 worrying appears to be executed until the person is distracted from the activity by competing processing priorities or until some internal goal is satisfied. When asked about internal stop signals, patients often report that they are represented by a "felt sense," which is interpreted as meaning they will be able to cope (e.g., "I feel my thinking is clear and I have a plan"). Alternatively, it may be an appraisal made by these individuals that they have generated all of the relevant threats and options, and therefore effective coping is likely.

Type 1 worrying exerts an effect on emotional responses that is mediated by the extent to which it achieves its goals. Worrying may initially produce anxiety responses, which subside as the goal of worrying is achieved. However, if emotional responses are themselves negatively interpreted (e.g., as a sign of not coping), this can fuel a need for continued worrying. This bidirectional relationship between Type 1 worry and emotion is represented by the dashed arrow in Figure 7.1. The model proposes that Type 1 worrying has other effects on emotion that are also represented by the dashed arrow in Figure 7.1. In particular, Type 1 worrying is predominantly verbal, and it can interfere with the emotional processing of other types of cognitive events (e.g., images). Therefore, in some circumstances, worrying exacerbates emotional symptoms that occur as a consequence of failures of habituation or emotional processing. Such negative effects of worrying are likely to contribute to negative beliefs about worry and one's ability to cope.

During the course of a worry episode, individuals with GAD activate negative metacognitive beliefs about the worry process and the consequences of worrying. During exacerbation of GAD (i.e., during distressing worry episodes), negative beliefs or appraisals of worry are always activated. However, if persons with GAD can worry within "safe limits," as determined by their appraisals or the use of coping behaviors, or the goal of worrying is rapidly achieved, full negative belief activation may be avoided. Two domains of negative belief are particularly salient: (1) beliefs about the uncontrollability of worry; and (2) beliefs about the mental, physical, and/or social dangers of worrying. Examples of negative beliefs include "My worrying is uncontrollable" and "Worrying could make me go crazy." The activation of negative beliefs leads to a negative appraisal of worrying, or Type 2 worry (meta-worry). Type 2 worry is the situational conscious appraisal of worry-related processes, and in GAD it reflects the situational readout of negative metacognitive beliefs. Once Type 2 worry occurs, threat appraisals are accentuated, leading to escalations in anxiety as depicted by the feedback cycle between Type 2 worry and emotion in Figure 7.1. Rapid escalations of anxiety are possible. For instance, if an individual appraises his or her worrying or anxious symptoms as a sign of immediate loss of control or mental breakdown, rapid increases of anxiety in the form of panic attacks may occur. Rising anxiety is often interpreted as a sign of likely failure of coping efforts, and this contributes to the need for continued Type 1 worrying in order to achieve internal goals signaling that it is safe to terminate the worry process. Therefore, the development of Type 2 worry (and negative metacognitive beliefs) prolongs worrying and interferes with the individual's ability to achieve internal goal states signaling that it is appropriate to stop worrying. In order to provide the reader with examples of the worry and metacognitive beliefs involved in the model, Table 7.1 summarizes the Type 1 worry, Type 2 worry, and metacognitive beliefs of three consecutive referrals to our clinic.

Two further mechanisms associated with Type 2 worrying and negative beliefs are involved in problem maintenance. In this model, these are labeled "behavior" and "thought control" (see Figure 7.1). Typically, behavioral responses and thought control strategies are problematic, because they lead to a failure to have experiences that can disconfirm Type 2 worry and negative metacognitive beliefs about the uncontrollability and dangers of worrying.

Behavior and Thought Control

Behavior varies, but often includes avoidance of situations, reassurance seeking, distraction, self-talk, and the like. The difficulty in using self-control strategies is compounded by the fact that people with GAD use worrying as a coping strategy and are therefore ambivalent about completely giving up the process of worry once it is initiated. The resulting ineffectiveness in worry control is interpreted as evidence of loss of control, thereby reinforcing meta-worry and negative beliefs. Unfortunately, when strategies are helpful at control, the nonoccurrence of catastrophes can be

TABLE 7.1. Characteristics of a Worry Episode and Metacognitions in Three Consecutive Clients with GAD

Patient number and sex	Type 1 worry	Type 2 worry	Negative metacognitive beliefs	Positive metacognitive beliefs
1F	Worry about writing an essay: Review all negative outcomes, try to answer them, and rationalize.	"Oh, God, I'm doing it again [worry]." "It will get worse and I'll go crazy."	"Worrying could make me go crazy." "If I don't control my worries, people will reject me."	"Worrying makes things turn out OK." "Worrying saves face."
2F	Worry about health and work: Dwell on negative side of things to try to work out worries until "mentally feel" can move on.	"I'm losing control." "I'm not normal to worry." "I'm harming myself with worry."	"Worrying is uncontrollable." "Worrying is harmful." "I could go crazy with worry." "If I don't control worry, it will control me."	"If I worry, I'll be prepared." "Worrying stops bad things from happening."
3F	Worry about work: Think of everything that can go wrong and plan action.	"I'm losing control." "I'm unable to function." "I'm losing my judgment, and people will think I'm incompetent." "I'm cracking up."	"Worrying is harmful." "I could go crazy with worry." "My worrying is uncontrollable."	"If I worry, I'll be thorough." "If I worry, I won't miss anything." "Worrying keeps me in control." "Worry helps me cope."

attributed to use of these behaviors, and negative beliefs about the dangers of worrying are maintained. "Thought control" in this context denotes that patients rarely decide not to worry once a trigger is encountered (since this would be like not coping); they instead attempt to suppress thoughts that trigger the need to worry in the first place. This suppression is inefficient and thereby reinforces meta-worry about loss of control. Deciding to interrupt the worry process, but allowing a negative thought to occur without catastrophizing, would provide evidence of control; however, it would not challenge negative meta-beliefs about the potential dangers of worrying. Thus some thought control strategies and behaviors may be helpful in challenging some negative beliefs, but they do not provide an unambiguous test of both domains of negative meta-cognitions (uncontrollability and danger) underlying problematic worry. In summary, thought control attempts can be both good and bad; some strategies may provide evidence of effective control, while others do not. Even if they do, they are likely to prevent individuals from directly challenging beliefs about the dangers of worrying.

The Development of Metacognitive Beliefs in GAD

Metacognitive beliefs are reinforced through various means, such as life events, information, and the effects of worry itself on thinking and feeling. The role of life events is illustrated by a patient attending our GAD clinic who reported that she had always been a "worrier." Her father was a worrier and had emphasized that it was helpful to worry (a factor contributing to positive beliefs about worry). She reported that worrying had not been a problem for her until her father was admitted to a hospital suffering from depression. Her father's "emotional breakdown" was attributed to the fact that he had been a worrier most of his life. At this point she appraised her worrying as potentially harmful, and she began to believe that worrying was dangerous. Her resulting worry about worry and coping strategies contributed to her worrying becoming excessive, uncontrollable, and distressing. In another case, a patient reported that it was the occurrence of intense physical sensations culminating in a panic attack during a worry episode that contributed to an evaluation of worrying as mentally and physically harmful.

EMPIRICAL SUPPORT FOR THE MODEL

Research conducted on worry-prone nonpatients and on individuals suffering from GAD has provided support for central aspects of this model of GAD (see also Wells, 1999). In this section, a brief summary of research is presented.

Metacognitive Beliefs and Pathological Worrying

The present model proposes that worrying is positively associated with both positive and negative beliefs about worrying. It also predicts that since negative beliefs are the predominant marker for the development of GAD worries, individuals with GAD should endorse greater negative beliefs than other anxious patients. Borkovec and Roemer (1995) conducted two studies exploring the reasons given for worrying by students. It is likely that such reasons correspond to beliefs about worrying. Individuals who met criteria for GAD, according to the Generalized Anxiety Disorder Questionnaire (GADQ, a self-report screening instrument; Roemer, Borkovec, Posa, & Borkovec, 1995) were asked to complete a six-item questionnaire about reasons for worrying. This questionnaire was based on reasons for worrying suggested by former patients with GAD and included motivation, problem solving, preparation for threat, avoidance, distraction from more upsetting topics, and superstitious reasons. Individuals meeting criteria for GAD rated using worry for distraction from more upsetting things significantly more than nonanxious subjects. In a second, larger study, subjects with GAD gave significantly more ratings than nonworried anxious or nonanxious subjects for distraction from more emotional topics. They also gave significantly higher ratings for superstitions and problem solving than nonanxious subjects. The nonworried anxious subjects did not differ significantly from either of these groups on these latter dimensions.

Tallis, Davey, and Capuzzo (1994) administered a battery of questionnaires to 128 subjects, and one of the measures was an instrument designed to elicit information on the phenomenology of worry. Two areas assessed in this study that are likely to reflect beliefs were the perceived negative and positive consequences of worrying. A little more than 71% of respondents thought that worrying made situations worse in general. Specific responses were used to generate a questionnaire that was administered to 127 undergraduate students, and the data were condensed with factor analysis. Four factors were obtained: pessimism and negative outlook (e.g., "Continued worry makes me lose track of all good things that happen"); problem exaggeration (e.g., "Worrying blows situations out of proportion"); performance disruption (e.g., "Worrying stalls decisive action"); and emotional discomfort (e.g., "Worry makes me focus on the wrong things"). In this study, 46% of respondents suggested that worrying was an attempt at problem solving between the ranges "definitely" and "always" on the rating scale provided. Subjects were asked to explain how they thought worry was a helpful process. Two factors emerged: (1) Worry acts as a motivator, and (2) worry facilitates preparation and analysis of situations. If these appraisals reflect individuals' beliefs about worrying, it appears that positive beliefs concerning worry as a motivational and preparatory strategy do exist.

Although these results are suggestive of the existence of positive beliefs about worrying in subjects with and without GAD, direct evidence of a relationship between metacognitive beliefs and worrying comes from work conducted by Cartwright-Hatton and Wells (1997). They developed the Meta-Cognitions Questionnaire (MCQ) to assess dimensions of positive and negative beliefs about worry and intrusive thoughts and individual differences in metacognitive processes. This questionnaire has five factorially derived subscales (with good psychometric properties) that reflect the following constructs:

1. Positive beliefs (e.g., "Worrying helps me cope"; alpha = .87)
2. Negative beliefs about uncontrollability and dangers of worrying (e.g., "When I start worrying I cannot stop," "Worrying is dangerous for me"; alpha = .89)
3. Cognitive confidence (e.g., "I have a poor memory"; alpha = .84)
4. General negative beliefs, including themes of need for control, weakness, punishment, superstition, and responsibility (e.g., "Not being able to control my thoughts is a sign of weakness"; alpha = .74)
5. Cognitive self-consciousness (e.g., "I pay close attention to the way my mind works"; alpha = .72)

In a series of studies, Cartwright-Hatton and Wells (1997) showed that all MCQ subscales were significantly and positively correlated with worry proneness and trait anxiety. Multiple-regression analyses demonstrated that when all these variables were entered, worry proneness remained positively and significantly associated with trait anxiety, positive worry beliefs, negative beliefs about uncontrollability and danger, and lack of cognitive confidence. In a further study, patients meeting DSM-III-R criteria for GAD or obsessive–compulsive disorder (OCD), patients with other anxiety or depressive disorders, and nonpatient controls were examined with the MCQ. No significant differences emerged in the endorsement of positive worry beliefs. However, patients with GAD and patients with OCD endorsed significantly greater negative beliefs concerning uncontrollability and danger than the other groups. The groups with GAD and OCD also reported significantly higher scores than nonpatients on general negative beliefs, including themes of need for control, superstition, punishment, and responsibility. The finding that patients with GAD and OCD responded similarly on the MCQ implies that both groups share negative metacognitive beliefs concerning thought processes.

We (Wells & Papageorgiou, 1998) tested for metacognitive predictors of pathological worry and obsessive–compulsive symptoms while controlling for the statistical interdependency of these variables. Pathological worry (assessed with the Penn State Worry Questionnaire; Meyer, Miller, Metzger, & Borkovec, 1990) and obsessive–compulsive symptoms were positively correlated with MCQ subscales in nonpatients. In this study, positive beliefs about worrying and negative beliefs concerning uncontrollability and danger were predictive of pathological worry when overlaps with obsessive–compulsive symptoms were controlled for. Of these two significant predictors, negative metacognitive beliefs concerning danger and uncontrollability made the greater contribution to the equation.

Davis and Valentiner (2000) tested aspects of the GAD model presented here using the MCQ in college students. In a regression analysis, they predicted Beck Anxiety Inventory scores from the MCQ after first controlling for worry measured by the Penn State Worry Questionnaire. Unfortunately, this is not a valid test of the present model, since the model is not a model of anxiety symptoms in the absence of pathological worry. However, in a subsequent set of analyses discriminating participants with GAD from nonanxious and nonworried anxious groups based on scores on the GADQ, these authors demonstrated that individuals classified as having GAD had higher negative beliefs (both on the uncontrollability and danger subscale and on the superstition, punishment, and responsibility subscale) than the other groups.

Investigations of metacognitive beliefs in patients with DSM-III-R GAD (which does not require worry to be uncontrollable) have produced results consistent with the model. We (Wells & Carter, 2001) compared metacognitive beliefs across individuals suffering from GAD, panic disorder, or social phobia, as well as nonpatients. There were no differences among groups for positive beliefs about worrying; however, the patients with GAD differed from other anxious patients and control subjects in reporting significantly higher negative beliefs concerning danger and uncontrollability. These results support the centrality given to negative beliefs in the present model. Moreover, the findings are consistent with the decision to include uncontrollability as a characteristic of GAD worry in DSM-IV (American Psychiatric Association, 1994). When Type 1 worrying (social and health) was treated as a covariate in this study, differences remained between patients with GAD on the one hand, and patients with panic disorder, patients with social phobia, and nonpatients on the other, in negative beliefs concerning uncontrollability and danger. This result suggests that differences in negative metacognitions among patients are not merely a function of differences in the frequency of Type 1 worry.

Type 2 Worry

A central concept in the present GAD model is the idea that pathological worrying like that characteristic of GAD is linked more to the activation of negative beliefs and Type 2 worry than it is to Type 1 worry content. Specifically, the model predicts that Type 2 worry should be positively associated with pathological worrying, independently of the frequency of Type 1 worries. In a test of this hypothesis, we (Wells & Carter, 1999) showed that among nonpatient subjects, Type 2 worry was significantly and positively associated with pathological worry proneness when trait anxiety and Type 1 worries were controlled for. However, Type 1 worrying did not remain a significant independent predictor of pathological worry proneness. A similar pattern emerged when participants were asked to rate "How much is worry a problem for you?" Once again, Type 2 worry and trait anxiety significantly predicted problem level, but social and health worries did not. In subsequent studies that additionally controlled for the uncontrollability of worrying, trait anxiety and Type 2 worry remained as significant predictors of pathological worry measured by the Penn State Worry Questionnaire. These data suggest that independently of the content of Type 1 worries, and of the uncontrollability of worry, Type 2 worry is significantly associated with pathological worrying. Nassif (1999, Study 1) tested the contribution of Type 2 worry to pathological worry in a Lebanese sample, while controlling for trait anxiety and two categories of Type 1 worry (social and health). Here trait anxiety, social worry, and meta-worry remained significant, with the largest independent contributions to pathological worry made by meta-worry and trait anxiety.

Nassif (1999, Study 2) screened nonpatients for the presence of DSM-III-R GAD, based on the GADQ screening instrument. Of 104 people tested, 19 were identified as meeting criteria for GAD and 50 as nonanxious. A comparison of these two subgroups showed that participants meeting criteria for GAD had significantly higher Type 2 worry scores than nonanxious participants (note that those with GAD also had significantly greater negative beliefs on the two MCQ subscales: uncontrollability and danger, and general negative beliefs).

In summary, the results of cross-sectional studies of metacognitive beliefs and Type 2 worry are consistent with the model. However, these data are unable to provide support for a causal role of metacognitions in the development of GAD. For this purpose, it is necessary to examine additional studies.

Causal Status of Metacognitions in GAD

Is there any evidence that negative metacognitive beliefs or Type 2 worry are causally linked to the development of GAD and pathological worry? Nassif (1999, Study 2) examined the longitudinal metacognitive predictors of pathological worry and GAD. Participants completed measures of pathological worry and metacognitions and the GADQ on two occasions, 12–15 weeks apart. Logistic regression analyses predicting group membership (DSM-III-R GAD vs. nonanxious) at Time 2 from the Time 1 measures showed that in separate equations, (1) Type 2 worry, but not Type 1 worry, was significantly and positively associated with the presence of GAD at Time 2, when GAD status at Time 1 was controlled for; (2) MCQ negative beliefs about uncontrollability and danger significantly predicted the presence of GAD at Time 2, when GAD status, trait anxiety, and Type 1 worry at Time 1 were controlled for.

Further prospective analyses, focusing on predictors of pathological worry at Time 2 rather than GAD status, showed significant positive associations between negative metacognitive beliefs (uncontrollability and danger, and general negative beliefs) assessed at Time 1 and pathological worry at Time 2 when pathological worry at Time 1 was controlled for.

Consequences of Worrying

The present model suggests that worrying as a predominant mode of processing/coping may contribute to problems of self-regulation of cognition and emotion. These problems, in turn, could strengthen negative metacognitive beliefs and meta-worry. Several studies have explored the negative effects of worry on emotion and thinking processes. Two lines of research are relevant to evaluating this hypothesis. The first has examined the effect of worrying on subsequent thinking; the second has explored the effects of worrying on intrusive images following stress. Borkovec, Robinson, and colleagues (1983) manipulated worry exposure in participants who were high and low in worrying, and showed that negative thought distractions increased following a 15-minute worry period, whereas distractions decreased for no worry and a 30-minute worry exposure. York, Borkovec, Vasey, and Stern (1987) showed that subjects had more negative thought intrusions after the induction of worry than after a neutral condition. These results suggest that brief periods of worrying may increase subsequent negative thinking.

In a different line of research, two studies have investigated the effects of worrying styles of thinking on intrusive images following exposure to stress. These studies tested the hypothesis that verbal worrying would block emotional processing of images. We (Butler, Wells, & Dewick, 1995) found that after watching a gruesome film, subjects who were asked to worry about it reported significantly more intrusive images during the following 3 days than subjects who were asked to image the film or "settle down" for 4 minutes after exposure. In a study replicating this effect and testing for possible mechanisms underlying the incubation effect of worry on intrusive images (Wells & Papageorgiou, 1995), we found that a brief period of worry following exposure to a stressful film produced the highest frequency of intrusive images during a subsequent 3-day period.

These results suggest that worrying may create its own problems that lead to further instances of intrusive thought and may block emotional processing following stress. Thus individuals who worry in response to stress and/or use worrying as a predominant coping strategy may be disadvantaged in terms of cognitive and emotional self-regulation.

Ineffective Thought Control Strategies

There is little available research on the nature of thought control strategies used by individuals with GAD. However, evidence from other sources suggests that some such strategies may be ineffective and perhaps counterproductive. Research with the Thought Control Questionnaire (Wells & Davies, 1994) suggests that worry and punishment, when conceptualized as thought control strategies, are associated with emotional disturbances (e.g., Reynolds & Wells, 1999; Warda & Bryant, 1998). The literature on thought suppression shows that asking individuals to attempt not to think about a particular target is often ineffective, and there is some mixed support for the idea that it may actually increase the frequency of thoughts about the target (Purdon, 1999; Wegner, Schneider, Carter, & White, 1987).

Two studies have examined the effects of suppressing worry. Becker, Rinck, Roth, and Margraf (1998) reported that patients with GAD experienced an enhancement effect when suppressing thoughts of their main worry. However, Mathews and Milroy (1994) found no effects of suppression in participants classified as high or low in worrying by the Penn State Worry Questionnaire. The results of studies of thought control are mixed, but overall they do suggest that some control strategies can be ineffective or negative in their effects. Although it seems likely that these effects would apply to individuals with GAD, firm conclusions await future studies of the effects of worry suppression in this group. Suppression studies will need to take a more sophisticated view and explore the effects of different types of thought control strategies and the possible complex interaction of strategy with beliefs.

The metacognitive model of GAD suggests that due to incompatible positive and negative beliefs about worry, patients are likely to vacillate between (unsuccessful) attempts to control and permit worry. A study by Purdon (2000) has produced evidence that appears to support the suggestion that positive and negative metacognitions are linked to different and potentially incompatible thought control responses. In an examination of *in vivo* negative appraisal of worrying in nonpatients, such appraisals were associated with greater attempts at thought control. However, positive beliefs about worrying emerged as concurrent predictors of a reduced motivation to get rid of thoughts.

IMPLICATIONS FOR TREATMENT: A METACOGNITION-FOCUSED THERAPY

The model presented here has several implications for treating GAD. It helps to explain the modest response of patients following other cognitive-behavioral therapy (CBT) interventions. Previous approaches have not been based on a specific model of the processes involved in the maintenance of GAD. The model implies that the modest effects obtained in other treatments result from a failure to understand and modify underlying psychological mechanisms responsible for generalized and excessive worry. The grounding of treatment in general cognitive theory or in anxiety management methods leads to a therapeutic focus on challenging and restructuring Type 1 worries and corresponding beliefs that are not metacognitions. This approach will be of limited value, because it does not substantially change patients' metacognitions concerning worry and associated coping behaviors. The present model suggests that the effectiveness of CBT could be improved by formulating cases in terms of the maintenance processes outlined in the model. In particular, it will be helpful to help patients become aware of the role of metacognitions and maladaptive behavioral responses in maintaining the problem, and to target these processes during the course of treatment.

A specialized form of cognitive therapy based on these principles has been developed (see Wells, 1997, 2000). Some of the central aspects of this type of treatment are outlined below.

Treatment Sequence

Treatment begins by constructing an idiosyncratic case formulation based on the cognitive model. This is followed by socialization to the model and by cognitive and behavioral reattribution strategies aimed at modifying negative metacognitive beliefs and appraisals. Beliefs and appraisals concerning the uncontrollability of worry are targeted first; later, strategies for modifying negative beliefs and appraisals concerning the dangers of worrying are introduced. Following modification of negative beliefs, positive beliefs concerning the use of worry as a coping strategy are addressed, and alternative strategies for appraisal and coping with threat are explored. The modification of uncontrollability beliefs early in therapy increases compliance with subsequent experiments, such as deliberate attempts to lose control of worrying and evoke the negative consequences of worry. The practice of alternative strategies for processing threat should be introduced after metacognitive belief change, so that alternative strategies do not become behaviors that prevent the disconfirmation of dysfunctional beliefs about worrying.

At the start of treatment, the therapist and patient review recent episodes of worry, with the aim of eliciting each component of the model and developing an individualized case conceptualization like that in Figure 7.2. The next step is to help the patient understand how negative and positive beliefs about worry, and the use of (or failure to use) behavioral and thought control strategies, maintain the problem. A central message to convey is the idea that excessive worrying is maintained by a range of

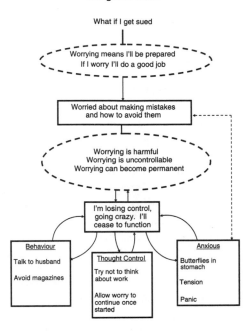

FIGURE 7.2. An idiosyncratic case conceptualization based on the GAD model. From Emotional Disorders and Metacognition: *Innovative Cognitive Therapy* (p. 143) by A. Wells, 2000, Chichester, UK: Wiley. Copyright 2000 by John Wiley & Sons Ltd. Reproduced with permission.

unhelpful beliefs about thinking. Therapist-directed questions offer an effective means of selling the model. For instance, to introduce the idea that beliefs about worrying are a central component of the problem, the therapist asks a number of hypothetical questions:

- "If you believed that your life depended on worrying, how much of a problem would worrying be?"
- "If you no longer believed that your worrying was uncontrollable, how much of a problem would you have?"

This type of questioning introduces the concept that beliefs and appraisals concerning worrying are central to problem maintenance. The therapist should emphasize the dissonance that exists between positive and negative beliefs about worrying, and ask how the patient thinks this could contribute to the maintenance of the problem.

Socialization to the model usually involves behavioral experiments aimed at illustrating the role of unhelpful thought control strategies in problem maintenance. In particular, patients are asked to engage in thought suppression to illustrate how some strategies are ineffective.

Modifying Negative Appraisals and Beliefs about Uncontrollability

Since patients with GAD believe that worrying is uncontrollable, several strategies have been developed to help them challenge this belief. First, a therapist explores with a patient modulating influences on worry. Situations can be identified in which worrying was interrupted by competing goals or distracting activities. For instance, the therapist may ask, "Can you think of a time when you were worrying and then something happened to distract you from worrying, such as the telephone ringing or someone visiting?" Such events can be used as evidence that worrying can be displaced and is therefore amenable to control.

Evidence and counterevidence concerning uncontrollability can be elicited. Patients often state that their past attempts at controlling worry have failed, and therefore this is evidence that their worrying is uncontrollable. However, it is important to elucidate whether such patients have ever actually tried in a fully committed way to give up the worry process once it is initiated. Typically, patients report that once a worry is initiated, they attempt to reason with their worry and feel that they must worry through a topic in order to feel better able to cope. The fact that patients do not unambiguously know whether worry can be postponed by using more appropriate strategies should be highlighted.

Indispensable strategies for challenging uncontrollability appraisals and beliefs are "worry postponement experiments." Worry postponement was first developed by Borkovec, Wilkinson, Folensbee, and Lerman (1983) as part of a stimulus control treatment. Here, patients were first asked to set aside a worry period. They then learned to monitor worry, to postpone it and focus on "present moment experience," and to engage in worry and problem solving only during the worry period. This earlier technique differs in several respects from the worry postponement *experiments* advocated by the present model. The only point of similarity is that both strategies ask patients to postpone worry. However, postponement experiments are presented with a rationale that emphasizes testing beliefs about uncontrollability, and they do not require patients to problem-solve during the worry period. Patients are instructed to use the allotted worry period only if they feel they "must" worry. Later in treatment, the worry period is actively used as an opportunity to attempt deliberately to lose control of worry. As a homework assignment, patients are asked to notice the onset of a worry and to postpone the worry sequence until a specified time period later in the day. Once the specified time arrives, the patient can decide either not to worry or to worry for a fixed time period (as a further test that worrying can be controlled). This experiment should be repeated for homework across several sessions as necessary. Ratings of belief in uncontrollability of worrying are tracked across the use of experiments and verbal reattribution methods as an index of their effectiveness.

When therapists are introducing this experiment to patients, it is helpful to emphasize that the aim is not to remove worries from consciousness (suppression), but merely to interrupt the catastrophizing (Type 1 worry) process. Patients may use a self-statement to facilitate this activity—for instance, "I'm not going to engage in this worry now. I will engage in this worry later."

Modifying Negative Appraisals and Beliefs Concerning the Dangers of Worrying

Several verbal reattribution strategies for challenging beliefs about the dangers of worrying have been developed. It is often helpful to question the mechanism by which worrying can lead to dangerous consequences, such as physical or mental harm. Some patients equate worrying with stress, and because they have learned that stress can be harmful, they assume that worrying must also be harmful. Several possibilities are available for weakening beliefs based on this type of reasoning. First, the differences between worrying and stress can be highlighted. Second, the mechanisms by which stress can have detrimental personal effects can be questioned. For instance, it may be suggested that stress in itself may not be harmful, but that the appraisal of and responses to stress may be important mediating factors. When therapists are challenging distorted beliefs based on "stress mechanisms," education is an effective tool. Highlighting the dissonance that exists between positive and negative worry beliefs provides a means of weakening one set of these beliefs. If patients believe that worrying facilitates coping, how can it be that worrying is also dangerous and can lead to mental breakdown?

Negative beliefs that worrying can cause mental or physical catastrophe are most amenable to modification through behavioral experiments. In one experiment, patients with GAD are asked to make active efforts to lose control or cause mental/physical harm by deliberately increasing the intensity of their worry. This can be practiced during an allotted postponed worry period and is followed by asking individuals to worry more, and to try to lose control of worrying next time a worry episode occurs, rather than postponing this attempt. Some patients are initially reluctant to engage in this type of experiment. Compliance is facilitated by ensuring that patients have a clear understanding of the model, by challenging uncontrollability beliefs before attempting such an experiment, and by first running this experiment in the therapy session.

Positive Beliefs and Strategy Shifts

Positive metacognitive beliefs are challenged later in treatment as a prerequisite to increasing patients' flexibility in the use of thinking strategies.

This is achieved by reviewing the evidence and counterevidence in support of positive beliefs and by the use of "mismatch strategies." Such a strategy consists of asking a patient to write out a detailed description of the events portrayed in a worry scenario. These events are then compared with the events that actually transpired in a worried-about situation. This technique can be implemented for situations that are avoided and in combination with exposure as a behavioral experiment. For instance, a patient was worrying about asking a work colleague for assistance. A worry narrative was written out, in which the negative consequences of engaging in this behavior were described in detail. The patient was then asked to engage in the behavior and to write a summary of the events that actually transpired in the situation. The strategy was used to illustrate how worry distorts reality. This procedure allows the therapist to raise the question: "If worry does not accurately depict reality, how helpful is it?"

One of the most powerful strategies for challenging positive metacognitive beliefs consists of the deliberate experimental increase and then decrease of worrying. Here, patients are asked to engage in daily activities that are normally associated with worrying while first deliberately increasing and then decreasing worry. If worrying enhances coping or positive outcomes, it should be possible to detect better outcomes when worry is increased and worse outcomes when the activity is decreased in intensity. Patients who engage in this experiment find that there is usually no difference in outcomes across high-worry and low-worry periods, and most often lowered worrying is associated with feeling better.

Toward the end of treatment, greater attention is given to reviewing alternative ways of thinking about threat and dealing with negative intrusions or triggers for worrying. Many patients with GAD report having been "worriers" for most of their lives. Worrying has become a predominant and inflexible means of dealing with potential threat. It is therefore helpful to discuss and practice alternative strategies for dealing with "what if" triggers for worrying. One strategy is to encourage patients to use positive endings for "what if" thoughts, rather than contemplating the worst consequences in response to these triggers and attempting to generate a wide range of coping options until some tenuous internal criterion is met. Patients should be encouraged to generate immediate positive outcomes (e.g., in the form of images) for initial worrying thoughts and to use evidence (e.g., knowledge of coping in the past) other than a "felt sense" to make predictions about competency and coping in the future.

At this stage of treatment, it is important to ensure that residual avoidance of situations that might trigger worrying is reversed. Exposure to worry-eliciting stimuli can be undertaken in conjunction with implementation of new thinking strategies (e.g., choosing not to worry, using new positive endings for old worries). In this way, a new cognitive and behavioral repertoire or "Plan B" for dealing with worry triggers can be formulated to replace the original "Plan A" characterized by Type 1 worry sequences.

Relapse Prevention

Relapse prevention consists of generating a summary of the patient's understanding of the nature of GAD and a description of effective strategies for dealing with worry. This summary is written out as a "therapy blueprint," which the patient keeps for future reference. Residual negative beliefs are assessed and challenged when these continue to exist. Post-treatment booster sessions are typically scheduled for 3 and 6 months after the termination of weekly therapeutic contact. Booster sessions present an opportunity to monitor beliefs and behaviors, and to fine-tune and reimplement any necessary treatment strategies.

CONCLUSIONS

A cognitive model of pathological worry and GAD has been described in this chapter. It is proposed that worrying becomes pathological and persists because patients hold dysfunctional metacognitive beliefs about the meaning and significance of worrying. Individuals with GAD worry as a processing and coping strategy. The development of negative beliefs and negative appraisal of worrying is key to the escalation of distress and transformation of worrying into a problematic experience in GAD. Metacognitive beliefs lead to behavioral and thought control responses that have the counterproductive effects of enhancing intrusive thoughts and preventing disconfirmation of negative beliefs about worrying. The repeated use of worrying supported by positive beliefs may incubate intrusive thoughts, thus reinforcing negative meta-beliefs and interfering with self-regulatory mechanisms such as those supporting emotional processing. Negative beliefs lead to worry avoidance strategies, which fail to expose the individual to situations that can disconfirm negative beliefs about the danger or uncontrollability of worrying. In this model, the inflexible use of worrying as a processing/coping strategy and the subsequent development of negative metacognitive beliefs and appraisals lead to the excessive, generalized, and distressing worrying that is characteristic of GAD. A brief review of the literature and summary of empirical tests of the model provide supporting evidence for this approach. However, further research and development in the assessment and measurement of metacognitions are required. A specialized form of cognitive therapy based on this model has been devised.

The results of a recent open trial of community outpatients with GAD treated with metacognitive therapy (Wells & King, 2003) demonstrated large and highly significant improvements in worry, anxiety, and depression. Posttreatment gains were maintained over 6- to 12-month follow-up. Moreover, using Jacobsen norms for recovery in trait anxiety reported by Fisher and Durham (1999), 87.5% of patients were recovered at posttreatment, and the mean improvement in trait anxiety was 60.4%. These findings are encouraging and larger-scale evaluation of the treatment is underway.

REFERENCES

American Psychiatric Association. (1987). *Diagnostic and statistical manual of mental disorders* (3rd ed., rev.). Washington, DC: Author.

American Psychiatric Association. (1994). *Diagnostic and statistical manual of mental disorders* (4th ed.). Washington, DC: Author.

Barlow, D. H. (2002). *Anxiety and its disorders: The nature and treatment of anxiety and panic* (2nd ed.). New York: Guilford Press.

Beck, A. T. (1967). *Depression: Causes and treatment*. Philadelphia: University of Pennsylvania Press.

Beck, A. T. (1976). *Cognitive therapy and the emotional disorders*. New York: International Universities Press.

Becker, E. S., Rinck, M., Roth, W. T., & Margraf, J. (1998). Don't worry and beware of white bears: Thought suppression in anxiety patients. *Journal of Anxiety Disorders, 12*, 39–55.

Borkovec, T. D., & Inz, J. (1990). The nature of worry in generalized anxiety disorder: A predominance of thought activity. *Behaviour Research and Therapy, 28*, 153–158.

Borkovec, T. D., Robinson, E., Pruzinsky, T., & DePree, J. A. (1983). Preliminary exploration of worry: Some characteristics and processes. *Behaviour Research and Therapy, 21*, 9–16.

Borkovec, T. D., & Roemer, L. (1995). Perceived functions of worry among generalized anxiety disorder subjects: Distraction from more emotionally distressing topics? *Behavior Therapy and Experimental Psychiatry, 26*, 25–30.

Borkovec, T. D., Shadick, R. N., & Hopkins, M. (1991). The nature of normal and pathological worry. In R. M. Rapee & D. H. Barlow (Eds.), *Chronic anxiety: Generalized anxiety disorder and mixed anxiety depression* (pp. 29–51). New York: Guilford Press.

Borkovec, T. D., Wilkinson, L., Folensbee, R., & Lerman, C. (1983). Stimulus control applications to the treatment of worry. *Behaviour Research and Therapy, 21*, 247–251.

Butler, G., Wells, A., & Dewick, H. (1995). Differential effects of worry and imagery after exposure to a stressful stimulus: A pilot study. *Behavioural and Cognitive Psychotherapy, 23*, 45–56.

Cartwright-Hatton, S., & Wells, A. (1997). Beliefs about worry and intrusions: The Meta-Cognitions Questionnaire and its correlates. *Journal of Anxiety Disorders, 11*, 279–296.

Clark, D. A., & Claybourn, M. (1997). Process characteristics of worry and obsessive intrusive thoughts. *Behaviour Research and Therapy, 35*, 1139–1141.

Coles, M. E., Mennin, D. S., & Heimberg, R. G. (2001). Distinguishing obsessive features and worries: The role of thought–action fusion. *Behaviour Research and Therapy, 39*, 947–959.

Davis, R. N., & Valentiner, D. P. (2000). Does meta-cognitive theory enhance our understanding of pathological worry and anxiety? *Personality and Individual Differences, 29,* 513–526.

Durham, R. C., & Allan, T. (1993). Psychological treatment of generalized anxiety disorder: A review of the clinical significance of results in outcome studies since 1980. *British Journal of Psychiatry, 163,* 19–26.

Eysenck, M. W. (1992). *Anxiety: The cognitive perspective.* Hove, UK: Erlbaum.

Fisher, P. L., & Durham, R. C. (1999). Recovery rates in generalized anxiety disorder following psychological therapy: An analysis of clinically significant change in the STAI-T across outcome studies since 1990. *Psychological Medicine, 29,* 1425–1434.

Flavell, J. M. (1979). Metacognition and cognitive monitoring: A new area of cognitive-developmental inquiry. *American Psychologist, 34,* 906–911.

Mathews, A., & Milroy, R. (1994). Effects of priming and suppression of worry. *Behaviour Research and Therapy, 32,* 843–850.

Meyer, T. J., Miller, M. L., Metzger, R. L., & Borkovec, T. D. (1990). Development and validation of the Penn State Worry Questionnaire. *Behaviour Research and Therapy, 28,* 487–495.

Nassif, Y. (1999). *Predictors of pathological worry.* Unpublished master's thesis, University of Manchester, Manchester, UK.

Papageorgiou, C., & Wells, A. (1999). Process and meta-cognitive dimensions of depressive and anxious thoughts and relationships with emotional intensity. *Clinical Psychology and Psychotherapy, 6,* 156–162.

Purdon, C. (1999). Thought suppression and psychopathology. *Behaviour Research and Therapy, 37,* 1029–1054.

Purdon, C. (2000, July). *Metacognition and the persistence of worry.* Paper presented at the annual conference of the British Association of Behavioural and Cognitive Psychotherapy, Institute of Education, London.

Rapee, R. M. (1991). Generalized anxiety disorder: A review of clinical features and theoretical concepts. *Clinical Psychology Review, 11,* 419–440.

Reynolds, M., & Wells, A. (1999). The Thought Control Questionnaire: Psychometric properties in a clinical sample, and relationships with PTSD and depression. *Psychological Medicine, 29,* 1089–1099.

Roemer, L., & Borkovec, T. D. (1993). Worry: Unwanted cognitive activity that controls unwanted somatic experience. In D. M. Wegner & J. W. Pennebaker (Eds.), *Handbook of mental control* (pp. 220–238). Englewood CLiffs, NJ: Prentice Hall.

Roemer, L., Borkovec, M., Posa, P., & Borkovec, T. D. (1995). A self diagnostic measure of generalized anxiety disorder. *Journal of Behaviour Therapy and Experimental Psychiatry, 26,* 345–350.

Sarason, I. G. (1972). Experimental approaches to test-anxiety: Attention and the uses of information. In C. D. Spielberger (Ed.), *Anxiety: Current trends in theory and research* (Vol. 2). New York: Academic Press.

Spielberger, C. D., Gorsuch, R. L., Lushene, R., Vagg, P. R., & Jacobs, G. A. (1983). *Manual for the State–Trait Anxiety Inventory: STAI (Form Y).* Palo Alto, CA: Consulting Psychologists Press.

Tallis, F., Davey, G. C. L., & Bond, A. (1994). The Worry Domains Questionnaire. In G. C. L. Davey & F. Tallis (Eds.), *Worrying: Perspectives on theory, assessment, and treatment* (pp. 285–297). Chichester, UK: Wiley.

Tallis, F., Davey, G. C. L., & Capuzzo, N. (1994). The phenomenology of nonpathological worry: A preliminary investigation. In G. C. L. Davey & F. Tallis (Eds.), *Worrying: Perspectives on theory, assessment, and treatment* (pp. 61–89). Chichester, UK: Wiley.

Warda, G., & Bryant, R. A. (1998). Cognitive bias in acute stress disorder. *Behaviour Research and Therapy, 36*, 1177–1183.

Wegner, D. M., Schneider, D. J., Carter, S. R., & White, T. L. (1987). Paradoxical effects of thought suppression. *Journal of Personality and Social Psychology, 53*, 5–13.

Wells, A. (1994a). Attention and the control of worry. In G. C. L. Davey & F. Tallis (Eds.), *Worrying: Perspectives on theory, assessment, and treatment* (pp. 91–114). Chichester, UK: Wiley.

Wells, A. (1994b). A multidimensional measure of worry: Development and preliminary validation of the Anxious Thoughts Inventory. *Anxiety, Stress, and Coping, 6*, 289–299.

Wells, A. (1995). Meta-cognition and worry: A cognitive model of generalized anxiety disorder. *Behavioural and Cognitive Psychotherapy, 23*, 301–320.

Wells, A. (1997). *Cognitive therapy of anxiety disorders: A practice manual and conceptual guide*. Chichester, UK: Wiley.

Wells, A. (1999). A metacognitive model and therapy for generalized anxiety disorder. *Clinical Psychology and Psychotherapy, 6*, 86–95.

Wells, A. (2000). *Emotional disorders and metacognition: Innovative cognitive therapy*. Chichester, UK: Wiley.

Wells, A., & Carter, K. (1999). Preliminary tests of a cognitive model of generalized anxiety disorder. *Behaviour Research and Therapy, 37*, 585–594.

Wells, A., & Carter, K. (2001). Further tests of a cognitive model of generalized anxiety disorder: Metacognitions and worry in GAD, panic disorder, social phobia, depression, and nonpatients. *Behavior Therapy, 32*, 85–102.

Wells, A., & Davies, M. (1994). The Thought Control Questionnaire: A measure of individual differences in the control of unwanted thoughts. *Behaviour Research and Therapy, 32*, 871–878.

Wells, A., & King, P. (2003). *Metacognitive therapy for generalized anxiety disorder: An open trial*. Manuscript submitted for publication.

Wells, A., & Matthews, G. (1994). *Attention and emotion: A clinical perspective*. Hove, UK: Erlbaum.

Wells, A., & Morrison, A. P. (1994). Qualitative dimensions of normal worry and normal intrusive thoughts: A comparative study. *Behaviour Research and Therapy, 32*, 867–870.

Wells, A., & Papageorgiou, C. (1995). Worry and the incubation of intrusive images following stress. *Behaviour Research and Therapy, 33*, 579–583.

Wells, A., & Papageorgiou, C. (1998). Relationships between worry and obsessive-compulsive symptoms and meta-cognitive beliefs. *Behaviour Research and Therapy, 36*, 899–913.

Wine, J. D. (1971). Test anxiety and the direction of attention. *Psychological Bulletin, 76*, 92–104.

York, D., Borkovec, T. D., Vasey, M., & Stern, R. (1987). Effects of worry and somatic anxiety induction on thoughts, emotion and physiological activity. *Behaviour Research and Therapy, 25*, 523–526.

CHAPTER 8

Neurobiology

SMIT S. SINHA
JAN MOHLMAN
JACK M. GORMAN

The neurobiology of generalized anxiety disorder (GAD) is a nascent research area. This is in part due to the comparatively recent recognition of GAD as a distinct nosological entity, rather than a residual diagnostic category for otherwise unexplained anxiety (Rickels & Rynn, 2001; see also Mennin, Heimberg, & Turk, Chapter 1, this volume).

It is difficult to draw firm conclusions regarding GAD neurobiology from the existing research. This literature consists largely of unreplicated studies utilizing relatively small samples and disparate methodologies, rendering interpretation difficult. Nevertheless, it does appear that the neurobiological substrates involved in GAD reflect abnormalities in neurochemical and neurophysiological systems that are implicated in animal models of anxiety, as well as the pathogenesis of human anxiety (e.g., Davis, 1997; LeDoux, 1998).

Moreover, as noted by Noyes and Hoehn-Saric (1998) and others (e.g., Sullivan, Coplan, Kent, & Gorman, 1999), indices of both the central nervous system (CNS) and the peripheral nervous system (PNS) reflect prolonged and blunted activity. This may be a unique and distinguishing biological feature of GAD as compared to other anxiety disorders.

This chapter reviews and summarizes research to date on the neurobiology of GAD. First, we provide an overview of the potential brain areas mediating GAD. Second, roles of the major neurotransmitter, neuropeptide, and neurohormonal systems are explored. Third, several measures of CNS and PNS functioning are reviewed, including the respiratory system, abnormalities of which are likely to play an important role in the production of generalized anxiety. Fourth, the negative impact of persistent anxiety and chronic worry on overall health, particularly immune system function and coronary heart disease, is discussed. Throughout the chapter, findings are discussed in relation to prevailing theoretical models of anxiety pathophysiology. We conclude by discussing limitations in the existing research, as well as recommending future directions.

POTENTIAL NEUROANATOMICAL AREAS IN GAD: A BRIEF OVERVIEW

Comprehensive neuroanatomical models of fear and anxiety have been developed through extensive preclinical research. Their specific relationship to GAD is presently unclear and probably imperfect. However, they provide an important basis from which to delineate potential brain structures mediating generalized anxiety and worry in humans.

The amygdala is a small structure within the temporal lobe that plays a major role in the attribution of emotional and motivational valence to a diverse range of stimuli. More recently, it has been shown to be central to an elaborate neural network subserving conditioned fear responses in animals, which may have relevance to understanding human anxiety states and disorders (LeDoux, 1996). The amygdala is uniquely situated to receive information from several brain areas involved in the detection of threat. To coordinate a response, it maintains important reciprocal connections to specific brain regions that generate the many physiological manifestations of arousal and anxiety.

The hippocampus, another temporal lobe structure that has a prominent role in emotion and memory, has been primarily implicated in contextual fear memory (Gorman, Kent, Sullivan, & Coplan, 2000) and coordinates responses to more complex fear cues than does the amygdala. The septo-hippocampal area has also been shown to be critical to an animal model of anxiety, behavioral inhibition, which involves freezing and cessation of activity during anxiety-provoking situations (Gray & McNaughton, 2000). Such behaviors are reminiscent of the generalized anxious apprehension seen in GAD.

The amygdala and hippocampus act in concert to generate complex negative emotional states, such as anxiety. These areas are capable of bidirectional communication with the frontal cortex, which can lead to incorrect appraisals of relatively benign situations as threatening. Persistent and pervasive threat directs the frontal cortex to formulate cognitions of apprehension and worry. Thus a complex interplay between lower centers (the amygdala and hippocampus) and higher centers (the frontal cortex) may serve to generate and maintain anxiety and worry in GAD (Davis, 1997).

NEUROTRANSMITTERS, NEUROMODULATORS, AND THE NEUROENDOCRINE SYSTEM

Gamma-Aminobutyric Acid

Gamma-aminobutyric acid (GABA) is an amino acid that functions as the major inhibitory neurotransmitter in the CNS. Receptors for GABA are ubiquitous in the CNS and have dense distribution in several brain areas responsible for the production of fear and anxiety, such as the frontal cortex, hippocampus, and amygdala (Petrovich & Swanson, 1997).

Some of the most commonly used anxiolytic therapeutic agents for GAD are the benzodiazepines (e.g., diazepam). These drugs act at the benzodiazepine receptor, which functionally are coupled to the GABA receptors. Binding of a benzodiazepine to its receptors increases the GABA receptors' affinity for available GABA. Thus the net effect of benzodiazepine administration is overall facilitation of GABA-ergic inhibitory neurotransmission (Goddard & Charney, 1997), with concomitant reduction in anxiety. Conversely, activation of the benzodiazepine receptors by an antagonist (a substance that decreases the action of a neurotransmitter) induces significant anxiety.

Substantial preclinical evidence demonstrates that GABA is one of the most important neurochemical systems mediating anxiety (Charney & Deutch, 1996), and that it may be implicated in the pathogenesis of the major anxiety disorders (Goddard & Charney, 1997). In addition, the GABA system is linked to immune system functioning. Peripheral benzodiazepine receptors modulate cytokine production of monocytes (cells that ingest dead or damaged cells), lymphocytes (cells that attack pathogens), and chemotaxis (the ability of a monocyte to migrate toward chemo-attracting substances).

Investigation of the benzodiazepine–GABA system in GAD is limited to a few studies. In general, these studies point to decreased benzodiazepine function in GAD. Weizman, Tenne, and Granek (1987) demonstrated decreased platelet benzodiazepine receptor binding in patients with GAD compared to nonanxious controls. Ferrarese and colleagues (1990) found that 40 outpatients with GAD showed decreased benzodiazepine binding on lymphocytes, compared with 20 controls—an effect that was reversed with benzodiazepine treatment. A later study (Sacerdote, Paneral, Frattola, & Ferrarese, 1999) replicated these findings, and additionally indicated a diminished chemotaxic response that was not restored after pharmacological treatment. Rocca and colleagues (1991) found that benzodiazepine receptor density on lymphocytes was significantly decreased in 15 patients with GAD and 10 patients with obsessive–compulsive disorder (OCD), but not in patients with panic disorder. Interestingly, this effect normalized following treatment with diazepam, suggesting altered benzodiazepine receptor functioning and density with pharmacological intervention.

Roy-Byrne, Cowley, Greenblatt, Shader, and Hommer (1990) demonstrated that patients with GAD have decreased benzodiazepine–GABA receptor sensitivity. They found a reduced sensitivity to diazepam (as measured by the degree to which diazepam slowed the velocity of saccadic eye movements) in patients with GAD compared to controls. Cowley, Roy-Byrne, Greenblatt, and Hommer (1993) also found a significant positive correlation between sensitivity to benzodiazepines (as reflected by velocity of saccadic eye movements) and scores on a self-report measure of novelty seeking in patients with GAD.

Tiihonen, Kuikka, and Rasanen (1997) investigated central benzodiazepine receptor binding and distribution in GAD, utilizing single-photon emission computerized tomography (SPECT) imaging with NNC 13-8241, a benzodiazepine receptor radioligand. Ten female patients with GAD and 10 age-matched female controls were studied. Benzodiazepine receptor binding was significantly reduced in the left temporal pole in patients as compared to controls. Furthermore, there was significantly greater homogeneity in benzodiazepine receptor density in the patient group. Increased homogeneity in the benzodiazepine system indicates decreased capacity for healthy, adaptive anxiety-related responses that can be executed by normal individuals with more heterogeneous benzodiazepine receptor distribution.

Benzodiazepines, as well as endogenous substances that bind to the GABA receptor (e.g., diazepam-binding inhibitor, or DBI), may be less effective in patients with GAD than in patient groups with normal GABA-binding rates. Moreover, benzodiazepine receptors and DBI play a major role in regulating CNS steroid production and may be involved in activation of the limbic–hypothalamic–pituitary–adrenal (LHPA) axis (Ferrarese et al., 1993). Decreased receptor density also implies reduced capacity of the benzodiazepine–GABA system to regulate anxiety and has been associated with a decrease in the content of messenger ribonucleic acid for peripheral benzodiazepine receptor coding (Rocca, 1998), which modulates chemotaxis and production of mono- and lymphocytes. Though it is currently unknown whether the effects discussed here have an impact on immune system functioning in GAD, this may be an important avenue for future studies.

Norepinephrine

Norepinephrine (NE) is the primary neurotransmitter mediating the sympathetic nervous system and becomes markedly more active during periods of stress and anxiety. The key neuroanatomical origin of NE is the locus ceruleus in the brain stem. The locus ceruleus sends diffuse projections to major brain regions that subserve anxiety, and it is critical to fear, arousal, and stress responses (Charney & Deutsch, 1996).

Several studies have shown that NE function is abnormally increased in anxiety disorders, particularly panic disorder (Ballenger, 2001; Charney & Deutsch, 1996). It has similarly been suggested that NE plays a role in chronic anxiety and GAD (e.g., Brawman-Mintzer et al., 1997). Unfortunately, studies of NE function to date have been largely inconclusive.

Studies of baseline levels of catecholamines and an NE metabolite, 3-methoxy-4-hydroxyphenethylene glycol (MHPG), have yielded mixed results. Sevy, Papadimitriou, Surmont, Goldman, and Mendlewicz (1989) examined the plasma levels of NE and MHPG in controls, patients with GAD, and patients with major depressive disorder (MDD). The patients with GAD had levels of NE and MHPG higher than those of controls, but lower than those found in the group with MDD. Mathew, Ho, Francis, Taylor, and Weinman (1982) found elevated levels of catecholamines and MHPG in patients with GAD compared to controls. However, a replication failed, leading the authors to conclude that stress resulting from venipuncture caused the elevation found in their prior investigation. Munjack and colleagues (1990) used an indwelling catheter and blood draw 20 minutes after insertion to control for the immediate effects of venipuncture and found no differences between controls and patients with GAD in NE levels at rest. They found significantly increased plasma MHPG in the group with GAD; however, the difference was small and did not significantly predict diagnosis. Garvey, Noyes, Woodman, and Laukes (1995) found that levels of urinary vanillylmandelic acid, another NE metabolite, significantly predicted severity of clinician-rated anxiety symptoms (tension, intellectual difficulties, muscular symptoms, and genitourinary symptoms) in a sample of 45 patients with GAD.

Cowley and Roy-Byrne (1991) note that studies of catecholamine function are generally not well controlled, and negative results could be accounted for by methodological difficulties. For example, no studies have controlled for diet or exercise, both of which can affect catecholamine assays. Moreover, all studies drew blood from the forearm region, where the venous bed causes variability even in the absence of other confounds (Best & Halter, 1982). Thus the results of catecholamine studies should be interpreted with caution.

Indirect assessment of NE receptor function can be achieved by measuring the growth hormone (GH) response to clonidine, an alpha-adrenergic agonist (a substance that increases the action of a neurotransmitter). Blunted GH response suggests reduced alpha-2 receptor sensitivity secondary to chronically increased NE drive. Cameron and colleagues (1990) found reduced NE receptor binding following a clonidine challenge in patients with GAD and patients with panic disorder as compared to controls. However, no differences were found between the groups in blood pressure, pulse, or plasma NE. Abelson and colleagues (1991) also found blunting of the GH response to clonidine in patients with GAD versus controls, suggesting increased NE activity. Plasma MHPG, heart rate, blood pressure, and psychological responses to clonidine did not differ between groups.

Charney, Woods, and Heninger (1989) found a trend for the MHPG response to yohimbine, a presynaptic alpha-2 receptor antagonist, to be lower in patients with GAD than in controls, again suggesting adrenoreceptor subsensitivity secondary to NE overdrive. However, behavioral and cardiovascular responses to yohimbine were similar for patients and controls. Thus the evidence for increased NE activity in GAD is mixed.

Recent evidence from treatment studies of venlafaxine, a serotonin–NE reuptake inhibitor (SNRI), may shed light on NE's role in GAD (see Lydiard & Monnier, Chapter 14, this volume, for a review of pharmacological treatments for GAD). In several trials including young and older adults with GAD, venlafaxine performed significantly better than placebo (Katz, Reynolds, Alexopoulos, & Hackett, 2002; Meoni, Salinas, Brault, & Hackett, 2001), suggesting a possible etiological role for NE. Further studies are needed before the role of NE in GAD will be clearly understood.

Serotonin

The neurotransmitter serotonin (5-HT) is currently recognized as important in the pathophysiology of diverse anxiety states. This has been largely due to the demonstrable efficacy of several serotonergic agents (e.g., buspirone, paroxetine) across the entire anxiety disorder spectrum (Sinha, Kent, & Gorman, 1999).

5-HT has also been identified as a key contributor to anxiety pathophysiology in preclinical models (e.g., Eison, 1990; Graeff, 1996; Gray & McNaughton, 2000). Serotonergic pathways arise from the raphe nuclei and project to diverse areas of the brain that are involved in the regulation of anxiety, including the amygdala and septo-hippocampal areas. Lesions along this substrate or the administration of agonists such as buspirone result in anxiolytic effects (e.g., Tye, Iversen, & Green, 1979; Van der Maelen, Matheson, Wilderman, & Patterson, 1986).

Though low levels of 5-HT have been linked to anxiety (Goddard & Charney, 1997), aggression, and impulsivity (Mann, Brent, & Arango, 1997), studies attempting to determine whether there are abnormalities in the 5-HT system in GAD have produced mixed results. Garvey and colleagues (1995) found that urinary levels of 5-hydroxyindoleacetic acid, a 5-HT metabolite, significantly predicted severity of clinician-rated anxiety symptoms (tension, somatosensory, genitourinary, and total severity) in a sample of 45 patients with GAD. Germine, Goddard, Woods, Charney, and Heninger (1992) found that m-chlorophenylpiperazine (mCPP), a nonspecific 5-HT$_1$ and 5-HT$_2$ agonist, elicited increased anxiety and anger behaviors in patients with GAD but not controls. An earlier study found that mCPP had little or no effect in patients with panic disorder or nonanxious controls (Charney, Woods, Goodman, & Heninger, 1987). Den Boer (1990) found that administration of ritanserin, a 5-HT antagonist, reduced anxiety in patients with GAD. Though these results suggest that patients with GAD are hypersensitive to such serotonergic agents, da Roza Davis, Sharpley, and Cowen (1992) found no difference between patients with GAD and controls in increase of slow-wave sleep after administration of ritanserin. This issue remains unclear.

Brewerton, Lydiard, and Johnson (1995) found reduced cerebrospinal fluid levels of 5-HT in patients with GAD compared to a control group. In addition, reduced platelet binding of the selective serotonin reuptake inhibitor (SSRI) paroxetine has been observed in GAD compared to controls (Iny et al., 1994). However, Schneider, Munjack, Severson, and Palmer (1987) found no differences in platelet binding of imipramine, an antidepressant with significant serotonergic activity, between patients and controls. Thus, although the precise nature of serotonin abnormalities is presently unclear, these studies suggest that low levels of 5-HT may characterize and contribute to GAD.

Cholecystokinin

The neuropeptide cholecystokinin (CCK) has been implicated in the etiology of both normal and pathological anxiety. Two CCK receptors have been identified in the CNS, CCK-a and CCK-b; CCK-b has the highest density in brain regions that mediate anxiety. To date, the preponderance of clinical evidence links CCK to the production of panic attacks—most robustly in patients with panic disorder, but also in patients with other anxiety disorders, as well as nondisordered individuals (Bradwejn & Koszcyki, 1994).

The involvement of CCK in GAD pathophysiology is an understudied area. Brawman-Mintzer and colleagues (1997) induced panic attacks with the CCK-b agonist compound pentagastrin in 71% of subjects with GAD compared to 14% of nonanxious controls. This rate of panic is very similar to that found in patients with panic disorder in response to sodium lactate and CO$_2$ challenge; it raises the possibility that CCK may contribute to the genesis of panic symptoms in GAD. CCK also induced substantial anxiety in the group with GAD.

Preclinical studies demonstrate that CCK has pronounced anxiogenic effects both alone and in interaction with other neurotransmitters implicated in the pathogenesis of anxiety, such as 5-HT. This has led to the development of CCK receptor antagonists as novel anxiolytic agents (Bradwejn & Koszcyki, 1994). A study by Goddard and colleagues (1999) evaluated the effects of a CCK-b antagonist, CI-988, on behavioral, neuroendocrine, and physiological changes to the mixed postsynaptic 5-HT agonist mCPP (an anxiogenic compound) in 16 patients with GAD. CI-988 was not found to be anxiolytic, nor could it affect biochemical or physiological changes induced by mCPP. This study suggests that mCPP-induced anxiety in GAD may not be related to 5-HT effects or to interactions between 5-HT and CCK activity. Further research is needed to delineate more clearly how CCK relates to anxiety production in GAD.

Limbic–Hypothalamic–Pituitary–Adrenal Axis

The LHPA axis is the main neuroendocrine system regulating stress and anxiety in humans. Information about fear and anxiety signals are relayed from limbic areas to the paraventricular nucleus of the hypothalamus, which produces corticotropin-releasing factor (CRF). CRF then stimulates the pituitary gland to release adrenocorticotropin-releasing hormone (ACTH), which in turn acts on the adrenal gland with the net effect of stimulating cortisol production. An increase in cortisol is the hallmark of the human stress response; it functions to maintain homeostasis and prepare an individual's defenses in the face of threat and danger (Levine, 1993). Function of the LHPA axis has been studied extensively in the anxiety disorders; however, few studies have evaluated this system in GAD.

Fossey and colleagues (1996) found no significant difference in the cerebrospinal fluid levels of CRF in patients with GAD, panic disorder, or OCD, as well as nonanxious controls. Rosenbaum and colleagues (1983) and Hoehn-Saric, McLeod, Lee, and Zimmerli (1991) found no differences in basal urinary free or plasma cortisol in patients with GAD compared to nonanxious controls. However, patients with GAD demonstrate an elevated dexamethasone suppression test (DST) nonsuppression rate (Avery et al., 1985; Schweizer, Swenson, Winokur, Rickels, & Maislin, 1986). Nonsuppression on the DST is one of the most consistent findings in melancholic depression (Young et al., 1994) and suggests increased drive of the LHPA axis. Interestingly, nonsuppression in GAD was unrelated to scores on the Hamilton Rating Scale for Depression (Hamilton, 1960). Tiller, Biddle, Maguire, and Davies (1988) also found DST nonsuppression in GAD that normalized with effective treatment. Thus at least some evidence links GAD to overproduction of cortisol, which is probably secondary to increased central LHPA function.

Though there is a strong association between thyroid system dysfunction and anxiety symptoms, evidence to date does not implicate thyroid abnormalities in GAD pathophysiology. Munjack and Palmer (1988) did not find differences in total serum thryoxine, free thyroxine index, triiodothyronine resin uptake, or thyroid-stimulating hormone between patients with GAD and controls. Similarly, Fossey and colleagues (1993) found no abnormalities in the level of thyrotropin-releasing hormone in patients with GAD. No differences have been found between patients with GAD and controls in plasma thyroid hormone (Kelly & Cooper, 1998); levels of the catecholaminergic enzymes catechol-O-methyl transferase or dopamine-beta-hydroxylase (both of which are agents that break down catecholamines) (Mathew et al., 1982; Mathew, Ho, Taylor, & Semchuk, 1981); or serum prolactin levels (Mathew, Ho, & Kralik, 1979).

CENTRAL AND PERIPHERAL NERVOUS SYSTEM PHYSIOLOGY

Brain Activity Patterns and Cerebral Metabolism

A small number of brain imaging studies have been carried out in GAD. DeBellis and colleagues (2000), using magnetic resonance imaging (MRI), found significantly larger right and total amygdala volumes in a group of children and adolescents with GAD as compared to controls matched on age, sex, height, and handedness. Groups did not differ in size of several other comparison regions, including the hippocampus and basal ganglia, or on global brain morphology. Because some have speculated that different brain regions are implicated in different anxiety disorders (e.g., Charney & Deutch, 1996), it may be that this difference is specific to GAD. However, amygdala volumes were not significantly correlated with clinical measures of anxiety. Thus other unidentified areas may also be involved in the generation or maintenance of anxiety and worry. It is notable, however, that a subset of participants had additional diagnoses of mood or anxiety disorders. The authors also construed GAD as a disorder characterized by "autonomic hyperactivity" (p. 55), which is not entirely consistent with current diagnostic criteria (e.g., Marten et al., 1993).

A recent extension of this work by DeBellis, Keshavan, Schifflett, and colleagues (2002) indicated that superior temporal gyrus (STG) volumes (both white and gray matter) were larger in children and adolescent patients with GAD than in controls. In addition, the authors found greater overall and white matter STG asymmetry in the group with GAD, but no differences in basal ganglia or thalamus volumes—two areas implicated in pediatric OCD (Gilbert et al., 2000; Rosenberg et al., 1997). These findings diverged from those obtained by the same researchers with posttraumatic stress disorder (PTSD) using the same methodology in a pediatric sample (DeBellis, Keshavan, Frustaci, et al., 2002); the group with PTSD showed larger gray matter STG volume only, and greater asymmetry in gray but not white matter, after total cerebral and gray matter volumes were controlled for. Therefore, structurally, the brains of pediatric patients with GAD are characterized by size deviations in the amygdala and STG areas, and by white and gray matter asymmetry.

It is unclear whether there are accompanying functional differences in these and other areas of the brain, however. Several studies show that overall levels of cerebral metabolism and regional blood flow in GAD do not diverge from those of nonanxious controls (Harris & Hoehn-Saric, 1995; Tiller et al., 1988; Wilson & Mathew, 1993). However, Wu and colleagues (1991) posit that patients with GAD show significant differences in patterns of absolute brain metabolism. According to positron emission tomography (PET) data, metabolic rates were lower in the basal ganglia and white matter in patients with GAD as compared to controls. Relative metabolism was increased in the left inferior area 17 in the occipital lobe, right posterior temporal lobe, and right precentral frontal gyrus. After treatment with benzodiazepines, the group with GAD showed a reduction in metabolism in the basal ganglia, cortical lobes, and limbic system as compared to the control group. Wu and colleagues found that changes in basal ganglia and limbic system glucose metabolism correlated with changes in anxiety levels, implicating the role of these structures in the process of GAD.

There is evidence that SSRIs such as paroxetine may be effective in disrupting repetitive intrusive cognitions in OCD by acting on the "loop" formed by the prefrontal cortex, thalamus, caudate, and limbic regions (Rosenberg et al., 2000). Data from this investigation may demonstrate whether the same areas are involved in frequent, uncontrollable worrying in GAD.

Respiration

Anxiety disorders are closely linked to abnormalities in respiration. Challenge studies with sodium lactate and CO_2 (agents with pronounced stimulatory effects on the respiratory system, such as hyperventilation) have reliably demonstrated that panic disorder, in particular, is associated with robust behavioral and physiological hypersensitivity to respiratory provocation (Sinha, Papp, & Gorman, 2000).

Three studies have examined differences in respiration between patients with GAD and controls at rest. Munjack, Brown, and McDowell (1993) found lower mean venous CO_2 pressure and higher mean rate of respiration in patients with GAD versus controls. Kollai and Kollai (1992) found that the length of the respiratory cycle and amplitude of respiratory sinus arrhythmia were significantly reduced in patients with GAD compared to nonanxious controls. Wilhelm, Trabert, and Roth (2001) examined respiratory, cardiovascular, and electrodermal measures in 16 patients with panic disorder, 15 patients with GAD, and 19 nonclinical control subjects. Both patient groups reported greater anxiety and more cardiac symptoms than control subjects. With respect to respiratory indices, respiratory rate, minute volume, and pCO_2 showed significantly greater instability in both patient groups than in the control group. The group with panic disorder had greater instability in tidal volume than the group with GAD.

In a study of voluntary breath holding in panic and GAD, Roth, Wilhelm, and Trabert (1998) studied 19 patients with panic disorder, 17 patients with GAD, and 22 nonclinical controls. All subjects were instructed to hold their breath for 12 consecutive 30-second trials, with each trial separated by 60 seconds of normal breathing. Increases in self-rated anxiety during the breath-holding periods were similar across the three groups. However, heart rate accelerations after cessation of breath holding were greater in the group with GAD. Level of end-tidal pCO_2 in patients with GAD was significantly lower than in controls, but higher than in the group with panic disorder. Since end-tidal CO_2 reflects chronic hyperventilation, it is likely that patients with GAD have a level of chronic hyperventilation intermediate between patients with panic disorder and controls.

Pine and colleagues (2000) examined the responses of children with separation anxiety disorder, GAD, or social anxiety disorder, and of nondisordered controls, to 5% CO_2 inhalation. They found that CO_2 induced panic responses most robustly in the group with separation anxiety, consonant with certain longitudinal studies suggesting that this disorder can antecede the development of adult panic disorder (Klein, 1993). However, the group with GAD also experienced significant increases in anxiety during the CO_2 inhalation compared to the children with social anxiety, who were indistinguishable from the healthy comparison group. The group with GAD did not experience shortness of breath to the extent of the group with separation anxiety. In terms of overall response severity, the group with GAD fell between the group with separation anxiety and the other two groups.

In a randomized, double-blind, crossover study, Perna, Bussi, Allevi, and Bellodi (1999) studied the response of 15 patients with panic disorder, 13 patients with GAD, 10 patients with comorbid panic disorder and GAD, and 12 healthy controls. The patients with GAD responded with significantly less panic and anxiety to 35% CO_2 inhalation than the patients with panic disorder and were relatively indistinct from the controls. Patients with panic disorder and with comorbid panic disorder and GAD had similar responses to CO_2. Rapee (1986) found that 15 minutes of 5.5% CO_2 inhalation caused a subjective anxiety response in patients with GAD that was intermediate between the responses of patients with panic disorder and nonclinical controls.

Cowley, Dager, and McClellan (1988) infused intravenous sodium lactate into patients with GAD and panic disorder, as well as nonclinical controls. The patients with panic disorder had a higher rate of panic attacks (41%) to the infusion than the patients with GAD (11%). However, the patients with GAD responded with more subjective anxiety than either the patients with panic disorder or the controls.

In three challenge studies using either 5% or 35% CO_2, panic attacks were not experienced by patients with GAD (Gorman et al., 1988; Holt & Andrews, 1989; Verburg, Griez, & Meijer, 1995). In addition, patients with GAD consistently reported lower subjective levels of anxiety than patients with panic disorder, but higher levels than nonclinical controls, following respiratory challenges. This effect is independent of increases in somatic symptoms, which are typically equivalent to those reported by patients with panic (e.g., Verburg et al. 1995).

In summary, the available evidence suggests that patients with GAD have a respiratory sensitivity less than that seen in patients with panic disorder, but still significantly higher than that of nonpatients.

Electroencephalography and Electromyography

In an early analogue study, Carter, Johnson, and Borkovec (1986) assessed undergraduate "worriers" and "nonworriers" using electroencephalography (EEG) during a cognitive task, a worry period, and a brief relaxation period. During the cognitive task, worriers showed less activation in the parietal lobes than nonworriers. During worry, they exhibited more left-than right-hemisphere low and high beta activity, which was a reversal of the nonworriers' pattern. This effect in the worrier group was attenuated with relaxation, suggesting that it is particularly relevant to worriers. The authors reported that this effect was the only one that discriminated the worriers from the nonworriers during the worry induction task.

EEG has also been used to study responses to novel illuminated visual stimuli in vigilance tasks. Patients with GAD showed less decrease in alpha activity than controls during the task, suggesting less neural activity during the task (Grillon & Buchsbaum, 1987). Individuals with GAD also showed less general variability in EEG under task demands (Borkovec & Inz, 1990) than controls.

A recent study utilizing event-related potentials indicated that patients with GAD showed normal P300 latency and magnitude in an auditory "oddball" discrimination task, which measures neural activity during detection of novel stimuli (Turan et al., 2002). Because habituation to novelty is partly mediated by the benzodiazepine–GABA system (Bodnoff, Suranyi-Cadotte, Quirion, & Meaney, 1989), which may be disrupted in GAD, it may be that abnormalities in neural mechanisms of habituation will emerge. This hypothesis has yet to be tested.

Studies of patients with GAD using electromyography (EMG) show elevated baseline muscle tension at rest (Hoehn-Saric & Masek, 1981; Hoehn-Saric, McLeod, & Zimmerli, 1989a), particularly in the lower frontalis region, as compared to controls. Hoehn-Saric et al. (1989a) found that different muscle groups showed divergent activity under task demands; frontalis tension was higher in patients with GAD than controls at baseline and remained high during a stressor. Gastrocnemius tension was low at baseline but increased significantly during a risk-taking task. Following the risk-taking task, patients with GAD showed less pronounced skin conductance than controls. However, overall habituation and fluctuation rates in skin conductance have been found to be similar between patients with GAD and controls (Birket-Smith, Hasle, & Jensen, 1993).

Hazlett, McLeod, and Hoehn-Saric (1994) also found elevated levels of tension in frontalis and gastrocnemius muscles in patients with GAD as compared to a nonanxious control group at rest, but no differences in skin conductance, heart rate, blood pressure, or respiration. The authors reported that the EMG profile of GAD is characterized by "random walks around a stable mean, with occasional short bursts of EMG activity" (p. 193). There were no differences between the groups on the frequency or amplitude of EMG bursts. Hoehn-Saric and Masek (1981) also reported elevated muscle tension at rest but no differences in skin conductance or heart rate in a sample of patients retrospectively classified as having GAD.

Lyonfields, Borkovec, and Thayer (1995) and Thayer, Friedman, and Borkovec (1996) found lower vagal tone, increased heart rate, and lower heart rate variability in patients with GAD both at rest and during worry compared to controls. Thayer and colleagues also found shorter interbeat intervals and lower high-frequency spectral power across baseline, worry, and relaxation periods in the group with GAD than in controls, and, relative to baseline and relaxation, shorter interbeat intervals and lower vagal tone in the group with GAD. However, one study found no differences between patients with GAD and controls in vagal tone at rest (Kollai & Kollai, 1992). Low vagal tone has been associated with lowered attentional focus and distractibility (Richards, 1987) and shorter interbeat intervals with the shifting of attention away from external events (Porges, 1992).

EEG during Sleep

Sleep provides various measures of CNS arousal that have been used in the study of anxiety. Sleep abnormalities have a significant impact upon the clinical presentation of GAD and should continue to be systematically evaluated.

Saletu-Zyhlarz and colleagues (1997) and Saletu and colleagues (1997) examined the objective sleep and quality of awakening among patients with GAD compared to nonanxious controls. Objective measures were obtained by polysomnography. The patients demonstrated significantly increased wake time during the total sleep period, more early morning awakening, decreased total sleep time, and decreased sleep efficiency (defined as the ratio of time spent in bed to time spent actually sleeping). EEG mapping in the late morning hours demonstrated increased EEG indices of the tendency to fall asleep. These were positively correlated with scores on the Zung Self-Rated Anxiety Scale.

Papadimitriou, Linkowski, Kerkhofs, Kempenaers, and Mendlewicz (1988) used EEG to compare sleep patterns of patients with GAD (n = 10), GAD with comorbid MDD (n = 10), and MDD (n = 10). No difference was found between the groups with GAD and with GAD/MDD on any sleep-related variable; however, both of these groups showed significantly longer rapid-eye-movement (REM) latency, a lower number of awakenings, and fewer stage shifts than the group with MDD. Papadimitriou and colleagues also compared sleep polysomnographic recordings of patients with GAD, patients with MDD, and controls. The patients with GAD evidenced significantly fewer stage shifts and awakenings than the group with MDD during Night 1 and on a three-night average. The group with GAD also showed significantly longer REM latency and shorter total and Stage 2 duration than controls, although they did not differ from the group with MDD on these variables.

Reynolds, Shaw, Newton, Coble, and Kupfer (1983) found that patients with GAD showed longer REM latency, reduced REM sleep percentage and eye movement activity, and more consistent sleep patterns over two nights than patients with MDD. However, the groups did not differ significantly on sleep initiation or maintenance (both of which were difficult for both groups) or amount of slow-wave sleep, which was diminished in both groups. Lauer, Garcia-Borreguero, Pollmacher, Ozdaglar, and Krieg (1990) found increased Stage 1 sleep in patients with GAD, suggesting an increased time to deeper sleep as compared to controls; however, Saletu and colleagues (1994) found increases in Stages 3 and 4 as compared to controls, with no difference in Stage 1, REM latency, or total REM duration. However, data were collected from participants' own homes rather than a lab, which may have affected outcome.

Sleep-related variables (REM latency, sleep stage shifts, awakenings) thus differentiated patients with GAD from depressed groups and controls across these studies. It is unclear, however, whether the poor sleep quality found among patients with GAD is caused primarily by neurobiological phenomena, worrying, contextual variables (lab vs. home), or a combination thereof.

GAD AND HEALTH

Craske, Rapee, Jackel, and Barlow (1989) found that illness/health/injury was the most frequently endorsed category of worry domains among patients with GAD, whose severity of worry scores on this domain differed significantly from that of nonworried controls. A study by Katon and colleagues (1990) indicated that the diagnosis of GAD was assigned to more than 20% of individuals with high rates of utilizing outpatient medical care. It is unclear whether the overutilization bias is driven by excessive worrying about health or legitimate illness. However, because patients with GAD tend to overutilize primary health care services (e.g., Ormel et al., 1993; Roy-Byrne & Katon, 1997), it is important to ascertain whether the disorder has a negative impact on the body's ability to fight disease and infection. A small body of evidence indicating the deleterious effects of worry and GAD on immune system functioning is consistent with this possibility.

Immunosuppression

Maier and Watkins (2000) hypothesize that the immune system is a "sensory pathway for psychology" (p. 98) because the brain and immune system are connected by a bidirectional substrate, allowing cross-talk and feedback. Cytokine release is contingent upon brain–immune system communication via this bidirectional pathway. The authors argue that shortly after an external stressor, NE and 5-HT are released in the hippocampus and hypothalamus, leading to changes in behavior and neurochemistry that prepare the immune system to fight disease and infection. Interestingly, the authors also argue that psychological stressors (such as placing a rat in a novel cage) cause outcomes similar to those caused by infection, such as fever, increased white cell count, and metabolic shifts toward the production of acute-phase proteins. (A discussion of other immune system changes brought about by stressors can be found in Maier & Watkins, 1998.)

LaVia, Workman, and Lydiard (1992) examined the relationship between stress and immunosuppression in a sample of patients and found that those meeting criteria for GAD, panic disorder, or both had higher "stress intrusion" scores (p. 139) on the Impact of Event Scale (indicating the respondent's tendency to allow stress to overwhelm and dominate) and a higher frequency of upper respiratory infections than those who were free of psychiatric disorder. An extension of this work (LaVia et al., 1996) in a sample of 14 patients with GAD and 14 controls yielded concordant results. In cultures containing the same initial number of monocytes (cells that ingest dead or damaged cells), T-lymphocytes (cells that directly attack pathogens), and B-lymphocytes (cells that produce pathogen-attacking antibodies), stimulation with anti-CD3 (a substance that can activate cells in the immune system) over 72 hours induced significantly decreased immunodefensive activity in the group with GAD. This indicates that in the patients with GAD, lymphocytes were less able to mount a response to a mitogen (a substance that causes mitosis and cell division) than healthy controls. Moreover, the group with GAD evidenced a higher rate of upper respiratory infections and resultant sick days from work than the controls over an unspecified period of time.

Two studies (Segerstrom, Glover, Craske, & Fahey, 1998; Segerstrom, Solomon, Kemeny, & Fahey, 1998) have investigated the effects of frequent worry on the number and cytotoxicity of natural killer cells in peripheral blood in nonpatients. The authors were particularly interested in the activity of natural killer cells derived from bone marrow, which are specialized for targeting and killing infected cells and tumors through a poorly understood process. A wide variety of stressors (e.g., mental arithmetic, Stroop task) can lead to the release of natural killer cells (Kiecolt-Glaser, Cacioppo, Malarkey, & Glaser, 1992), whose action is believed to be mediated by the autonomic nervous system (ANS) (e.g., Bachen et al., 1995; Benschop et al., 1994). It is notable that a recent study of persons described as "emotional repressors" (Barger, Marsland, Bachen, & Manuck, 2000) showed that, compared to "nonrepressors," the number of circulating natural killer cells was attenuated following an acute stressor, even after possible confounds were controlled for (physical activity, age, smoking).

In the study by Segerstrom, Solomon, and colleagues (1998), natural killer cell count was investigated before and after a naturally occurring stressful event—the 1994 earthquake in Northridge, California. The authors compared those who scored below and above the median on the Penn State Worry Questionnaire (PSWQ; Meyer, Miller, Metzger, & Borkovec, 1990). Natural killer cell count was significantly lower in the high-worry group 11–24 days after the earthquake and 53–67 days after the earthquake compared to baseline. Immediately following the earthquake, high-worry individuals had fewer natural killer cells than expected, and the discrepancy became larger over time. Low-worry participants showed natural killer cell counts consistent with expected values and did not show a decrease until 105–130 days after the earthquake. No differences were found between the groups on cell cytotoxicity, T-cell count, or B-cell count.

In the study by Segerstrom, Glover, and colleagues (1998), immune system functioning following presentation of a phobic stimulus was studied in three groups of subjects: controls, low-worry individuals (below the mean on the PSWQ) who were fearful of either spiders or snakes, and high-worry persons (at least one standard deviation above the mean on the PSWQ) who were fearful of spiders or snakes. The low-worry/fearful group showed an increase in natural killer cell count in peripheral blood, an adaptive response to presentation of the phobic stimulus. The high-worry/fearful group responded much like the nonfearful control group; natural killer cell count was not elevated in response to the stressor, although autonomic indices were similar to those of the low-worry group, indicating autonomic arousal. Thus, in both of these studies, immune system functioning in worried subjects appeared to be dysregulated following a stressor, as indicated by decreased natural killer cell count. These effects await replication in samples of patients with GAD, for whom chronic worry is the prominent symptom.

Although Segerstrom, Glover, and colleagues ' (1998) study suggests that the actions of the immune system and the ANS may be partially independent, many have argued that the release of cytokines is contingent upon certain ANS-driven signals. If this is the case, then it is plausible that ANS dysregulation could be involved in immune system dysfunction in those who chronically worry. Borkovec, Shadick, and Hopkins (1991) have speculated that the profile of ANS activity in GAD seems to deviate from the nonspecific stress response often discussed in the literature. Because increased rates of worry have been associated with autonomic inflexibility and natural killer cell activity is believed to be mediated by the ANS, patients with GAD might be expected to have a dysregulation of the natural killer cell system. However, others have suggested that the immunosuppressive effects of an activated stress response system may be driven by mechanisms other than the ANS, such as the CNS (e.g., Sullivan et al., 1997). Thus it appears that chronic worry may interfere with an adaptive response to an external stressor such as an earthquake or phobic stimulus; however, further studies are needed before the definitive role played by the ANS, CNS, and subsequent effects on the immune system can be strongly argued.

Worry and Coronary Heart Disease

Kubzansky and colleagues (1997) noted that worry can either facilitate problem solving or lead to perceived lack of control and ineffective strategizing. The latter have been linked to cardiovascular illness in general and to coronary heart disease (CHD) in particular (Ewart, 1990), although these effects also depend on personality and situational factors (e.g., Hubbs-Tait & Blodgett, 1989). Kubzansky and colleagues hypothesized that worrying is related to risk of CHD. Participants were interviewed initially in 1975 and were followed for 20 years, with comprehensive interviews about frequency and domains of worry (i.e., social conditions, health, financial, self-definition, aging) and medical examinations completed every 3–5 years. Categories of CHD were nonfatal myocardial infarction (MI), angina pectoris, fatal CHD, total CHD (nonfatal MI plus fatal CHD), combined angina pectoris and total CHD, and sudden cardiac death. Social conditions worry (defined as worry about general world conditions, economic depression, world war, and the future of the world) was associated with nonfatal MI and total CHD, but not with fatal CHD. Health worry was associated with increased risk of angina and sudden cardiac death. Financial worry was associated with increased risk of combined CHD and angina. Multiple comparisons were made without adjusting the error rate; thus some results could have occurred by chance, and all await replication. Furthermore, those with high scores on social conditions worry were also more likely to smoke, to have at least two alcoholic drinks per day, and to report a family history of CHD, as compared to those with low scores. It is unclear whether these variables were controlled for in the analysis. Kubzansky and colleagues did not test interactions between worry and other potentially important variables (e.g., stressful life events) in elucidating CHD risk. However, this study provides one avenue for future investigations into GAD and its consequences.

SUMMARY OF FINDINGS

In summary, the neurobiological profile of GAD probably involves abnormalities in diverse neurotransmitter and neuropeptide systems, including GABA (e.g., Ferrarese et al., 1990; Sacerdote et al., 1999; Weizman et al., 1987), NE (e.g., Garvey et al., 1995; Sevy et al., 1989), 5-HT (e.g., Den Boer, 1990; Germine et al., 1992), CCK (e.g., Brawman-Mintzer et al., 1997), and CRF (e.g., Avery et al., 1985; Schweizer et al., 1986). Many of the studies reviewed herein have indicated that patients with GAD show blunted CNS and PNS activity, especially in response to challenge agents (e.g., Abelson et al., 1991; Cameron et al., 1990; Lyonfields et al., 1995; Thayer et al., 1996). This overall picture suggests general nervous system dysregulation and, in some cases, a disruption of the adaptive stress response. Furthermore, these patients may require a longer period of time to return to baseline after a stressor (e.g., Hoehn-Saric et al., 1989a), suggesting prolonged hyporesponsiveness. Markers of this effect include decreased neurotransmitter activity and sensitivity (e.g., Abelson et al., 1991; Brewerton et al., 1995; Charney et al., 1989; Ferrarese et al., 1990, 1993; Weizman et al., 1987); lower mean venous CO_2 pressure (Munjack et al., 1993); reduced length of the respiratory cycle (Kollai & Kollai, 1992); more dramatic response (but less dramatic than that of patients with panic disorder) to respiratory challenge agents (e.g., Perna et al., 1999), decreased skin conductance, heart rate, EEG, and frontalis EMG (Borkovec & Inz, 1990; Grillon & Buchsbaum, 1987; Hazlett et al., 1994; Hoehn-Saric et al., 1989a; Lyonfields et al., 1995; Thayer et al., 1996); and decreased activity of natural killer cells (Segerstrom, Glover, et al., 1998; Segerstrom, Solomon, et al., 1998), monocytes, and lymphocytes (LaVia et al., 1996) than in nonclinical controls.

No differences among patients with GAD, nonclinical controls, and other patient groups have been found with regard to cerebral metabolism (Harris & Hoehn-Saric, 1995); cerebrospinal levels of CRF (Fossey et al.,

1996); thyrotropin-releasing hormone (Fossey et al., 1993); plasma thyroid hormone (Kelly & Cooper, 1998); catecholaminergic enzymes (e.g., Mathew et al., 1980); and blood pressure, heart rate, or interbeat interval (Hoehn-Saric & Masek, 1981; Hoehn-Saric et al., 1989a) at rest. Therefore, whereas blunting does appear to occur in patients with GAD as compared to other patient groups or nonclinical controls, the effect does not occur across the entire nervous system, and additional mediators of blunting are currently unknown.

Borkovec was the first to suggest that patients with GAD use worrying instrumentally as a strategy for avoiding or suppressing emotion-laden mental imagery (see Borkovec, Alcaine, & Behar, Chapter 4, this volume). Since Borkovec's initial hypothesis, this notion has been repeatedly tested (e.g., Borkovec & Inz, 1990; Borkovec, Lyonfields, Wiser, & Diehl, 1993; Borkovec et al., 1991). Aikens and Craske (2001) suggest that patients with GAD find negative affective states intolerable and use worrying as a strategy to suppress arousal (perhaps brought about by aversive mental images), which subsequently reinforces the use of worry as an emotion regulation strategy. This model views worry in GAD as somewhat akin to a repressive coping style (e.g., Weinberger, Schwartz, & Davidson, 1979), which has also been known to bring about autonomic blunting (e.g., Boden & Dale, 2001).

This model is gaining popularity, due to its ability to explain both symptoms and physiological consequences of GAD; it emphasizes worry and its consequences as the hallmark elements of the disorder. Perhaps this model can inform future biological studies of GAD. For instance, one possible neural circuit for the intentional suppression of emotion has been shown to include right prefrontal areas (superior gyrus, anterior cingulate gyrus; Beauregard, Levesque, & Bourgouin, 2001). However, Noyes and Hoehn-Saric (1998) caution that autonomic blunting is not necessarily characteristic of GAD, but is associated with a range of states—such as partial attention to a stimulus, an anxiety disorder predisposition, or a partial adaptation to chronic stress.

LIMITATIONS AND FUTURE DIRECTIONS

Few investigations of brain structure and function in GAD as compared to other anxiety disorders (e.g., OCD) have been performed. However, the small number of studies that do exist indicate structural differences in pediatric patients; low rates of cerebral metabolism in the basal ganglia and white matter at rest; less alpha decrease during presentation of illuminated stimuli; higher metabolic rates in the cerebellum, thalamus, and occipital, temporal, and frontal lobes during a viewing task; and increased basal ganglia metabolism during a hypervigilance task. It is also possible that abnormalities in the GABA system disrupt the process of habituation to novelty in GAD. These findings should be replicated and extended.

Careful use of diagnostic criteria in GAD is warranted, because we found a lingering assumption that the disorder includes sympathetic arousal and hyperactivity. We also found that few studies of GAD neurobiology or physiology utilize theory as a basis for investigation, and that many studies appeared to be focused too broadly, rather than testing specific hypotheses. Use of any of the excellent animal models of anxiety (e.g., Davis, 1997; LeDoux, 1996) as a basis for future work should result in results that are more interpretable than many reviewed herein, whose implications were unclear in the absence of a relevant theoretical framework.

Many studies of GAD have relied primarily on peripheral measures of biological activity, such as plasma or urinary metabolites. Peripheral measurements should not be considered direct measurements of central neurochemical activity (e.g., Garvey et al., 1995), and results of such studies must be interpreted with caution. Moreover, studies using peripheral measures should implement better controls. For instance, in studies of catecholamine activity, confounds such as exercise and diet must be taken into account in interpreting results. Similarly, studies of vagal tone must control or directly manipulate attentional focus.

Manipulation checks for laboratory stressors are needed to ensure that adequate levels of anxiety are being induced and effectively measured. Few studies have investigated biological activity during periods of induced worry in GAD. None have studied biological aspects of naturalistic worry. Studies of neurobiological consequences of naturalistic worrying in GAD are needed, especially if worrying is used as an emotion regulation strategy. There may be unique characteristics of this strategy that will not be tapped by induced worrying in the laboratory. Furthermore, many of the studies reviewed herein await replication, as activities in neurobiological and physiological systems are strongly influenced by situational and intraindividual factors (e.g., Dimsdale, 1984; Garwood, Engel, & Capriotti, 1982).

The next wave of studies of GAD should seek to fill gaps in the literature, as well as to replicate and extend prior findings. In studies of neurotransmitters and neuromodulators, additional challenge studies are needed, especially for NE. Because there is considerable evidence of reduced binding to GABA receptor sites, studies of central versus peripheral binding would add to our understanding of this characteristic. Additional studies of the role of 5-HT are also needed.

In physiological studies of GAD, indices of GABA-ergic activity, immune system functioning (e.g., natural killer cell count and activity), frequency of illnesses (e.g., the common cold and other upper respiratory infections), and exacerbation of existing disease should be included. It will be important to look more closely at the tendency of patients with GAD to overutilize medical care. Could this be the result of needless worry about health, or is it a legitimate difference caused by immunosuppression in GAD?

Although a number of investigations have probed worry domains, not many have found differential effects of worry themes. However, Kubzansky and colleagues (1997) raise interesting questions about the impact of worry domains on cardiovascular health. This is an important line of inquiry that should be pursued.

Hoehn-Saric, McLeod, and Zimmerli (1989b) argue for subtypes of GAD, perhaps based on affected organ groups; this is an avenue that must be explored further. When they divided a sample of patients with GAD into subgroups with predominant versus few cardiac complaints, the group with high cardiac complaints showed more heart interbeat interval variability following stress. The heterogeneity of the disorder may account for the low interrater reliability ratings for GAD (e.g., Barlow & DiNardo, 1991; Marten et al., 1993) and may confound studies of nervous system activity. Cloninger (1986) has attempted to identify subtypes based on prominent symptomatology (somatic vs. psychic). Borkovec and colleagues (1991) noted that patients with GAD who report cognitive symptoms as most prominent also show the least autonomic reactivity and flexibility in response to stressors. Evidence for differential response to medication was reported by Hoehn-Saric, McLeod, and Zimmerli (1988): Patients with somatic GAD responded to alprazolam, and those with psychic GAD responded to imipramine. Hoehn-Saric, Hazlett, and McLeod (1993) have also investigated early- versus late-onset GAD and concluded that those with the early-onset form were more likely to have a constitutional vulnerability to anxiety and more severe impairment, whereas those with the late-onset form were more likely to report a precipitating event. These possibilities, as well as other possible subtyping schemes, warrant further empirical investigation.

GAD is a disorder that has very high rates of comorbidity with other mood and anxiety disorders (e.g., Bakish, 1999; Ballenger et al., 2001; Brawman-Mintzer et al., 1993) and is sometimes viewed as a vulnerability factor for the development of other psychiatric problems (e.g., Brown, Barlow, & Liebowitz, 1994; Noyes, 2001). Perhaps the neurobiological consequences of chronic worry in GAD contribute to the development of additional disorders. Researchers are beginning to comprehend the mutual influence of psychosocial variables and neurobiology more fully, and collaborative research over the next decade should focus on these important issues specific to GAD.

REFERENCES

Abelson, J. L., Glitz, D., Cameron, O. G., Lee, M. A., Bronzo, M., & Curtis, G. C. (1991). Blunted growth hormone response to clonidine in patients with generalized anxiety disorder. *Archives of General Psychiatry, 48,* 157–162.

Aikens, D. E., & Craske, M. G. (2001). Cognitive theories of generalized anxiety disorder. *Psychiatric Clinics of North America, 24,* 57–74.

Avery, D. H., Osgood, T. B., Ishiki, D. M., Wison, L. G., Kenny, M., & Dunner, D. L. (1985). The DST in psychiatric outpatients with generalized anxiety disorder, panic disorder, or primary affective disorder. *American Journal of Psychiatry, 142,* 844–848.

Bachen, E. A., Manuck, S. B., Cohen, S., Muldoon, M. F., Raible, R., Herbert, T. B., & Rabin, B. S. (1995). Adrenergic blockade ameliorates cellular immune response to mental stress in humans. *Psychosomatic Medicine, 57,* 366–372.

Bakish, D. (1999). The patient with comorbid depression and anxiety: The unmet need. *Journal of Clinical Psychiatry, 60*(Suppl. 6), 20–24.

Ballenger, J. C. (2001). Overview of different pharmacotherapies for attaining remission in generalized anxiety disorder. *Journal of Clinical Psychiatry, 62*(Suppl. 19), 11–19.

Ballenger, J. C., Davidson, J. R., Lecrubier, Y., Nutt, D. J., Borkovec, T. D., Rickels, K., Stein, D. J., & Wittchen, H. U. (2001). Consensus statement on generalized anxiety disorder from the International Consensus Group on Depression and Anxiety. *Journal of Clinical Psychiatry, 62*(Suppl. 11), 53–58.

Barger, S. D., Marsland, A. L., Bachen, E. A., & Manuck, S. B. (2000). Repressive coping and blood measures of disease risk: Lipids and endocrine and immunological responses to a laboratory stressor. *Journal of Applied Social Psychology, 30,* 1619–1638.

Barlow, D. H., & DiNardo, P. A. (1991). The diagnosis of generalized anxiety disorder: Development, current status, and future directions. In R. Rapee & D. H. Barlow (Eds.), *Chronic anxiety: Generalized anxiety disorder and mixed anxiety–depression* (pp. 95–118). New York: Guilford Press.

Beauregard, M., Levesque, J., & Bourgouin, P. (2001). Neural correlates of conscious self-regulation of emotion. *Journal of Neuroscience, 21,* 6993–7000.

Benschop, R. J., Brosschot, J. F., Godaert, G. L. R., deSmet, M. B. M., Geenen, R., Olff, M., Heijnen, C. J., & Ballieux, R. E. (1994). Chronic stress affects immunologic but not cardiovascular responsiveness to acute psychological stress in humans. *American Journal of Physiology, 266,* 75–80.

Best, J. D., & Halter, J. B. (1982). Release and clearance rates of epinephrine in man: Importance of arterial measurements. *Journal of Clinical Endocrinology and Metabolism, 55,* 263–268.

Birket-Smith, M., Hasle, N., & Jensen, H. H. (1993). Electrodermal activity in anxiety disorders. *Acta Psychiatrica Scandinavica, 88,* 350–355.

Boden, J. M., & Dale, K. (2001). Cognitive and affective consequences of repressive coping. *Current Psychology: Developmental, Learning, Personality, Social, 20,* 122–137.

Bodnoff, S. R., Suranyi-Cadotte, B. E., Quirion, R., & Meaney, M. (1989). Role of the central benzodiazepine receptor system in behavioral habituation to novelty. *Behavioral Neuroscience, 103,* 209–212.

Borkovec, T. D., & Inz, J. (1990). The nature of worry in generalized anxiety disorder: A predominance of thought activity. *Behaviour Research and Therapy, 28,* 153–158.

Borkovec, T. D., Lyonfields, J. D., Wiser, S. L., & Diehl, L. (1993). An examination of image and thought processes in generalized anxiety. *Behaviour Research and Therapy, 31,* 321–324.

Borkovec, T. D., Shadick, R. N., & Hopkins, M. (1991). The nature of normal and pathological worry. In R. Rapee & D. H. Barlow (Eds.), *Chronic anxiety: Generalized anxiety disorder and mixed anxiety–depression* (pp. 29–51). New York: Guilford Press.

Bradwejn, J., & Koszcyki, D. (1994). The cholecystokinin hypothesis of panic and anxiety. *Annals of the New York Academy of Sciences, 713,* 273–282.

Brawman-Mintzer, O., Lydiard, R. B., Emmanuel, N., Payeur, R., Johnson, M., Roberts, J., Jarrell, M. P., & Ballenger, J. C. (1993). Rates of psychiatric comorbidity in patients with generalized anxiety disorder. *American Journal of Psychiatry, 150,* 1216–1218.

Brawman-Mintzer, O., Lydiard, R. B., Brandwein, J., Villarreal, G., Knapp, R., Emmanuel, N., Ware, M. R., He, Q., & Ballenger, J. C. (1997). Effects of cholecystokinin agonist pentagastrin in patients with generalized anxiety disorder. *American Journal of Psychiatry, 154,* 700–702.

Brewerton, T., Lydiard, R. B., & Johnson, M. R. (1995, May). *CSF serotonin: Diagnostic and seasonal differences.* Paper presented at the annual meeting of the American Psychiatric Association, Miami, FL.

Brown, T. A., Barlow, D. H., & Liebowitz, M. R. (1994). The empirical basis of generalized anxiety disorder. *American Journal of Psychiatry, 151,* 1272–1280.

Cameron, O. G., Smith, C. B., Lee, M. A., Hollingsworth, P. J., Hill, E. M., & Curtis, G. C. (1990). Adrenergic status in anxiety disorders: Platelet alpha$_2$–adrenergic receptor binding, blood pressure, pulse, and plasma catecholamines in panic and generalized anxiety disorder patients and in normal subjects. *Biological Psychiatry, 28,* 3–20.

Carter, W. R., Johnson, M. C., & Borkovec, T. D. (1986). Worry: An electrocortical analysis. *Advances in Behaviour Research and Therapy, 8,* 193–204.

Charney, D. S., & Deutch, A. (1996). A functional neuroanatomy of anxiety and fear: Implications for the treatment and pathophysiology of anxiety disorders. *Critical Reviews in Neurobiology, 10,* 419–446.

Charney, D. S., Woods, S. W., Goodman, W., & Heninger, G. R. (1987). Serotonin function in anxiety: Effects of the serotonin agonist MCPP in panic disorder patients and healthy subjects. *Psychopharmacology, 92,* 14–24.

Charney, D. S., Woods, S. W., & Heninger, G. R. (1989). Noradrenergic function in generalized anxiety disorder: Effects of yohimbine in healthy subjects and patients with generalized anxiety disorder. *Psychiatry Research, 27,* 173–182.

Cloninger, C. R. (1986). A unified biosocial theory of personality and its role in the development of anxiety states. *Psychiatric Developments, 4,* 167–226.

Cowley, D. S., Dager, S., & McClellan, J. (1988). Response to lactate infusion in GAD. *Biological Psychiatry, 24,* 409–414.

Cowley, D. S., & Roy-Byrne, P. P. (1991). The biology of GAD and chronic anxiety. In R. Rapee & D. H. Barlow (Eds.), *Chronic anxiety: Generalized anxiety disorder and mixed anxiety–depression* (pp. 52–75). New York: Guilford Press.

Cowley, D. S., Roy-Byrne, P. P., Greenblatt, D. J., & Hommer, D. (1993). Personality and benzodiazepine sensitivity in anxious patients and control subjects. *Psychiatry Research, 47,* 151–162.

Craske, M. G., Rapee, R. M., Jackel, L., & Barlow, D. H. (1989). Qualitative dimensions of worry in DSM-III-R generalized anxiety disorder subjects and nonanxious controls. *Behaviour Research and Therapy, 27,* 397–402.

da Roza Davis, J. M., Sharpley, A. L., & Cowen, P. J. (1992). Slow wave sleep and 5HT2 receptor sensitivity in generalized anxiety disorder: A pilot study with ritanserin. *Psychopharmacology, 108,* 387–389.

Davis, M. (1997). Neurobiology of fear responses: The role of the amygdala. *Journal of Neuropsychiatry and Clinical Neuroscience, 9,* 382–402.

DeBellis, M. D., Casey, B. J., Dahl, R. E., Birmaher, B., Williamson, D. E., Thomas, K. M., Axelson, D. A., Frustaci, K., Boring, A., Hall, J., & Ryan, N. D. (2000). A pilot study of amygdala volumes in pediatric generalized anxiety disorder. *Biological Psychiatry, 48,* 51–57.

DeBellis, M. D., Keshavan, M. S., Frustaci, K., Schifflett, H., Iyengar, S., Beers, S. R., & Hall, J. (2002). Superior temporal gyrus volumes in maltreated children and adolescents with PTSD. *Biological Psychiatry, 51,* 544–552.

DeBellis, M. D., Keshavan, M. S., Schifflett, H., Iyengar, S., Dahl, R., Axelson, D. A., Birmaher, B., Hall, J., Moritz, G., & Ryan, N. D. (2002). Superior temporal gyrus volumes in pediatric GAD. *Biological Psychiatry, 51,* 553–562.

Den Boer, J. A. (1990). Serotonin function in panic disorder: A double-blind placebo study with fluvoxamine and ritanserin in patients with panic disorder. *Psychopharmacology, 102,* 85–94.

Dimsdale, J. E. (1984). Generalizing from laboratory studies to field studies of human stress physiology. *Psychosomatic Medicine, 46,* 463–469.

Eison, M. S. (1990). Serotonin: A common neurobiologic substrate in anxiety and depression. *Journal of Clinical Psychopharmacology, 10*(Suppl.), 26–30.

Ewart, C. (1990). A social problem-solving approach to behavior change in coronary heart disease. In S. A. Shumaker, E. B. Schron, J. K. Ockene, & W. McBee (Eds.), *The handbook of health behavior change* (pp. 153–190). New York: Springer.

Ferrarese, C., Appollonio, I., Bianchi, G., Frigo, M., Marzorati, C., Pecora, N., Perego, M., Pierpaoli, C., & Frattola, L. (1993). Benzodiazepine receptors and diazepam binding inhibitor: A possible link between stress, anxiety, and the immune system. *Psychoneuroendocrinology, 18,* 3–22.

Ferrarese, C., Appollonio, I., Frigo, M., Perego, M., Piolti, R., Trabucchi, M., & Frattola, L. (1990). Decreased density of benzodiazepine receptors in lymphocytes of anxious patients: Reversal after chronic diazepam treatment. *Acta Psychiatrica Scandinavica, 82,* 169–173.

Fossey, M. D., Lydiard, R. B., Ballenger, J. C., Laraia, M. T., Bissette, G., & Nemeroff, C. B. (1993). Cerebrospinal fluid thyrotropin-releasing hormone concentrations in patients with anxiety disorders and normal comparison subjects. *Journal of Neuropsychiatry and Clinical Neuroscience, 4,* 335–337.

Fossey, M. D., Lydiard, R. B., Ballenger, J. C., Laraia, M. T., Bissette, G., & Nemeroff, C. B. (1996). Cerebrospinal fluid corticotropin-releasing hormone concentrations in patients with anxiety disorders. *Biological Psychiatry, 39,* 703–707.

Garvey, M. J., Noyes, R., Jr., Woodman, C., & Laukes, C. (1995). Relationship of generalized anxiety symptoms to urinary 5–hydroxyindoleacetic acid and vanillylmandelic acid. *Psychiatry Research, 57,* 1–5.

Garwood, M., Engel, B. T., & Capriotti, R. (1982). Autonomic nervous system function and aging: Response specificity. *Psychophysiology, 19,* 378–385.

Germine, M., Goddard, A. W., Woods, S. W., Charney, D. S., & Heninger, G. R. (1992). Anger and anxiety responses to *m*-chlorophenylpiperazine in generalized anxiety disorder. *Biological Psychiatry, 32,* 457–461.

Gilbert, A. R., Moore, G. J., Keshavan, M. S., Paulson, L. A., Narula, V., & Mac Master,

F. P. (2000). Decrease in thalamic volumes of pediatric patients with obsessive–compulsive disorder who are taking paroxetine. *Archives of General Psychiatry, 57,* 449–456.

Goddard, A. W., & Charney, D. S. (1997). Toward an integrated neurobiology of panic disorder. *Journal of Clinical Psychiatry, 58*(Suppl.), 4–11.

Goddard, A. W., Woods, S. W., Money, R., Pande, A. C., Charney, D. S., Goodman, W. K., Heninger, G. R., & Price, L. H. (1999). Effects of CCKb antagonist CI-988 on responses to mCPP in generalized anxiety disorder. *Psychiatry Research, 85,* 225–240.

Gorman, J. M., Fyer, M., Goetz, R., Askenazi, J., Liebowitz, M. R., Fyer, A. J., Kinney, J., & Klein, D. F. (1988). Ventilatory physiololgy of patients with panic disorder. *Archives of General Psychiatry, 45,* 31–39.

Gorman, J. M., Kent, J. M., Sullivan, G., & Coplan, J. D. (2000). Neuroanatomical hypothesis of panic disorder, revised. *American Journal of Psychiatry, 157,* 493–505.

Graeff, F. (1996). Role of 5–HT in stress, anxiety, and depression. *Pharmacology, Biochemistry, and Behavior, 54,* 129–141.

Gray, J. A., & McNaughton, M. (2000). *The neuropsychology of anxiety* (2nd ed.). Oxford: Oxford University Press.

Grillon, C., & Buchsbaum, M. S. (1987). EEG topography of response to visual stimuli in generalized anxiety disorder. *Electroencephalography and Clinical Neurophysiology, 66,* 337–348.

Hamilton, M. (1960). A rating scale for depression. *Journal of Neurology, 23,* 56–61.

Harris, G. J., & Hoehn-Saric, R. (1995). Functional neuroimaging in biological psychiatry. In J. Panksepp (Ed.), *Advances in biological psychiatry* (pp. 113–160). Greenwich, CT: JAI Press.

Hazlett, R. L., McLeod, D. R., & Hoehn-Saric, R. (1994). Muscle tension in generalized anxiety disorder: Elevated muscle tonus or agitated movement? *Psychophysiology, 31,* 189–195.

Hoehn-Saric, R., Hazlett, R. L., & McLeod, D. R. (1993). Generalized anxiety disorder with early and late onset of symptoms. *Comprehensive Psychiatry, 34,* 291–298.

Hoehn-Saric, R., & Masek, B. (1981). Effects of naloxone on normals and chronically anxious patients. *Biological Psychiatry, 16,* 1041–1050.

Hoehn-Saric, R., McLeod, D. R., Lee, Y. B., & Zimmerli, W. D. (1991). Cortisol levels in generalized anxiety disorder. *Psychiatry Research, 38,* 313–315.

Hoehn-Saric, R., McLeod, D. R., & Zimmerli, W. D. (1988). Differential effects of alprazolam and imipramine in generalized anxiety: Somatic versus psychic symptoms. *American Journal of Psychiatry, 146,* 854–859.

Hoehn-Saric, R., McLeod, D. R., & Zimmerli, W. D. (1989a). Somatic manifestations in women with generalized anxiety disorder. *Archives of General Psychiatry, 46,* 1113–1119.

Hoehn-Saric, R., McLeod, D. R., & Zimmerli, W. D. (1989b). Symptoms and treatment responses of generalized anxiety disorder patients with high versus low levels of cardiovascular complaints. *Journal of Clinical Psychiatry, 49,* 293–301.

Holt, P., & Andrews, G. (1989). Provocation of panic: Three elements of the panic reaction in four anxiety disorders. *Behaviour Research and Therapy, 27,* 253–261.

Hubbs-Tait, L., & Blodgett, C. J. (1989). The mediating effects of self-esteem and coronary-prone behavior on problem solving and affect under low and high stress. *Behavioral Medicine, 15,* 101–110.

Iny, L. J., Pecknold, J., Suranyi-Cadotte, B E., Bernier, B., Luthe, L., Nair, N. P. V., &

Meaney, M. J. (1994). Studies of a neurochemical link between depression, anxiety, and stress. *Biological Psychiatry, 36,* 281–291.

Katon, W., Von Korff, M., Lin, E., Lipscomb, P., Russo, J., Wagner, E., & Polk, E. (1990). Distressed high utilizers of medical care: DSM-III-R diagnoses and treatment needs. *General Hospital Psychiatry, 12,* 355–362.

Katz, I. R., Reynolds, C. F., Alexopoulos, G. S., & Hackett, D. (2002). Venlafaxine ER as a treatment for generalized anxiety disorder in older adults: Pooled analysis of five randomized placebo-controlled clinical trials. *American Journal of Geriatric Psychiatry, 50,* 18–25.

Kelly, C. B., & Cooper, S. J. (1998). Differences in variability in plasma noradrenaline between depressive and anxiety disorders. *Journal of Psychopharmacology, 12,* 161–167.

Kiecolt-Glaser, J. K., Cacioppo, J. T., Malarkey, W. B., & Glaser, R. (1992). Acute psychological stressors and short-term immune changes: What, why, for whom, and to what extent? *Psychosomatic Medicine, 54,* 680–685.

Klein, D. (1993). False suffocation alarms, spontaneous panics and related conditions: An integrative hypothesis. *Archives of General Psychiatry, 50,* 306–317.

Kollai, M., & Kollai, B. (1992). Cardiac vagal tone in generalized anxiety disorder. *British Journal of Psychiatry, 151,* 831–835.

Kubzansky, L. D., Kawachi, I., Spiro, A., Weiss, S. T., Vokonas, P. S., & Sparrow, D. (1997). Is worrying bad for your heart?: A prospective study of worry and coronary heart disease in the Normative Aging Study. *Circulation, 95,* 818–824.

LaVia, M. F., Munno, I., Lydiard, R. B., Workman, E. W., Hubbard, J. R., Michel, Y., & Paulling, E. (1996). The influence of stress intrusion on immunodepression in generalized anxiety disorder patients and controls. *Psychosomatic Medicine, 58,* 138–142.

LaVia, M. F., Workman, E. W., & Lydiard, R. B. (1992). Subtype response to stress-induced immunodepression. *Functional Neurology, 7,* 19–22.

Lauer, C. J., Garcia-Borreguero, D., Pollmacher, T., Ozdaglar, A., & Krieg, J. C. (1990). All-night EEG sleep in anxiety disorders and major depression. In J. Horne (Ed.), *Sleep '90* (pp. 229–231). Basel: Karger.

LeDoux, J. (1996). *The emotional brain.* New York: Simon & Schuster.

LeDoux, J. (1998). Fear and the brain: Where have we been, where are we going? *Biological Psychiatry, 44,* 1229–1238.

Levine, S. (1993). The psychoneuroendocrinology of stress. *Annals of the New York Academy of Sciences, 697,* 61–69.

Lyonfields, J. D., Borkovec, T. D., & Thayer, J. F. (1995). Vagal tone in generalized anxiety disorder and the effects of aversive imagery and worrisome thinking. *Behavior Therapy, 26,* 457–466.

Maier, S. F., & Watkins, L. R. (1998). Cytokines for psychologists: Implications of bidirectional immune-to-brain communication for understanding behavior, mood, and cognition. *Psychological Review, 105,* 2239–2246.

Maier, S. F., & Watkins, L. R. (2000). The immune system as a sensory system: Implications for psychology. *Current Directions in Psychological Science, 9,* 98–102.

Mann, J. J., Brent, D., & Arango, V. (1997). The neurobiology and genetics of suicide and attempted suicide: A focus on the serotonergic system. *Neuropsychopharmacology, 24,* 467–477.

Marten, P. A., Brown, T. A., Barlow, D. H., Borkovec, T. D., Shear, M. K., & Lydiard, R. B. (1993). Evaluation of the ratings comprising the associated symptom criterion of DSM-III-R generalized anxiety disorder. *Journal of Nervous and Mental Disease, 181,* 676–682.

Mathew, R. J., Ho, B. T., Francis, D. J., Taylor, D. L., & Weinman, M. L. (1982). Dopamine-beta-hydroxylase response to epinephrine injection in anxious patients and normals. *Biological Psychiatry, 17,* 393–397.

Mathew, R. J., Ho, B. T., & Kralik, P. (1979). Anxiety and serum prolactin. *American Journal of Psychiatry, 5,* 716–718.

Mathew, R. J., Ho, B. T., Taylor, D. L., & Semchuk, K. M. (1981). Catecholamine and dopamine-ß-hydroxylase in anxiety. *Journal of Psychosomatic Research, 25,* 499–504.

Meoni, P., Salinas, E., Brault, & Hackett, D. (2001). Pattern of symptom improvement following treatment with venlafaxine XR in patients with generalized anxiety disorder. *Journal of Clinical Psychiatry, 62,* 888–893.

Meyer, T. J., Miller, M. L., Metzger, R. L., & Borkovec, T. D. (1990). Development and validation of the Penn State Worry Questionnaire. *Behaviour Research and Therapy, 28,* 487–495.

Munjack, D. J., Baltazar, P. L., DeQuattro, V., Sobin, P., Palmer, R., Zulueta, A., Crocker, B., Uusigli, R., Buckwallter, G., & Leonard, M. (1990). Generalized anxiety disorders: Some biochemical aspects. *Psychiatry Research, 32,* 35–43.

Munjack, D. J., Brown, R. A., & McDowell, D. E. (1993). Existence of hyperventilation in panic disorder with and without agoraphobia, GAD, and normals: Implications for the cognitive theory of panic. *Journal of Anxiety Disorders, 7,* 37–48.

Munjack, D. J., & Palmer, R. (1988). Thyroid hormones in panic disorder, panic disorder with agoraphobia and generalized anxiety disorder. *Journal of Clinical Psychiatry, 6,* 223–229.

Noyes, R. (2001). Comorbidity in generalized anxiety disorder. *Psychiatric Clinics of North America, 24,* 41–55.

Noyes, R., & Hoehn-Saric, R. (1998). *The anxiety disorders.* Cambridge, UK: Cambridge University Press.

Ormel, J., Von Korff, M., Van den Brink, W., Katon, W.. Brilman, E., & Oldehinkel, T. (1993). Depression, anxiety, and social disability show synchrony of change in primary care patients. *American Journal of Public Health, 83,* 385–390.

Papadimitriou, G. N., Linkowski, P., Kerkhofs, M., Kempenaers, C., & Mendlewicz, J. (1988). Sleep EEG recordings in generalized anxiety disorder with significant depression. *Journal of Affective Disorders, 15,* 113–118.

Perna, G., Bussi, R., Allevi, L., & Bellodi, L. (1999). Sensitivity to 35% carbon dioxide in patients with GAD. *Journal of Clinical Psychiatry, 62,* 379–84.

Petrovich, G. D., & Swanson, L. W. (1997). Projections from the lateral part of the central amygdalar nucleus to the postulated fear conditioning circuit. *Brain Research, 763,* 247–254.

Pine, D. S., Klein, R. G., Coplan, J. D., Papp, L. A., Hoven, C. W., Martinez, J., Kovalenko, P., Mandell, D. J., Moreau, D., Klein, D. F., & Gorman, J. M. (2000). Differential carbon dioxide sensitivity in childhood anxiety disorders and nonill comparison group. *Archives of General Psychiatry, 57,* 960–967.

Porges, S. W. (1992). Autonomic regulation and attention. In B. A. Campbell & H. Hayne (Eds.), *Attention and information processing in infants and adults* (pp. 201–223). Hillsdale, NJ: Erlbaum.

Rapee, R. (1986). Differential response to hyperventilation in panic disorder and generalized anxiety disorder. *Journal of Abnormal Psychology, 95,* 24–28.

Reynolds, C., Shaw, D., Newton, T., Coble, P. A., & Kupfer, D. J. (1983). EEG sleep in outpatients with generalized anxiety: A preliminary comparison with depressed outpatients. *Psychiatry Research, 8,* 81–89.

Richards, J. E. (1987). Infant visual sustained attention and respiratory sinus arrythmia. *Child Development, 58,* 488–496.

Rickels, K., & Rynn, M. (2001). Overview and clinical presentation of generalized anxiety disorder. *Psychiatric Clinics of North America, 24,* 19–40.

Rocca, P. (1998). Peripheral benzodiazepine receptor messenger RNA is decreased in lymphocytes of generalized anxiety disorder patients. *Biological Psychiatry, 43,* 767–773.

Rocca, P., Ferrero, P., Gualerzi, A., Zanalda, E., Maina, G., Bergamasco, B., & Ravizza, L. (1991). Peripheral-type benzodiazepine receptors in anxiety disorders. *Acta Psychiatrica Scandinavica, 84,* 537–544.

Rosenbaum, A. H., Schatzberg, A. F., Jost, F. A., Cross, P. D., Wells, L. A., Jiang, N. S., & Maruta, T. (1983). Urinary free cortisol levels in anxiety. *Psychosomatics, 24,* 835–837.

Rosenberg, D. A., Averbach, D. H., O'Hearn, K. M., Seymour, A. B., Birmaher, B., & Sweeney, J. A. (1997). Oculomotor response inhibition abnormalities in pediatric obsessive–compulsive disorder. *Archives of General Psychiatry, 54,* 831–838.

Rosenberg, D. R., MacMaster, F. P., Keshavan, M. S., Fitzgerald, K. D., Stewart, C. M., & Moore, G. J. (2000). Decrease in caudate glutamatergic concentrations in pediatric obsessive-compulsive disorder patients taking paroxetine. *Journal of the American Academy of Child and Adolescent Psychiatry, 39,* 1096–1103.

Roth, W., Wilhelm, F., & Trabert, W. (1998). Voluntary breath holding in panic and GAD. *Psychosomatic Medicine, 60,* 671–679.

Roy-Byrne, P. P., Cowley, D. S., Greenblatt, D. J., Shader, R. I., & Hommer, D. (1990). Reduced benzodiazepine receptor sensitivity in panic disorder. *Archives of General Psychiatry, 47,* 534–538.

Roy-Byrne, P. P., & Katon, W. (1997). Generalized anxiety disorder in primary care: The precursor/modifier pathway to increased health care utilization. *Journal of Clinical Psychiatry, 58,* 34–40.

Sacerdote, P., Paneral, A. E., Frattola, L., & Ferrarese, C. (1999). Benzodiazepine-induced chemotaxis is impaired in monocytes from patients with generalized anxiety disorder. *Psychoneuroendocrinology, 24,* 243–249.

Saletu, B., Anderer, P., Brandstatter, N., Frey, R., Grunberger, J., Klosch, G., Mandl, M., Wetter, T., & Zeithofer, J. (1994). Insomnia in generalized anxiety disorder: Polysomnographic, psychometric, and clinical investigations before, during, and after therapy with a long- versus short-half-life benzodiazepine. *Pharmacopsychiatry, 29,* 69–90.

Saletu, B., Saletu-Zyhlarz, G., Anderer, P., Brandstaetter, N., Frey, R., Gruber, G., Kloesch, G., Mandl, M., Grunberger, J., & Linzmayer, L. (1997). Nonorganic insomnia in generalized anxiety disorder: 2. Comparative studies on sleep, awakening and daytime vigilance and anxiety under lorazepam plus diphenhydramine (Somnium®) versus lorazepam alone, utilizing clinical, polysomnographic and EEG methods. *Neruopsychobiology, 36,* 130–152.

Saletu-Zyhlarz, G., Saletu, B., Anderer, P., Brandstaetter, N., Frey, R., Gruber, G., Kloesch, G., Mandl, M., Gruenberger, J., & Linzmayer, L. (1997). Nonorganic insomnia in generalized anxiety disorder: 1. Controlled studies on sleep, awakening and daytime vigilance utilizing polysomnography and EEG mapping. *Neuropsychobiology, 36,* 117–129.

Schneider, L. S., Munjack, D., Severson, J. A., & Palmer, R. (1987). Platelet (-3H)imipramine binding in generalized anxiety disorder, panic disorder, and agoraphobia with panic attacks. *Biological Psychiatry, 22,* 59–66.

Schweizer, E. E., Swenson, D. M., Winokur, A., Rickels, K., & Maislin, G. (1986). The dexamethasone suppression test in generalized anxiety disorder. *British Journal of Psychiatry, 149,* 320–322.

Segerstrom, S. C., Glover, D. G., Craske, M. G., & Fahey, J. L. (1998). Worry affects the immune response to phobic fear. *Brain, Behavior, and Immunity, 13,* 80–92.

Segerstrom, S. C., Solomon, G. F., Kemeny, M. E., & Fahey, J. L. (1998). Relationship of worry to immune sequelae of the Northridge earthquake. *Journal of Behavioral Medicine, 21,* 433–450.

Sevy, S., Papadimitriou, G. N., Surmont, D. W., Goldman, S., & Mendlewicz, J. (1989). Noradrenergic function in generalized anxiety disorder, major depressive disorder, and healthy subjects. *Biological Psychiatry, 25,* 141–152.

Sinha, S., Kent, J., & Gorman, J. M. (1999). Pharmacotherapy of panic disorder. In *Psychopharmacology: The fourth generation of progress* [CD-ROM]. Nashville, TN: American College of Neuropsychopharmacology.

Sinha, S., Papp, L. A., & Gorman, J. M. (2000). How respiratory physiology helped our understanding of panic disorder. *Journal of Affective Disorders, 16,* 191–200.

Sullivan, G. M., Canfield, S. M., Lederman, S., Xiao, E., Ferin, M., & Wardlaw, S. L. (1997). Intracerebroventricular injection of interleukin-1 suppresses peripheral lymphocyte function in the primate. *Neuroimmunomodulation, 4,* 12–18.

Sullivan, G. M., Coplan, J. D., Kent, J. M., & Gorman, J. M. (1999). The noradrenergic system in pathological anxiety: A focus on panic with relevance to generalized anxiety and phobias. *Biological Psychiatry, 46,* 1205–1218.

Thayer, J. F., Friedman, B. H., & Borkovec, T. D. (1996). Autonomic characteristics of generalized anxiety disorder and worry. *Biological Psychiatry, 39,* 255–266.

Tiihonen, J., Kuikka, J., & Rasanen, P. (1997). Cerebral benzodiazepine receptor binding and distribution in GAD: A fractal analysis. *Molecular Psychiatry, 2,* 463–471.

Tiller, J. W., Biddle, N., Maguire, K. P., & Davies, B. M. (1988). The dexamethasone suppression test and plasma dexamethasone in generalized anxiety disorder. *Biological Psychiatry, 23,* 261–270.

Turan, T., Esel, E., Karaasian, F., Basturk, M., Oguz, A., & Yabanoglu, I. (2002). Auditory event-related potentials in panic and generalized anxiety disorders. *Progress in Neuropsychopharmacology and Biological Psychiatry, 26,* 123–126.

Tye, N. C., Iversen, S D., & Green, A. R. (1979). The effects of benzodiazepines and serotonergic manipulations on punished responding. *Neuropharmacology, 18,* 689–695.

Van der Maelen, C. P., Matheson, G. K., Wilderman, R. C., & Patterson, L. A. (1986). Inhibition of serotonergic dorsal raphine neurons by systemic and iontophoretic administration of buspirone, a non-benzodiazepine anxiolytic drug. *European Journal of Pharmacology, 129,* 123–130.

Verburg, K., Griez, E., & Meijer, J. (1995). Discrimination between panic disorder and GAD by 35% CO_2 challenge. *American Journal of Psychiatry, 152,* 1081–1083.

Weizman, R., Tanne, Z., & Granek, M. (1987). Peripheral benzodiazepine binding sites on platelet membranes are increased during diazepam treatment of anxious patients. *European Journal of Pharmacology, 138,* 289–292.

Weinberger, D. A., Schwartz, G. E., & Davidson, R J. (1979). Low-anxious, high-anxious, and repressive coping styles: Psychometric patterns and behavioral and physiological response to stress. *Journal of Abnormal Psychology, 88,* 369–380.

Wilhelm, F. H., Trabert, W., & Roth, W. T. (2001). Physiological instability in panic disorder and generalized anxiety disorder. *Biological Psychiatry, 49,* 596–605.

Wilson, W. H., & Mathew, R. J. (1993). Cerebral blood flow and metabolism in anxiety disorders. In R. Hoehn-Saric & D. R. McLeod (Eds.), *Biology of anxiety disorders* (pp. 1–59). Washington DC: American Psychiatric Press.

Wu, J. C., Buchsbaum, M. S., Hershey, T. G., Hazlett, E., Sicotte, N., & Johnson, J. C. (1991). PET in generalized anxiety disorder. *Biological Psychiatry, 29,* 1181–1189.

Young, E. A., Haskett, R. F., Grunhaus, L., Pande, A., Weinberg, V. M., & Akil, H. (1994) Increased evening activation of the HPA axis in depressed patients. *Archives of General Psychiatry, 51,* 701–707.

PART III
Assessment and Treatment

CHAPTER 9

Assessment

CYNTHIA L. TURK
RICHARD G. HEIMBERG
DOUGLAS S. MENNIN

As we have discussed in Chapter 1 of this volume, when generalized anxiety disorder (GAD) was introduced into the third edition of the *Diagnostic and Statistical Manual of Mental Disorders* (DSM-III; American Psychiatric Association [APA], 1980), it was a residual category that could not be diagnosed in the presence of any other anxiety or affective disorder. Subsequent changes in the diagnostic criteria made it difficult to maintain a consistent focus in the development of theoretical models of the disorder. Advances in the assessment of GAD also lagged as a result. Early attempts to diagnose GAD according to DSM-III criteria were characterized by low interrater reliability (Barlow, 1987), and only relatively limited, nonspecific tools were available to assess symptom severity and treatment response. Fortunately, in recent years, instruments have emerged that are based upon theoretical models of GAD and that specifically target its essential feature, worry.

Our review of the assessment literature focuses on diagnostic instruments, self-report and clinician-administered measures, and instruments that address constructs theoretically relevant to GAD. We also propose several domains that we believe are worthwhile to assess for individuals with GAD (e.g., depression, quality of life). Studies employing cognitive and psychophysiological methodologies in the assessment of GAD have greatly improved our understanding of this disorder. However, due to space limitations, assessment of these domains is not reviewed. This review is also limited to adults (see Albano & Hack, Chapter 15, and Beck &

Averill, Chapter 16, this volume, for reviews of the assessment of children and adolescents and of older adults, respectively).

DIAGNOSTIC MEASURES

Anxiety Disorders Interview Schedule

The Anxiety Disorders Interview Schedule for DSM-IV (ADIS-IV; Brown, DiNardo, & Barlow, 1994) and the ADIS-IV Lifetime Version (ADIS-IV-L; DiNardo, Brown, & Barlow, 1994) provide a thorough diagnostic assessment of the anxiety disorders. They also include modules for mood disorders, substance abuse and dependence, and other disorders that overlap with anxiety disorders either conceptually or in terms of presenting symptoms (e.g., hypochondriasis). In addition, there are screening questions for other major disorders (e.g., psychosis). For each disorder, a 0–8 clinical severity rating (CSR) is assigned to index the degree of distress and interference associated with that diagnosis. Disorders receiving a CSR of 4 or higher qualify as "official" DSM-IV diagnoses. When multiple disorders receive a CSR of 4 or higher, the disorder receiving the highest CSR is designated as the "principal" diagnosis, and the other disorders are designated as "additional."

In a major reliability study of the ADIS-IV-L, 362 individuals seeking treatment at an anxiety specialty clinic received two independent administrations by highly trained interviewers (Brown, DiNardo, Lehman, & Campbell, 2001). Seventy-six individuals received a principal diagnosis of GAD, and 113 received either a principal or an additional diagnosis of GAD according to both interviewers. GAD evidenced good reliability when examined as a principal diagnosis (kappa = .67) or as clinical diagnosis (kappa = .65).

Brown and colleagues (2001) examined sources of unreliability for all current diagnoses of DSM-IV GAD. In 35 of 47 (74%) cases, one interviewer assigned a diagnosis of GAD, while the other diagnosed another disorder with overlapping features. Of the disagreements involving another disorder, 22 of 35 (63%) involved a mood disorder. Another 10 of 35 (29%) involved anxiety disorder not otherwise specified (i.e., one interviewer judged that many but not all of the diagnostic criteria for GAD had been met). Interestingly, no disagreement involved obsessive–compulsive disorder, despite the similarity of worry and obsessions as unwanted, distressing cognitive activities. Furthermore, for 26 of 47 (55%) disagreements on the diagnosis of GAD, difference in patient report between the two interviews contributed to the unreliability. In future editions of the DSM, refinement of the GAD diagnostic criteria to improve differentiation from mood disorders and to increase patients' ability to consistently report on the subjective features of GAD may further improve reliability (Brown et al., 2001).

Key and associated features of disorders are assessed dimensionally by the ADIS-IV(-L), based on the assumption that symptoms exist on a continuum of severity, rather than simply being present or absent. For GAD, excessiveness and uncontrollability are assessed on 9-point scales for eight domains of worry (e.g., minor matters, health, finances). Good interrater reliability was found for composite scores for excessiveness of worry (r = .73), uncontrollability of worry (r = .78), and the associated symptoms of somatic tension and negative affect (r = .83). The CSR for GAD (r = .72) also evidenced good interrater reliability.

Overall, the ADIS-IV-L demonstrates good reliability for the diagnosis of GAD, good reliability for the features of GAD, and good to excellent reliability for the diagnosis of the other anxiety disorders (Brown et al., 2001). Its use of dimensional ratings for the clinical severity of disorders and their associated features increases its clinical and research utility, relative to other commonly used structured interviews. Lastly, its modular format makes it easy to administer only those sections of interest.

Structured Clinical Interview for DSM

The Structured Clinical Interview for DSM for Axis I disorders (Patient Edition) has been updated to conform to the DSM-IV-TR (APA, 2000) descriptions (SCID-I/P; First, Spitzer, Gibbon, & Williams, 2001). The SCID-I/P begins with an overview of education, work history, and present illness; this is followed by modules for the major diagnostic categories, including anxiety disorders, mood disorders, psychotic disorders, substance use disorders, somatoform disorders, eating disorders, and adjustment disorders. Its modular format makes it easy to administer only those sections of interest. Unlike the ADIS-IV and ADIS-IV(-L), the SCID-I/P does not provide dimensional severity ratings for diagnoses or symptoms, but it assesses a broader range of disorders.

In a mixed sample of 390 psychiatric patients from six sites, the reliability of the SCID for DSM-III-R (Spitzer et al., 1988) was calculated based on two independent interviews (Williams et al., 1992). Kappa was .56 for a current diagnosis of DSM-III-R (APA, 1987) GAD.

In a study using the DSM-IV version of the SCID, interrater reliability was determined using 27 videotapes of client interviews from the Collaborative Longitudinal Personality Disorder Study and 84 rater pairs (Zanarini et al., 2000). This procedure produced a median kappa of .63 for the diagnosis of GAD. Test–retest reliability was calculated based on two direct interviews of 52 patients from the same study. With this approach, the median kappa was .44 for the diagnosis of GAD.

In summary, more research is needed regarding the interrater reliability of the SCID-I/P, as no large-scale study has yet been conducted for this most recent version of the instrument. However, its coverage of a broad range of disorders may make it an attractive choice for some investigators.

Mini International Neuropsychiatric Interview

The Mini International Neuropsychiatric Interview for DSM-IV, English Version 5.0.0 (MINI; Sheehan & Lecrubier, 2002) is a diagnostic interview that uses a modular format to assess for the presence of mood disorders, anxiety disorders, substance abuse/dependence, eating disorders, and psychotic disorders. With the goal of minimizing the duration of the interview, the interviewer instructs patients that they will be asked very precise questions about psychological problems that require yes or no answers. With a mean interview duration of 21 minutes (SD = 7.7) in one study (Lecrubier et al., 1997) and of 18.7 minutes (SD = 11.6) in another (Sheehan et al., 1997), the MINI is briefer than most other diagnostic interviews.

In a study using the Composite International Diagnostic Interview (CIDI) as the gold standard for DSM-III-R diagnoses, the MINI was found to have poor agreement for the diagnosis of GAD (kappa = .36), with the MINI yielding a high number of false positives (Lecrubier et al., 1997). In another study using the SCID as the gold standard for DSM-III-R diagnoses, the MINI was found to have good agreement for the diagnosis of GAD (kappa = .70) (Sheehan et al., 1997). A limitation of both these studies is that the same interviewer administered both the MINI and the gold standard interview. Test–retest reliability calculated based on MINIs conducted 1–2 days apart by different interviewers indicated good agreement for the diagnosis of GAD (.78)(Sheehan et al., 1997).

The structure and wording of the GAD section have been changed since the versions of the MINI administered in the studies reviewed above. Additional research is needed to evaluate the adequacy of the current MINI as a diagnostic tool appropriate for the assessment of GAD.

Generalized Anxiety Disorder Questionnaire

The original Generalized Anxiety Disorder Questionnaire (GADQ; Roemer, Borkovec, Posa, & Borkovec, 1995) was a self-report measure assessing DSM-III-R criteria for GAD. It was productively used in multiple studies to create analogue samples with and without GAD, in order to study constructs of interest to theoretical models of GAD (e.g., Lyonfields, Borkovec, & Thayer, 1995). The GADQ has recently been revised so that it is now consistent with DSM-IV criteria (GADQ-IV; Newman et al.,

2002). The GADQ-IV consists of nine items. Most items are dichotomous and measure the excessiveness and uncontrollability of worry (e.g., "Do you experience excessive worry?") and severity of related physical symptoms (e.g., muscle tension). One item is open-ended and asks for a list of the most frequent worry topics. Two items are rated on a scale of 0 ("none") to 8 ("very severe") and measure functional impairment and subjective distress, respectively. Thus all DSM-IV criteria for GAD are assessed, with the exception of the exclusion criteria (criteria D and F; APA, 1994). The GADQ was scored by relating the items to DSM-III-R criteria, so that individuals endorsing all but one critical item (e.g., excessiveness of worry) did not receive a diagnosis. In contrast, the authors of the GADQ-IV recommend using a total score rather than matching item responses to specific DSM-IV criteria (Newman et al., 2002). Cutoff scores are then used to determine presence or absence of GAD. Thus an individual may fail to endorse an GADQ-IV item required by DSM-IV (e.g., excessive worry more days than not during the past 6 months), but will still receive a diagnosis of GAD according to the new GADQ-IV scoring system.

In a preliminary examination of the reliability and validity of the GADQ-IV, three studies were conducted (Newman et al., 2002). In Study 1, 143 undergraduate students completed the GADQ-IV. A trained interviewer administered the ADIS-IV or ADIS-IV-L at least 10 days later. A receiver operating characteristic analysis was used to compare GADQ-IV dimensional scores to ADIS-IV diagnosis. A cutoff score of 5.7 was identified as achieving the optimal balance between sensitivity and specificity. With this cutoff score, 25 of 30 cases of GAD were correctly identified (83% sensitivity), and 101 of 113 cases without GAD were correctly classified (89% specificity). The kappa between the ADIS-IV and the GADQ-IV was .67, with 88% of participants correctly classified. In Study 2, the GADQ-IV was more highly correlated ($r = .66$) with the Penn State Worry Questionnaire (PSWQ; Meyer, Miller, Metzger, & Borkovec, 1990) than with the PTSD Checklist (Weathers, Huska, & Keane, 1991) ($r = .45$) or the Social Interaction Anxiety Scale (Mattick & Clarke, 1998) ($r = .34$) among a sample of 391 undergraduates. In Study 3, 148 undergraduates completed the GADQ-IV during sessions 2 weeks apart. Kappa was .64, with 136 of 148 cases (92%) showing stability across time for their categorization.

In another study, 31 treatment-seeking individuals with a primary diagnosis of GAD and 53 nonanxious community participants were assessed with the GADQ-IV and the ADIS-IV-L (Luterek, Turk, Heimberg, Fresco, & Mennin, 2002). The GADQ-IV was internally consistent (alpha = .93). Of the nonanxious community participants, 50 of 53 (94.3%) were correctly classified as not having a diagnosis of GAD with the current dimensional scoring system. All participants with GAD according to the ADIS-IV-L were correctly classified as having GAD by the GADQ-IV.

Within the entire sample, the GADQ-IV total score was highly correlated with the PSWQ ($r = .92$) and the Worry Domains Questionnaire (WDQ; Tallis, Eysenck, & Mathews, 1992) ($r = .74$). The GADQ-IV was more highly correlated with the PSWQ and the WDQ than a measure of fear of observation by others.

Some recent data raise questions regarding the validity of using the dimensional scoring system to identify cases of GAD in populations different from the population used to derive the original cutoff score of 5.7. In the predominantly European American sample of undergraduates used in the original validation study of the GADQ-IV (Newman et al., 2002), a relatively small percentage of students (14%) was identified by the GADQ-IV as having GAD. However, in another study using an ethnically diverse sample of women, a cutoff score of 5.7 resulted in 32% of the sample being classified as positive for GAD (Roemer, Salters, Raffa, & Orsillo, in press). Similarly, among an ethnically diverse sample of 766 undergraduates from an urban college, a cutoff score of 5.7 resulted in 33% of individuals being classified as positive for GAD (Turk, Heimberg, Luterek, Mennin, & Fresco, in press). In this study, matching item responses to specific DSM-IV criteria, as was done for the original version of the scale, resulted in a more modest 14.5% of the sample being classified as positive for GAD. The discrepancy between the two scoring systems was due to the fact that the cutoff score of 5.7 identified 146 more cases of GAD than the criteria-based scoring system. The criteria-based scoring system did not classify any participant as having GAD that the cutoff score system did not. Importantly, in these studies, GADQ-IV diagnoses were not compared against structured clinical interview.

In summary, the GADQ-IV is a quick and easy way to screen for GAD. It will prove to be a valuable tool for creating analogue samples for research (e.g., Mennin, Turk, Fresco, & Heimberg, 2003). Future research should address the validity of the GADQ-IV dimensional scoring method versus the original categorical scoring method, and should also assess the sensitivity of the GADQ-IV as a measure of treatment outcome.

ASSESSMENT OF WORRY

Penn State Worry Questionnaire

The PSWQ (Meyer et al., 1990) assesses the extent to which worry is excessive, uncontrollable, and pervasive (e.g., "I know I should not worry about things, but I just cannot help it"). The PSWQ was developed to assess clinically significant worry without focusing on particular domains of worry. It contains 16 items rated on a 5-point scale (1 = "not at all typical of me," 5 = "very typical of me"). Five items inquire about the absence of worry and are reverse-scored. A weekly version has been developed for use during treatment (Stöber & Bittencourt, 1998).

The PSWQ has been shown to have good internal consistency not only for individuals with a primary DSM-III-R diagnosis of GAD (alpha = .86), but also for patients with primary DSM-III-R diagnoses of social phobia (alpha = .94), simple phobia (alpha = .95), obsessive–compulsive disorder (alpha = .94), panic disorder (alpha = .93), and panic disorder with agoraphobia (alpha = .91) (Brown, Antony, & Barlow, 1992). Good internal consistency has also been demonstrated for community controls (alpha = .90; Brown et al., 1992) and undergraduates (alphas = .91–.95 across five different samples; Meyer et al., 1990). Among college students, the PSWQ has also demonstrated good test–retest reliability over periods as long as 8–10 weeks (Study 3, r = .92; Meyer et al., 1990).

The PSWQ has demonstrated significant positive correlations with other self-report measures of worry (Davey, 1993; van Rijsoort, Emmelkamp, & Vervaeke, 1999). When the PSWQ was used to define groups high, medium, and low in worry, the high-worry group generated more worrisome topics during an interview and reported spending more time worrying during the preceding week (Meyer et al., 1990). The PSWQ has also been shown to be related to other constructs theoretically related to worry, such as perfectionism (Meyer et al., 1990) and intolerance of uncertainty (Freeston, Rhéaume, Letarte, Dugas, & Ladouceur, 1994). Stöber (1998) asked participants to complete the PSWQ and have three peers make ratings with the PSWQ regarding the target individual (e.g., "He/she is always worrying about something"). Self-ratings and aggregate peer ratings were significantly correlated (r = .55).

The findings regarding the relationship of the PSWQ to measures of anxiety and depression have varied, depending upon the nature of the sample under study. Among undergraduate and community samples, moderate correlations between the PSWQ and measures of anxiety and depressive symptoms have been observed. We (Fresco, Heimberg, Mennin, & Turk, 2002) found that the PSWQ correlated significantly with several subscales of the Mood and Anxiety Symptom Questionnaire (Watson & Clark, 1991): Anxious Arousal (r = .27), General Distress–Anxiety (r = .43), Anhedonic Depression (r = .39), and General Distress–Depression (r = .50). The PSWQ has also demonstrated significant correlations with the Trait Anxiety version of the State–Trait Anxiety Inventory (STAI; Spielberger, Gorsuch, Lushene, Vagg, & Jacobs, 1983) in college student (r's = .64–.74; Davey, 1993; Meyer et al., 1990) and community (r = .75; van Rijsoort et al., 1999) samples, and with the Beck Depression Inventory (BDI; Beck, Rush, Shaw, & Emery, 1979) in undergraduate (r's = .36–.45; Fresco et al., 2002; Meyer et al., 1990) and community (r = .62; van Rijsoort et al., 1999) samples.

Interestingly, within samples consisting exclusively of individuals with GAD, the correlations between the PSWQ and measures of anxiety and depression are attenuated. In a sample of 55 patients with GAD, Molina and Borkovec (1994) found that the PSWQ was moderately associated with the STAI Trait Anxiety version ($r = .44$), but bore little relationship to the Zung (1971) Self-Rating Anxiety Scale, the Hamilton (1959) Anxiety Rating Scale (HARS), the Hamilton (1960) Rating Scale for Depression (HSRD), or the BDI. In contrast, 7 of 10 correlations among these symptom measures were significant. Similarly, among the 50 patients with a primary diagnosis of GAD in the Brown and colleagues (1992) study, the PSWQ was not significantly related to the HARS, the HRSD, or Lovibond's (1983) Self-Analysis Questionnaire Anxiety and Depression subscales.

Individuals with a primary diagnosis of GAD scored higher on the PSWQ than nonclinical controls and individuals with another anxiety disorder (Brown et al., 1992). Based on the results of a receiver operating characteristic analysis, we (Fresco, Mennin, Heimberg, & Turk, 2003) have recommended a PSWQ cutoff score of 53 to maximize both sensitivity and specificity in identifying individuals with GAD relative to community persons with no Axis I diagnosis. A PSWQ cutoff score of 65 has been recommended to maximize both sensitivity and specificity in identifying individuals with GAD relative to individuals with a diagnosis of social anxiety disorder. However, in one study, the PSWQ failed to discriminate between patients with a primary diagnosis of GAD and patients with a primary diagnosis of major depression (Starcevic, 1995).

Three studies have used exploratory factor analysis to examine whether the PSWQ represents a unidimensional construct. Brown and colleagues (1992) reported a unifactorial solution based on the responses of 436 patients with anxiety disorders. van Rijsoort and colleagues (1999) also retained a unifactorial solution based on the responses of 161 Dutch citizens. Stöber (1995), however, chose to retain a two-factor solution based on the responses of 224 German college students and community members. One factor assessed the tendency to worry, and the other assessed absence of worry.

We (Fresco et al., 2002) administered the PSWQ to 788 undergraduates. Confirmatory factor analyses indicated that a two-factor model, with one factor consisting of the 11 positively worded items (Worry Engagement) and one factor consisting of the five reverse-scored items (Absence of Worry), provided a better fit to the data than a unifactorial model. There was also evidence for a higher-order General Worry Factor. Examination of the association of the lower-order factors and the higher-order factor with measures of depression and anxiety symptoms indicated that the lower-order factor of Worry Engagement made the largest unique contribution to the prediction of symptom measures. Worry Engagement (alpha = .94) was considerably more internally consistent than Absence of Worry (alpha = .70) and slightly more internally consistent than the PSWQ total score (alpha = .90). We concluded that using an 11-item Worry Engagement scale would probably be no worse than and possibly superior to using the 16-item PSWQ total score to measure the component of worry most highly associated with anxiety and depression.

More recently, Brown (in press) conducted confirmatory factor analyses of the PSWQ with 1,200 outpatients seeking treatment at a clinic for anxiety and related disorders. Brown criticized the two-factor model accepted by Fresco and colleagues (2002), suggesting that the Absence of Worry factor lacked substantive meaning and pointing out that error theory, which reflects method effects from the negatively worded items, was not taken into account. Brown replicated that Fresco and colleagues' model provided a good fit to the data but noted that the two factors were highly correlated, suggesting poor discriminant validity. Brown then demonstrated that a one-factor model, which took method effects into account, provided a fit that was superior to the two-factor model. Based on these findings, he concluded that the covariances among the items on the PSWQ are best explained by a single underlying construct. Brown noted, however, that since most studies will not take the complex error structure of the PSWQ into account, it may be justifiable to use the five reverse-worded items to assess potential response bias, but then not include them in the final scoring of the scale. This approach, however, needs further evaluation.

The PSWQ appears to be sensitive to change in response to therapeutic interventions. For example, Borkovec and Costello (1993) compared the efficacy of a cognitive-behavioral treatment package, applied relaxation, and a nondirective control therapy in the treatment of GAD. Significant pretreatment-to-posttreatment decreases were observed on the PSWQ for the groups receiving cognitive-behavioral treatment and applied relaxation, but not for the group receiving the nondirective control therapy.

In summary, the PSWQ has good psychometric properties and sensitivity to treatment change. It is a good choice for research and clinical studies with a goal of assessing the intensity of pathological worry.

Worry Domains Questionnaire

The WDQ (Tallis et al., 1992) provides a global total score, which indicates how much an individual worries in general, and five domain scores, which reflect amount of worry in specific content areas. The WDQ is intended to measure worry as it occurs among adults with no psychological disorder. The five domains assessed by the WDQ are (1) Relationships (e.g., "I worry that I am not loved"), (2) Lack of Confidence (e.g., "I worry that I feel insecure"), (3) Aimless Future (e.g., "I worry that I'll never achieve my ambitions"), (4) Work Incompetence (e.g., "I worry that I make mistakes at work"), and (5) Financial (e.g., "I worry that my money will run out"). For each of the 25 items (5 items per domain), participants indicate how much they worry on a 5-point scale (0 = "not at all," 4 = "extremely"). Stöber and Joormann (2001a) have created a 10-item short form of the WDQ (WDQ-SF), which is highly correlated with the original ($r = .97$).

The WDQ appears to be a reliable measure. The total score has demonstrated good internal consistency with a sample of 136 college students (alpha = .92; Davey, 1993). Similar results were obtained with a sample of 224 German college students and community members (alpha = .91), although the five subscales were somewhat less internally consistent (alphas = .75–.86) than the total score (Stöber, 1995). Joormann and Stöber (1997) found similar results with two additional large samples. Tallis, Davey, and Bond (1994) reported test–retest correlations of $r = .79$ for the total score and r's = .46–.86 for the subscale scores with a sample of 16 individuals assessed over an interval of 2–4 weeks. Stöber (1998) reported test–retest correlations of $r = .85$ for the total score and r's = .71–.86 for the subscale scores with a larger sample of 148 German college students assessed twice over 4 weeks.

The WDQ correlates highly with other measures of worry. It has been shown to be highly correlated with the PSWQ in several studies (r's = .62–.68; Davey, 1993; Stöber, 1998; Stöber & Joormann, 2001b). It has also demonstrated significant correlations with the Student Worry Scale ($r = .68$; Davey, Hampton, Farrell, & Davidson, 1992), which assesses worry about 10 areas relevant to college students (Davey, 1993). The WDQ domains of Relationships, Lack of Confidence, and Aimless Future are highly intercorrelated (r's = .71–.79) and are less strongly correlated with the Work Incompetence (r's = .42–.72) and Financial (r's = .22–.44) domains (Joormann & Stöber, 1997). Stöber (1995) found a similar pattern of subscale intercorrelations.

To further examine the validity of the WDQ, Stöber (1998) asked participants to complete the WDQ and have three friends make WDQ ratings from an observer's perspective (e.g., "The target person worries that he/she will lose close friends"). The correlations between self-ratings and aggregate peer ratings were $r = .49$ for the total score and r's = .32–.53 for the subscale scores. All correlations were significant.

In another study relevant to the validity of the WDQ, Dugas, Freeston, Doucet, Lachance, and Ladouceur (1995) asked 154 university students to list their worries as part of a modified French translation of the GADQ and then to complete the WDQ. WDQ items and free-response items were then classified using the Categorization Grid for Worries (Lachance, Doucet, Freeston, & Ladouceur, 1993), which consisted of 18 worry themes. A rank-ordering of worry themes was created for the WDQ by using the mean of item scores for each theme, and for the free-response measure by using the proportion of participants reporting each theme. A significant correlation was found between ranks of worry themes on the WDQ and the free-response measure (tau = .61). For both measures, worries about finances and work were ranked first and second, respectively. However, some worry themes captured by the free-response measure were not represented on the WDQ.

Although the PSWQ and WDQ have been found to be correlated in several studies, the measures do not appear to tap identical aspects of the worry process. Davey (1994) has proposed that worry can be conceptualized as existing along a continuum from the nonpathological worry experienced by individuals with no psychological disorder to the pathological worry experienced by individuals with GAD. Davey (1993) has also suggested that nonpathological worry has adaptive aspects, such as facilitating constructive problem solving. Davey proposed that a content-based measure of everyday worries such as the WDQ should tap into the problem-focused, constructive features of worry, while a measure of clinical worry, such as the PSWQ should not. Partial-correlation analyses in which the PSWQ was correlated with measures of coping while holding trait anxiety constant revealed no significant findings. However, the same partial-correlation analyses with the WDQ revealed a significant correlation with a measure of active cognitive coping ($r = .26$). Thus the WDQ appears to capture some positive aspects of the worry process that the PSWQ does not.

Preliminary evidence suggests that the WDQ, unlike the PSWQ, may be sensitive to ethnic differences in worry (Scott, Eng, & Heimberg, 2002). Within a large unselected sample of college students, differences were observed among African Americans, European Americans, and Asian Americans for the total score and all WDQ subscales except for the Financial domain. African Americans endorsed less worry than European Americans and Asian Americans for the total score and on the Relationships, Lack of Confidence, and Work Incompetence subscales. For the aimless future domain, Asian Americans scored significantly higher than European Americans, who in turn scored higher than African Americans. Within ethnic groups, European Americans and African Americans experienced variations in intensity of worry across the specific domains, but Asian Americans did not.

Joormann and Stöber (1997) conducted a confirmatory factor analysis on the responses of 466 individuals completing the WDQ. Consistent with the original configuration of the scale, a model consisting of five intercorrelated yet distinct factors provided the best fit for the data. These findings were cross-validated with a second sample consisting of 503 participants.

Using a multiple-group method of confirmatory factor analysis on the WDQ responses obtained from 161 individuals from the community, van Rijsoort and colleagues (1999) found that some items had their highest loadings on a component that did not correspond to the domain to which that item was assigned. In addition, van Rijsoort and colleagues (1999) sought to expand the domains assessed by the WDQ and added five items addressing worry about health. After reassignment of items to the component on which they loaded most highly, a revised version of the WDQ (WDQ-R) was created that consists of the original five domains plus health worry as a sixth domain. Internal consistency for the total score (alpha = .94) and all subscales (alphas = .85–.88), except for the three-item Work Incompetence domain (alpha = .64), were good for this new scale.

In the nonclinical adult population for which it was developed, the WDQ appears to be a reliable and valid measure. In addition, it seems to capture aspects of the nonpathological worry process that the PSWQ does not. Therefore, the WDQ is well suited for use in research with nonclinical populations, as was intended by the measure's authors (Tallis et al., 1994). The authors also suggest that the WDQ may have utility as a supplemental clinical instrument (e.g., administered in conjunction with the PSWQ) as a means of providing a worry profile to identify important areas for intervention. Unfortunately, few data are available regarding the reliability and validity of the WDQ in clinical populations. In one study, patients with GAD and college students meeting criteria for GAD scored significantly higher on the WDQ than college students without GAD did (Ladouceur et al., 1998). In another study, patients with GAD had higher WDQ scores than patients with another primary anxiety disorder diagnosis (Ladouceur et al., 1999). However, Tallis and colleagues (1994) reported normative data in which patients with GAD and patients with obsessive–compulsive disorder attained very similar WDQ total and domain scores. Finally, the WDQ has been criticized as limited in terms of the domains of worry sampled (e.g., Dugas et al., 1995; van Rijsoort et al., 1999).

Anxious Thoughts Inventory

The Anxious Thoughts Inventory (AnTI; Wells, 1994) is a 22-item measure that includes three factor-analytically derived subscales: (1) Social Worry (e.g., "I worry about making a fool of myself"); (2) Health Worry (e.g., "I have thoughts about being seriously ill"); and (3) Meta-Worry, which captures negative thoughts about one's own worry (e.g., "I worry that I cannot control my thoughts as well as I would like to"). Respondents rate each item on a 4-point scale (1 = "almost never," 4 = "almost always").

In a sample of 239 undergraduates, acceptable internal consistency was observed for the Social Worry (alpha = .84), Health Worry (alpha = .81), and Meta-Worry (alpha = .75) subscales (Wells, 1994). In a sample of 64 college students, 6-week test–retest reliabilities were satisfactory for the total score (r = .80) as well as for the Social Worry (r = .76), Health Worry (r = .84), and Meta-Worry (r = .77) subscales (Wells, 1994). Positive correlations were observed between the PSWQ and the AnTI Social Worry (r = .60), Health Worry (r = .33), and Meta-Worry (r = .69) subscales in a sample of 140 undergraduate and postgraduate students (Wells & Carter, 1999). In relation to the cognitive model of GAD proposed by Wells, the Social Worry and Health Worry subscales of the AnTI represent relatively normal cognitive processes, whereas Meta-Worry is a central causal factor of pathological worry (see Wells, Chapter 7, this volume). Consistent with this model, Meta-Worry has been shown to be a significant predictor of pathological worry (as measured by the PSWQ) after controlling for trait anxiety, Social Worry, and Health Worry (Wells & Carter, 1999). Furthermore, social and health worries were not significant independent predictors of pathological worry in this final regression equation. Lastly, consistent with Wells's cognitive model, patients with GAD scored significantly higher on the Meta-Worry subscale than either community controls or patients with social phobia or panic disorder (Wells & Carter, 2001). As expected, patients with GAD were less likely to be differentiated from the other groups on the basis of frequency of Health and Social worries. Patients with GAD and patients with social phobia achieved similar scores on the Social Worry subscale, which were significantly higher than those of patients with panic disorder and community controls. Similarly, patients with GAD and patients with panic disorder achieved similar scores on the Health Worry subscale, which were significantly higher than those of patients with social phobia and community controls.

ASSESSMENT OF CONSTRUCTS THEORETICALLY RELEVANT TO GAD

Beliefs about Worrying

A number of theorists have proposed that people hold positive beliefs about the benefits of worry, and that such beliefs may contribute to the maintenance of worry (Borkovec, Alcaine, & Behar, Chapter 4; Davey, Tallis, & Capuzzo, 1996; Dugas, Buhr, & Ladouceur, Chapter 6; and Wells, Chapter 7, this volume). In addition, some researchers have suggested that simultaneously holding positive and negative beliefs about worry is associated with greater psychopathology than holding only negative beliefs (Davey et al., 1996) or only positive beliefs (Davey et al., 1996; Wells, Chapter 7, this volume) about worry.

Why Worry?

The Why Worry? questionnaire (Freeston et al., 1994) is a 20-item scale that was developed to assess positive beliefs about worry (e.g., "By worrying, I can stop bad things from happening," "I worry because if the worst happens, I wouldn't be able to cope"). Items are rated on a 5-point Likert-type scale (1 = "not at all characteristic of me," 5 = "entirely characteristic of me").

The scale demonstrated good internal consistency in two separate samples of college students (alphas = .87–.91; Freeston et al., 1994). Factor analysis suggested one factor referring to the idea that worry prevents or minimizes negative outcomes, and another factor referring to the idea that worry is a positive action for finding a solution to a problem. The scale has recently been revised and expanded to 25 items (Holowka, Dugas, Francis, & Laugesen, 2000). Preliminary examination of the psychometric properties of the Why Worry-II suggested good internal consistency (alpha = .93), good 6-week test–retest reliability (r = .80), and significant correlation with the PSWQ (r = .45; Holowka et al., 2000).

Consequences of Worrying Scale

The Consequences of Worrying Scale (Davey et al., 1996) is a 29-item measure that contains five factor-analytically derived subscales. Initial items were generated by asking college students to list ways that worry made things worse or better. Three subscales assess negative beliefs about worry: (1) Worry Disrupts Effective Performance (e.g., "Worry makes me focus on the wrong things"), (2) Worry Exaggerates the Problem (e.g., "Problems are magnified when I dwell on them"), and (3) Worry Causes Emotional Discomfort (e.g., "Worry causes me stress"). Two subscales assess positive beliefs about worry: (4) Worry Motivates (e.g., "In order to get something done I have to worry about it"), and (5) Worry Helps Analytic Thinking (e.g., "Worrying makes me reflect on life by asking questions I might not usually ask when happy"). Individuals are asked to rate the extent to which each item describes them on a 5-point Likert-type scale.

The subscales were found to be internally consistent (alphas = .72–.87). All three subscales assessing negative beliefs were significantly correlated with the PSWQ (r's = .44–.57) and the WDQ (r's = .46–.50). For the subscales assessing positive beliefs, the Worry Helps Analytic Thinking subscale was significantly correlated with the PSWQ (r = .19) and the WDQ (r = .25), but the Worry Motivates subscale was not. In general, the subscales assessing negative beliefs demonstrated stronger associates with measures of anxiety, depression, and poor psychological health than the ones assessing positive beliefs.

Meta-Cognitions Questionnaire

The Meta-Cognitions Questionnaire (Cartwright-Hatton & Wells, 1997) is a 65-item instrument developed to measure beliefs about worry specifically and intrusive thoughts more generally. In addition to a total score, five factor-analytically derived subscales may be scored. The Positive Beliefs subscale consists of items suggesting that worry improves functioning (e.g., "I need to worry in order to work well") and is a desirable personality trait (e.g., "People who do not worry have no depth"). The Uncontrollability and Danger subscale consists of items assessing the belief that worry is harmful (e.g., "I could make myself sick with worry") and that worry is impossible to control (e.g., "I cannot ignore my worrying thoughts"). The Cognitive Confidence subscale contains items suggesting a lack of confidence in one's attentional (e.g., "I am easily distracted") and memory (e.g., "I do not trust my memory") functioning. The Superstition, Punishment, and Responsibility (SPR) subscale assesses perceived negative consequences of worrying (e.g., "If I did not control a worrying thought, and then it happened, it would be my fault") and not worrying (e.g., "If a bad thing happens which I have not worried about, I feel responsible"). Lastly, the Cognitive Self-Consciousness subscale measures the extent to which an individual monitors his or her cognitive processes (e.g., "I think a lot about my thoughts"). Items are rated on a 4-point Likert-type scale (1 = "do not agree," 4 = "agree very much").

The subcales have shown good internal consistency (alphas = .72–.89) in a college student sample (Cartwright-Hatton & Wells, 1997). Good 5-week test–retest reliability has been demonstrated for the total score (r = .94) and subscale scores (r's = .76–.89) with a sample of university employees and postgraduate students (Cartwright-Hatton & Wells, 1997). The total and subscale scores are positively correlated with social worries, health worries, worry about worry, and obsessive–compulsive symptoms (Cartwright-Hatton & Wells, 1997). The Positive Beliefs subscale and the Uncontrollability and Danger subscale predict pathological worry, even after controlling for obsessive–compulsive symptoms (Wells & Papageorgiou, 1998). Similarly, the Positive Beliefs subscale and the Uncontrollability and Danger subscale predict obsessional thoughts, even after controlling for worry (Wells & Papageorgiou, 1998). Lastly, the subscales have been found to discriminate among individuals with and without GAD. Wells and Carter (2001) found that patients with GAD scored significantly higher on the Uncontrollability and Danger subscale and the SPR subscale than community controls and patients with social phobia and panic disorder; no significant group differences were observed for the Positive Beliefs subscale (the Cognitive Confidence and Cognitive Self-Consciousness subscales were not examined in this study). In another study, undergraduates meeting GAD criteria on the GADQ scored higher on all five subscales than nonanxious undergraduates, and higher on all subscales except the Positive Beliefs subscale than nonworried anxious undergraduates (Davis & Valentiner, 2000).

Intolerance of Uncertainty

Dugas and colleagues (Chapter 6, this volume) have proposed and provided empirical support for a model of GAD that features intolerance of uncertainty as a central component. Intolerance of uncertainty is characterized by an excessive tendency to consider it unacceptable that a negative event might occur, regardless of the probability of its occurrence (Dugas, Gosselin, & Ladouceur, 2001). In order to assess this construct, the Intolerance of Uncertainty Scale (IUS; Freeston et al., 1994; see also Appendix 6.1 in Chapter 6, this volume) was developed. It consists of 27 items that target how an individual responds to uncertainty on cognitive, emotional, and behavioral levels (e.g., "When I am uncertain, I can't go forward," "The ambiguities in life stress me"). Items are rated on a 5-point scale (1 = "not at all characteristic of me," 5 = "entirely characteristic of me"). Although five factors have been identified (reflecting the views that uncertainty is unacceptable, uncertainty reflects badly on a person, frustration is related to uncertainty, uncertainty causes stress, and uncertainty prevents action), the authors recommend that the total score be used, due to the correlation among these factors. The IUS has demonstrated good internal consistency with a sample of 110 college students (alpha = .91; Freeston et al., 1994). Test–retest correlations of $r = .78$ were observed with a sample of 78 college students assessed over an interval of 5 weeks (Dugas, Freeston, & Ladouceur, 1997). As expected, the IUS has been shown to be positively correlated with the PSWQ ($r = .63$) and WDQ ($r = .57$; Freeston et al., 1994). These correlations remained significant even after reasons for worrying and dysphoria were controlled for (Freeston et al., 1994). The IUS also has demonstrated stronger correlations with the PSWQ than a measure of obsessions/compulsions and a measure of panic symptoms (Dugas et al., 2001). Patients with GAD had higher IUS scores than patients with another primary anxiety disorder diagnosis (Ladouceur et al., 1999). The IUS has also been used to discriminate patients with GAD from nonclinical controls (Dugas, Gagnon, Ladouceur, & Freeston, 1998). Lastly, the IUS has been shown to be sensitive to the effects of a cognitive-behavioral treatment targeting intolerance of uncertainty (Ladouceur et al., 2000).

Interpersonal Functioning

Theoretical work regarding the interpersonal dynamics of individuals with GAD has led to the development of new psychosocial treatment protocols that are currently being evaluated (Crits-Christoph, Gibbons, & Crits-Christoph, Chapter 12, and Newman, Castonguay, Borkovec, & Molnar, Chapter 13, this volume). Indeed, research increasingly suggests that GAD is a disorder associated with interpersonal difficulties. A substantial number of individuals with GAD perceive their relationships with family, friends, and romantic partners as moderately to severely impaired (Turk, Mennin, Fresco, & Heimberg, 2000). The cognitions of persons with GAD are more likely to concern interpersonal conflict than the cognitions of individuals with panic disorder (Breitholtz, Westling, & Öst, 1998). In fact, individuals with GAD appear to have interpersonal styles that contribute to the relationship problems they perceive. Pincus and Borkovec (1994) conducted a cluster analysis on responses to the Inventory of Interpersonal Problems (IIP; Horowitz, Rosenberg, Baer, Ureno, & Villasenor, 1988). The majority of individuals with GAD were characterized as having interpersonal styles that were overly nurturant and intrusive. The remainder were characterized as socially avoidant/ nonassertive or cold/vindictive. Using the Inventory of Interpersonal Problems Circumplex Scales (IIP-C; Alden, Wiggins, & Pincus, 1990), Borkovec, Newman, Pincus, and Lytle (2002) found that interpersonal problems that remained untreated following cognitive-behavioral therapy for GAD predicted poor end-state functioning at follow-up assessment. Therefore, a measure that assesses interpersonal style, such as the IIP, is recommended in the assessment of GAD. Preliminary data suggest that the IIP is sensitive to the effects of treatment for GAD that addresses maladaptive patterns of relating (Crits-Christoph et al., Chapter 12, and Newman et al., Chapter 13, this volume).

Emotion Regulation

Recent theoretical work by our research group suggests that GAD may best be conceptualized as a multicomponent syndrome involving both significant deficits in the self-regulation of emotions and overreliance on cognitive control strategies such as worry (Mennin, Heimberg, Turk, & Fresco, 2002; Mennin, Turk, Heimberg, & Carmin, 2003). Preliminary studies conducted in our laboratory provide initial evidence for this conceptualization of GAD (Mennin, Turk, Fresco, & Heimberg, 2003; Turk et al., in press) and suggest that it is important to understand how patients with GAD regulate their emotions. Our initial work in this area has relied on a battery of self-report instruments, including the Affective Control Scale (Williams, Chambless, & Ahrens, 1997), the Toronto Alexithymia Scale (Bagby, Parker, & Taylor, 1994; Bagby, Taylor, & Parker, 1994), the Trait Meta-Mood Scale (Salovey, Mayer, Goldman, Turvey, & Palfai, 1995), and the Berkeley Expressivity Questionnaire (Gross & John, 1997). In general, we have found that, relative to controls, individuals with GAD are more fearful of their emotions, have greater difficulty identifying and describing their emotions, have more difficulty repairing a negative mood state, experience their emotions more intensely, and are more expressive of negative emotions (Mennin, Turk, Fresco, & Heimberg, 2003; Turk et al., in press). These findings suggest that assessing how individuals with GAD handle their emotions may provide insight into deficits that may be targets for treatment.

Some critics have suggested that self-report methods for the assessment of emotion regulation skills are subject to considerable bias (Davies, Stankov, & Roberts, 1998; Wagner & Waltz, 1998; Westen, 1994). Self-report measures assume that respondents are aware of their emotional experiences and are accurate in their observations of their own regulatory behavior. Although self-report measures are useful to the extent that they can assess patients' subjective experiences of emotion, it is also important to employ more objective methodology. One example of an objective methodology for assessing emotion regulatory skills is the Mayer–Salovey–Caruso Emotional Intelligence Test (Mayer, Salovey, & Caruso, 2001), which is a performance measure in which emotional skills are assessed by asking the individual to perform tasks and solve emotional problems. Items are scored by comparing the test taker's answer to each item to that of the standardization sample.

NONSPECIFIC ANXIETY MEASURES

Assessment of GAD typically involves an assessment of general levels of anxiety. Although many instruments are available for this purpose, those measures most commonly used in the GAD treatment outcome literature are the focus of this review.

State–Trait Anxiety Inventory

The STAI (Spielberger et al., 1983) consists of separate 20-item self-report scales that measure current (State Anxiety) and chronic (Trait Anxiety) levels of anxiety, respectively. In studies of GAD treatment outcome, the Trait Anxiety version of the scale, which measures characteristic tendencies to be anxious, is commonly used and appears sensitive to treatment-related change (Fisher & Durham, 1999). Items (e.g., "I get in a state of tension or turmoil as I think over my recent concerns and interests") are rated on a 4-point Likert-type scale based on how the individual generally feels. The STAI Trait Anxiety scale has been found to have excellent internal consistency (alphas = .86–.95 across samples of working adults, students, and military recruits) and levels of test–retest stability that would be expected for a trait measure (e.g., median test–retest correlations of

.77 for college students and .70 for high school students) (Spielberger et al., 1983).

The STAI has demonstrated both convergent and discriminant validity (Spielberger et al., 1983). Nevertheless, using confirmatory factor-analytic procedures to analyze the responses of anxiety disorder patients on the Trait scale, Bieling, Antony, and Swinson (1998) found separate lower-order factors assessing (1) dysphoric mood and (2) anxiety and worry. The anxiety factor was more highly correlated with other measures of anxiety than other measures of depression; the depression factor was more highly correlated with other measures of depression than other measures of anxiety.

Beck Anxiety Inventory

The Beck Anxiety Inventory (BAI; Beck, Epstein, Brown, & Steer, 1988) is a 21-item self-report measure designed to assess the severity of anxiety symptoms and to discriminate anxiety from depression. Consequently, the majority of items represent symptoms of autonomic arousal or panic (e.g., "heart pounding or racing," "sweating (not due to heat)") rather than the more diffuse anxiety characteristic of GAD. Research has shown that individuals with GAD frequently endorse symptoms of autonomic arousal (e.g., Brown, Marten, & Barlow, 1995), and elevated BAI scores have been observed among individuals with GAD (e.g., Butler, Fennell, Robson, & Gelder, 1991). However, worry, the central feature of GAD, has been shown to decrease autonomic arousal (e.g., Borkovec, Lyonfields, Wiser, & Diehl, 1993; Hoehn-Saric, McLeod, & Zimmerli, 1989). Brown, Chorpita, and Barlow (1998) have reconciled these apparently contradictory findings on the basis of structural equation modeling suggesting that GAD is associated with high levels of negative affect, which is in turn associated with increased autonomic arousal. However, after variance in anxious arousal due to negative affect was accounted for, the disorder-specific features of GAD (i.e., worry) were shown to be associated with a suppression of autonomic arousal. In summary, although the BAI has demonstrated good psychometric properties (for a review, see Roemer, 2001), its emphasis on symptoms of anxious arousal does not provide an adequate sampling of the anxiety symptoms most characteristic of GAD (e.g., restlessness, muscle tension).

Hamilton Anxiety Rating Scale

The HARS (Hamilton, 1959) is a clinician-administered instrument intended for use with patients already diagnosed with an anxiety disorder, and designed to assess symptoms characteristic of an anxious mood. The most widely used version of the scale contains 14 items (Hamilton, 1969).

The HARS employs a semistructured interview format that provides symptom categories (e.g., "intellectual (cognitive)") accompanied by a more detailed description of what is encompassed by each category (e.g., "difficulty in concentration, poor memory"). How best to inquire about each symptom category is left to the discretion of the interviewer, since no specific questions are provided to the interviewer to guide symptom assessment. Items are rated on a 5-point scale (0 = "none," 4 = "very severe; grossly disabling"). No guidelines beyond the Likert scale descriptors are provided for determining severity ratings for each symptom cluster. In addition to the total score, psychic (e.g., "anxiety," "intellectual (cognitive)") and somatic (e.g., "gastrointestinal," "cardiovascular") subscales may be scored. The HARS has become the gold standard for pharmacological treatment outcome studies for GAD (see Lydiard & Monnier, Chapter 14, this volume).

Across studies, reliability coefficients for the HARS have ranged from fair to excellent. For the HARS administered 10 days or fewer apart to anxiety patients by separate interviewers, the interrater reliability was .65 (Moras, DiNardo, & Barlow, 1992). The alpha coefficients were .77 and .81 for the first and second HARS administrations, respectively. In another study, interrater reliability obtained via live observation was .96 (Kobak, Reynolds, & Greist, 1993). The alpha coefficient was .92. For the HARS administered within 7 days of each other to patients with GAD by separate interviewers, interrater reliability as assessed by the intraclass correlation coefficient was .79 (Shear et al., 2001). When interrater reliability was calculated based on videotape review, the interclass correlation coefficient was .98 (Shear et al., 2001).

In order to minimize differences in how clinicians ask probe questions and assign severity ratings for HARS symptoms, structured interview guides have been developed. The HARS Interview Guide (Bruss, Gruenberg, Goldstein, & Barber, 1994) and the Structured Interview Guide for the HARS (SIGH-A; Shear et al., 2001) have shown good interrater reliability. Shear et al. (2001) concluded that the reliability and validity of the SIGH-A and the original HARS were similar across their entire sample of patients with anxiety disorders. However, they observed a slight advantage for the SIGH-A for interrater reliability for their subsample of patients with GAD.

The HARS has been found to correlate with other measures of anxiety (e.g., Beck & Steer, 1991). Individuals with an anxiety disorder and individuals with an affective disorder score higher on the HARS than individuals from the community with no diagnosis (Kobak et al., 1993). In a discriminant analysis using the HARS and the HRSD to classify anxiety patients with or without comorbid depression, 76.5% of patients were correctly classified (Moras et al., 1992).

A reconstructed version of the scale (R-HARS), consisting of 10 items from the 14-item HARS and 6 items from the HRSD-24 (Guy, 1976), was developed to eliminate item overlap and decrease shared variance between the HARS and HRSD (Riskind, Beck, Brown, & Steer, 1987). Subsequent research, however, suggests that the reconstructed versions of the scales share considerable variance (37%) and do not distinguish between anxiety patients with comorbid mood disorders and those without comorbid mood disorders better than the original scales do (Moras et al., 1992). In addition, interrater reliability and internal consistency for the R-HARS were similar to those of the original version.

ADDITIONAL DOMAINS

Several additional domains should be examined in a comprehensive assessment of GAD. We recommend also assessing depression, disability, and quality of life.

Depression

Depression is common among individuals with GAD (e.g., Kessler, DuPont, Berglund, & Wittchen, 1999). Therefore, we recommend administering an instrument to assess depression. One option is the BDI (Beck et al., 1979) or BDI-II (Beck, Steer, & Brown, 1996), both of which assess various symptoms of depression—including the affective, cognitive, behavioral, somatic, and motivational components, as well as suicidal wishes. See Beck, Steer, and Garbin (1988) for a more general review of the psychometric characteristics of the BDI.

Disability

The construct of "disability" captures how a disorder interferes with an individual's ability to act in the world and fulfill important roles, such as those of parent, worker, friend, partner, and student (Hambrick, Turk, Heimberg, Schneier, & Liebowitz, 2003). Thus, although disability is related to the presence and severity of symptoms, individuals with similar symptoms may exhibit different degrees of impairment. In a recent study in our clinic (Turk et al., 2000), patients seeking treatment for GAD reported meaningful levels of current disability when assessed with the Liebowitz Self-Rated Disability Scale (Schneier et al., 1994) and the Sheehan Disability Scale (Sheehan, 1983). Although these measures appear to be reasonable choices for assessing disability among individuals with GAD, other options exist (see Mendlowicz & Stein, 2000).

Quality of Life

Whether an individual manifests high or low levels of disability, the internal states of worry, anxiety, and physical tension characteristic of GAD may nevertheless interfere with quality of life. Frisch (1994) has defined "quality of life" as the extent to which a person perceives his or her most important needs, goals, and wishes as being fulfilled. Indeed, although individuals seeking treatment for GAD typically report moderate disability, they report profound dissatisfaction with the their quality of life (Turk et al., 2000). Perhaps more so than for other anxiety disorders with more obvious behavioral referents, one of the best standards by which to judge the impact of a treatment for GAD is in terms of its effect on a patient's quality of life. Therefore, we strongly recommend the inclusion of a measure of quality of life as part of a comprehensive assessment battery for GAD. Although other instruments are available, we routinely administer the Quality of Life Inventory, a self-report measure assessing the extent to which clients perceive themselves as satisfied in the areas of their lives that they deem important to their happiness (Frisch, 1994). The Quality of Life Inventory appears to have good psychometric properties, and normative data are available (Frisch, 1994; Frisch, Cornell, Villanueva, & Retzlaff, 1992).

CONCLUSION

In recent years, our ability to diagnose GAD reliably, assess its important features, and evaluate treatment response has improved considerably. Advances in theoretical models of GAD have led to the development of promising instruments that target constructs central to these models. Despite this progress, more basic psychometric work is needed, especially for new or newly revised measures. Ultimately, improved assessment may allow us to better understand GAD, to better customize our treatments to our patients, and to increase the effectiveness of our treatments.

REFERENCES

Alden, L. E., Wiggins, J. S., & Pincus, A. L. (1990). Construction of circumplex scales for the Inventory of Interpersonal Problems. *Journal of Personality Assessment, 55,* 521–536.

American Psychiatric Association (APA). (1980). *Diagnostic and statistical manual of mental disorders* (3rd ed.). Washington, DC: Author.

American Psychiatric Association (APA). (1987). *Diagnostic and statistical manual of mental disorders* (3rd ed., rev.). Washington, DC: Author.

American Psychiatric Association (APA). (1994). *Diagnostic and statistical manual of mental disorders* (4th ed.). Washington, DC: Author.

American Psychiatric Association (APA). (2000). *Diagnostic and statistical manual of mental disorders* (4th ed., text rev.). Washington, DC: Author.

Bagby, R. M., Parker, J. D. A., & Taylor, G. J. (1994). The twenty-item Toronto Alexithymia Scale: I. Item selection and cross-validation of the factor structure. *Journal of Psychosomatic Research, 38,* 23–32.

Bagby, R. M., Taylor, G. J., & Parker, J. D. A. (1994). The twenty-item Toronto Alexithymia Scale: II. Convergent, discriminant, and concurrent validity. *Journal of Psychosomatic Research, 38,* 33–40.

Barlow, D. H. (1987). The classification of anxiety disorders. In G. L. Tischler (Ed.), *Diagnosis and classification in psychiatry: A critical reappraisal of DSM-III* (pp. 223–242). Cambridge, UK: Cambridge University Press.

Beck, A. T., Epstein, N., Brown, G., & Steer, R. A. (1988). An inventory for measuring clinical anxiety: Psychometric properties. *Journal of Consulting and Clinical Psychology, 56,* 893–897.

Beck, A. T., Rush, J., Shaw, B. F., & Emery, G. (1979). *Cognitive therapy of depression.* New York: Guilford Press.

Beck, A. T., & Steer, R. A. (1991). Relationship between the Beck Anxiety Inventory and the Hamilton Anxiety Rating Scale with anxious outpatients. *Journal of Anxiety Disorders, 5,* 213–223.

Beck, A. T., Steer, R. A., & Brown, G. K. (1996). *Beck Depression Inventory manual* (2nd ed.). San Antonio, TX: Psychological Corporation.

Beck, A. T., Steer, R. A., & Garbin, M. G. (1998). Psychometric properties of the Beck Depression Inventory: Twenty-five years of evaluation. *Clinical Psychology Review, 8,* 77–100.

Bieling, P. J., Antony, M. M., & Swinson, R. P. (1998). The State–Trait Anxiety Inventory, Trait version: Structure and content re-examined. *Behaviour Research and Therapy, 36,* 777–788.

Borkovec, T. D., & Costello, E. (1993). Efficacy of applied relaxation and cognitive-behavioral therapy in the treatment of generalized anxiety disorder. *Journal of Consulting and Clinical Psychology, 61,* 611–619.

Borkovec, T. D., Lyonfields, J. D., Wiser, S. L., & Diehl, L. (1993). The role of worrisome thinking in the suppression of cardiovascular response to phobic imagery. *Behavior Research and Therapy, 31,* 321–324.

Borkovec, T. D., Newman, M. G., Pincus, A. L., & Lytle, R. (2002). A component analysis of cognitive behavioral therapy for generalized anxiety disorder and the role of interpersonal problems. *Journal of Consulting and Clinical Psychology, 70,* 288–298.

Breitholtz, E., Westling, B. E., & Öst, L.-G. (1998). Cognitions in generalized anxiety disorder and panic disorder patients. *Journal of Anxiety Disorders, 12,* 567–577.

Brown, T. A. (in press). Confirmatory factor analysis of the Penn State Worry Questionnaire: Multiple factors or method effects? *Behaviour Research and Therapy.*

Brown, T. A., Antony, M. M., & Barlow, D. H. (1992). Psychometric properties of the Penn State Worry Questionnaire in a clinical anxiety disorders sample. *Behaviour Research and Therapy, 30,* 33–37.

Brown, T. A., Chorpita, B. F., & Barlow, D. H. (1998). Structural relationships among dimensions of the DSM-IV anxiety and mood disorders and dimensions of negative affect, positive affect, and autonomic arousal. *Journal of Abnormal Psychology,* *107,* 179–192.

Brown, T. A., DiNardo, P. A., & Barlow, D. H. (1994). *Anxiety Disorders Interview Schedule for DSM-IV (ADIS-IV).* Albany, NY: Graywind.

Brown, T. A., DiNardo, P. A., Lehman, C. L., & Campbell, L. A. (2001). Reliability of DSM-IV anxiety and mood disorders: Implications for the classification of emotional disorders. *Journal of Abnormal Psychology, 110,* 49–58.

Brown, T. A., Marten, P. A., & Barlow, D. H. (1995). Discriminant validity of the symptoms constituting the DSM-III-R and DSM-IV associated symptom criterion of generalized anxiety disorder. *Journal of Anxiety Disorders, 9,* 317–328.

Bruss, G. S., Gruenberg, A. M., Goldstein, R. D., & Barber, J. P. (1994). Hamilton Anxiety Rating Scale Interview Guide: Joint interview and test–retest methods for interrater reliability. *Psychiatry Research, 53,* 191–202.

Butler, G., Fennell, M., Robson, P., & Gelder, M. (1991). Comparison of behavior therapy and cognitive behavior therapy in the treatment of generalized anxiety disorder. *Journal of Consulting and Clinical Psychology, 59,* 167–175.

Cartwright-Hatton, S., & Wells, A. (1997). Beliefs about worry and intrusions: The Meta-Cognitions Questionnaire and its correlates. *Journal of Anxiety Disorders, 11,* 279–296.

Davey, G. C. L. (1993). A comparison of three worry questionnaires. *Behaviour Research and Therapy, 31,* 51–56.

Davey, G. C. L. (1994). Pathological worry as exacerbated problem-solving. In G. C. L. Davey & F. Tallis (Eds.), *Worrying: Perspectives on theory, assessment, and treatment* (pp. 35–59). Chichester, UK: Wiley.

Davey, G. C. L., Hampton, J., Farrell, J., & Davidson, S. (1992). Some characteristics of worrying: Evidence for worrying and anxiety as separate constructs. *Personality and Individual Differences, 13,* 133–147.

Davey, G. C. L., Tallis, F., & Capuzzo, N. (1996). Beliefs about the consequences of worrying. *Cognitive Therapy and Research, 20,* 499–520.

Davies, M., Stankov, L., & Roberts, R. D. (1998). Emotional intelligence: In search of an elusive construct. *Journal of Personality and Social Psychology, 75,* 989–1015.

Davis, R. N., & Valentiner, D. P. (2000). Does meta-cognitive theory enhance our understanding of pathological worry and anxiety? *Personality and Individual Differences, 29,* 513–526.

DiNardo, P. A., Brown, T. A., & Barlow, D. H. (1994). *Anxiety Disorders Interview Schedule for DSM-IV: Lifetime Version (ADIS-IV-L).* Albany, NY: Graywind.

Dugas, M. J., Freeston, M. H., & Ladouceur, R. (1997). Intolerance of uncertainty and problem orientation in worry. *Cognitive Therapy and Research, 21,* 593–606.

Dugas, M. J., Freeston, M. H., Doucet, C., Lachance, S., & Ladouceur, R. (1995). Structured versus free-recall measures: Effect on report of worry themes. *Personality and Individual Differences, 18,* 355–361.

Dugas, M. J., Gagnon, F., Ladouceur, R., & Freeston, M. H. (1998). Generalized anxiety disorder: A preliminary test of a conceptual model. *Behaviour Research and Therapy, 36,* 215–226.

Dugas, M. J., Gosselin, P., & Ladouceur, R. (2001). Intolerance of uncertainty and worry: Investigating specificity in a nonclinical sample. *Cognitive Therapy and Research, 25,* 551–558.

First, M. B., Spitzer, R. L., Gibbon, M., & Williams, J. B. W. (2001). *Structured Clinical Interview for DSM-IV-TR Axis I Disorders, Research Version, Patient Edition (SCID-I/*

P). New York: Biometrics Research Department, New York State Psychiatric Institute.

Fisher, P. L., & Durham, R. C. (1999). Recovery rates in generalized anxiety disorder following psychological therapy: An analysis of clinically significant change in the STAI-T across outcome studies since 1990. *Psychological Medicine, 29,* 1425–1434.

Freeston, M. H., Rhéaume, J., Letarte, H., Dugas, M., & Ladouceur, R. (1994). Why do people worry? *Personality and Individual Differences, 17,* 791–802.

Fresco, D. M., Heimberg, R. G., Mennin, D. S., & Turk, C. L. (2002). Confirmatory factor analysis of the Penn State Worry Questionnaire. *Behaviour Research and Therapy, 40,* 313–323.

Fresco, D. M., Heimberg, R. G., Mennin, D. S., & Turk, C. L. (2003). *Using the Penn State Worry Questionnaire to identify individuals with generalized anxiety disorder: A receiver operating characteristic analysis.* Manuscript submitted for publication.

Frisch, M. B. (1994). *Quality of Life Inventory: Manual and treatment guide.* Minneapolis, MN: National Computer Systems.

Frisch, M. B., Cornell, J., Villanueva, M., & Retzlaff, P. J. (1992). Clinical validation of the Quality of Life Inventory: A measure of life satisfaction for use in treatment planning and outcome assessment. *Psychological Assessment, 4,* 92–101.

Gross, J. J., & John, O. P. (1997). Revealing feelings: Facets of emotional expressivity in self-reports, peer ratings, and behavior. *Journal of Personality and Social Psychology, 72,* 435–448.

Guy, W. (1976). *ECDEU assessment manual for psychopharmacology.* Washington, DC: U.S. Department of Health, Education and Welfare.

Hambrick, J. P., Turk, C. L., Heimberg, R. G., Schneier, F., & Liebowitz, M. (2003). *Psychometric properties of disability measures among patients with social anxiety disorder.* Manuscript submitted for publication.

Hamilton, M. (1959). The assessment of anxiety states by rating. *British Journal of Psychiatry, 32,* 50–55.

Hamilton, M. (1960). A rating scale for depression. *Journal of Neurology, Neurosurgery and Psychiatry, 23,* 56–62.

Hamilton, M. (1969). Diagnosis and rating of anxiety. *British Journal of Psychiatry,* Special Publication No. 3, 76–79.

Hoehn-Saric, R., McLeod, D. R., & Zimmerli, W. D. (1989). Somatic manifestations in women with generalized anxiety disorder: Psychophysiological responses to psychological stress. *Archives of General Psychiatry, 46,* 1113–1119.

Holowka, D. W., Dugas, M. J., Francis, K., & Laugesen, N. (2000, November). *Measuring beliefs about worry: A psychometric evaluation of the Why Worry II questionnaire.* Poster presented at the annual meeting of the Association for Advancement of Behavior Therapy, New Orleans, LA.

Horowitz, L. M., Rosenberg, S. E., Baer, B. A., Ureno, G., & Villasenor, V. S. (1988). Inventory of Interpersonal Problems: Psychometric properties and clinical applications. *Journal of Consulting and Clinical Psychology, 56,* 885–892.

Joormann, J., & Stöber, J. (1997). Measuring facets of worry: A LISREL analysis of the Worry Domains Questionnaire. *Personality and Individuals Differences, 23,* 827–837.

Kessler, R. C., DuPont, R. L., Berglund, P., & Wittchen, H.-U. (1999). Impairment in pure and comorbid generalized anxiety disorder and major depression at 12 months in two national surveys. *American Journal of Psychiatry, 156,* 1915–1923.

Kobak, K. A., Reynolds, W. M., & Greist, J. H. (1993). Computerized and clinical assessment of depression and anxiety: Respondent evaluation and satisfaction. *Journal of Personality Assessment, 63*, 173–180.

Lachance, S., Doucet, C., Freeston, M. H., & Ladouceur, R. (1993, November). *Thèmes d'inquiétudes par questionnaire structuré et par rappel libre [Worry themes by a structured questionnaire and by free recall].* Communication presented at the XVIth Congress of the Société Québécoise pour la Recherche en Psychologie, Québec.

Ladouceur, R., Dugas, M. J., Freeston, M. H., Léger, E., Gagnon, F., & Thibodeau, N. (2000). Efficacy of a new cognitive-behavioral treatment for generalized anxiety disorder: Evaluation in a controlled clinical trial. *Journal of Consulting and Clinical Psychology, 68*, 957–964.

Ladouceur, R., Dugas, M. J., Freeston, M. H., Rhéaume, J., Blais, F., Boisert, J. M., Gagnon, F., & Thibodeau, N. (1999). Specificity of generalized anxiety disorder symptoms and processes. *Behavior Therapy, 30*, 191–207.

Lecrubier, Y., Sheehan, D., Weiller, E., Amorim, P., Bonora, I., Sheehan, K., Janavs, J., & Dunbar, G. (1997). The MINI International Neuropsychiatric Interview (M.I.N.I.), a short diagnostic structured interview: Reliability and validity according to the CIDI. *European Psychiatry, 12*, 224–231.

Lovibond, S. H. (1983, May). *The nature and measurement of anxiety, stress, and depression.* Paper presented at the meeting of the Australian Psychological Society, University of Western Australia.

Luterek, J. A., Turk, C. L., Heimberg, R. G., Fresco, D. M., & Mennin, D. S. (2002, November). *Psychometric properties of the GADQ-IV among individuals with clinician-assessed generalized anxiety disorder: An update.* Poster presented at the annual meeting of Association for the Advancement of Behavior Therapy, Reno, NV.

Lyonfields, J. D., Borkovec, T. D., & Thayer, J. F. (1995). Vagal tone in generalized anxiety disorder and the effects of aversive imagery and worrisome thinking. *Behavior Therapy, 26*, 457–466.

Mattick, R. P., & Clarke, J. C. (1998). Development and validation of measures of social phobia scrutiny fear and social interaction anxiety. *Behaviour Research and Therapy, 36*, 455–470.

Mayer, J. D., Salovey, P., & Caruso, D. (2001). *The Mayer–Salovey–Caruso Emotional Intelligence Test (MSCEIT).* Toronto: Multi-Health Systems.

Mendlowicz, M., & Stein, M. (2000). Quality of life in individuals with anxiety disorders. *American Journal of Psychiatry, 157*, 669–682.

Mennin, D. S., Heimberg, R. G., Turk, C. L., & Fresco, D. M. (2002). Applying an emotion regulation framework to integrative approaches to generalized anxiety disorder. *Clinical Psychology: Science and Practice, 9*, 85–90.

Mennin, D. S., Turk, C. L., Fresco, D. M., & Heimberg, R. G. (2003). *Emotion regulation deficits as a key feature of generalized anxiety disorder: Testing a theoretical model.* Manuscript submitted for publication.

Mennin, D. S., Turk, C. L., Heimberg, R. G., & Carmin, C. (2003). Focusing on the regulation of emotion: A new direction for conceptualizing and treating generalized anxiety disorder. In M. A. Reinecke & D. A. Clark (Eds.), *Cognitive therapy over the lifespan: Theory, research and practice* (pp. 60–89). New York: Wiley.

Meyer, T. J., Miller, M. L., Metzger, R. L., & Borkovec, T. D. (1990). Development and validation of the Penn State Worry Questionnaire. *Behaviour Research and Therapy, 28*, 487–495.

Molina, S., & Borkovec, T. D. (1994). The Penn State Worry Questionnaire: Psychometric properties and associated characteristics. In G. C. L. Davey & F. Tallis (Eds.),

Worrying: Perspectives on theory, assessment, and treatment (pp. 265–283). Chichester, UK: Wiley.

Moras, K., DiNardo, P. A., & Barlow, D. H. (1992). Distinguishing anxiety and depression: Reexamination of the reconstructed Hamilton scales. *Psychological Assessment, 4,* 224–227.

Newman, M. G., Zuellig, A. R., Kachin, K. E., Constantino, M. J., Przeworski, A., Erickson, T., & Cashman-McGrath, L. (2002). Preliminary reliability and validity of the Generalized Anxiety Disorder Questionnaire–IV: A revised self-report diagnostic measure of generalized anxiety disorder. *Behavior Therapy, 33,* 215–233.

Pincus, A. L., & Borkovec, T. D. (1994, June). *Interpersonal problems in generalized anxiety disorder: Preliminary clustering of patients' interpersonal dysfunction.* Paper presented at the annual meeting of the American Psychological Society, New York.

Riskind, J. H., Beck, A. T., Brown, G., & Steer, R. A. (1987). Taking the measure of anxiety and depression: Validity of the reconstructed Hamilton scales. *Journal of Nervous and Mental Disease, 175,* 474–479.

Roemer, L. (2001). Measures of anxiety and related constructs. In M. M. Antony, S. M. Orsillo, & L. Roemer (Eds.), *Practitioner's guide to empirically based measures of anxiety* (pp. 49–83). New York: Kluwer Academic/Plenum Press.

Roemer, L., Borkovec, M., Posa, S., & Borkovec, T. D. (1995). A self-report diagnostic measure of generalized anxiety disorder. *Journal of Behavior Therapy and Experimental Psychiatry, 26,* 345–350.

Roemer, L., Salters, K., Raffa, S., & Orsillo, S. M. (in press). Fear and avoidance of internal experiences in GAD: Preliminary tests of a conceptual model. *Cognitive Therapy and Research.*

Salovey, P., Mayer, J. D., Goldman, S. L., Turvey, C., & Palfai, T. P. (1995). Emotional attention, clarity, and repair: Exploring emotional intelligence using the Trait Meta-Mood Scale. In J. W. Pennebaker (Ed.), *Emotion, disclosure, and health* (pp. 125–154). Washington, DC: American Psychological Association.

Schneier, F. R., Heckelman, L. R., Garfinkel, R., Campeas, R., Fallon, B. A., Gitow, A., Street, L., Del Bene, D., & Liebowitz, M. R. (1994). Functional impairment in social phobia. *Journal of Clinical Psychiatry, 55,* 322–331.

Scott, E. L., Eng, W., & Heimberg, R. G. (2002). Ethnic differences in worry in a nonclinical population. *Depression and Anxiety, 15,* 79–82.

Shear, K. M., Vander Bilt, J., Rucci, P., Endicott, J., Lydiard, B., Otto, M. W., Pollack, M. H., Chandler, L., Williams, J., Ali, A., & Frank, D. M. (2001). Reliability and validity of a Structured Interview Guide for the Hamilton Anxiety Rating Scale (SIGH-A). *Depression and Anxiety, 13,* 166–178.

Sheehan, D. V. (1983). *The anxiety disease.* New York: Scribner.

Sheehan, D. V., & Lecrubier, Y. (2002). *MINI International Neuropsychiatric Interview for DSM-IV* (English Version 5.0.0). Tampa: University of South Florida.

Sheehan, D. V., Lecrubier, Y., Harnett-Sheehan, K., Janavs, J., Weiller, E., Bonara, L. I., Keskiner, A., Schinka, J., Knapp, E., Sheehan, M. F., & Dunbar, G. C. (1997). Reliability and validity of the MINI International Neuropsychiatric Interview (M.I.N.I.): According to the SCID-P. *European Psychiatry, 12,* 232–241.

Spielberger, C. D., Gorsuch, R. L., Lushene, R., Vagg, P. R., & Jacobs, G. A. (1983). *Manual for the State–Trait Anxiety Inventory.* Palo Alto, CA: Consulting Psychologists Press.

Spitzer, R. L., Williams, J. B. W., Gibbon, M., & First, M. B. (1988). *Structured Clinical Interview for DSM-III-R–Patient Version (SCID-P 6/1/88).* New York: Biometrics Research Department, New York State Psychiatric Institute.

Starcevic, V. (1995). Pathological worry in major depression: A preliminary report. *Behaviour Research and Therapy, 33,* 55–56.

Stöber, J. (1995). Besorgnis: Ein Vergleich dreier Inventare zur Erfassung allgemeiner Sorgen [Worry: A comparison of three questionnaires concerning everyday worries]. *Zeitschrift f?r Differentielle und Diagnostische Psychologie, 16,* 50–63.

Stöber, J. (1998). Reliability and validity of two widely used worry questionnaires: Self-report and peer convergence. *Personality and Individual Differences, 24,* 887–890.

Stöber, J., & Bittencourt, J. (1998). Weekly assessment of worry: An adaptation of the Penn State Worry Questionnaire for monitoring changes during treatment. *Behaviour Research and Therapy, 36,* 645–656.

Stöber, J., & Joormann, J. (2001a). A short form of the Worry Domains Questionnaire: Construction and factorial validation. *Personality and Individual Differences, 31,* 591–598.

Stöber, J., & Joormann, J. (2001b). Worry, procrastination, and perfectionism: Differentiating amount of worry, pathological worry, anxiety, and depression. *Cognitive Therapy and Research, 25,* 49–60.

Tallis, F., Davey, G. C. L., & Bond, A. (1994). The Worry Domains Questionnaire. In G. C. L. Davey & F. Tallis (Eds.), *Worrying: Perspectives on theory, assessment, and treatment* (pp. 61–89). Chichester, UK: Wiley.

Tallis, F., Eysenck, M., & Mathews, A. (1992). A questionnaire for the measurement of nonpathological worry. *Personality and Individual Differences, 13,* 161–168.

Turk, C. L., Heimberg, R. G., Luterek, J. A., Mennin, D. S., & Fresco, D. M. (in press). Delineating the specific emotion regulation deficits in generalized anxiety disorder: A comparison with social anxiety disorder. *Cognitive Therapy and Research.*

Turk, C. L., Mennin, D. S., Fresco, D. M., & Heimberg, R. G. (2000, November). *Impairment and quality of life among individuals with generalized anxiety disorder.* Poster presented at the annual meeting of the Association for Advancement of Behavior Therapy, New Orleans, LA.

van Rijsoort, S., Emmelkamp, P., & Vervaeke, G. (1999). The Penn State Worry Questionnaire and the Worry Domains Questionnaire: Structure, reliability, and validity. *Clinical Psychology and Psychotherapy, 6,* 297–307.

Wagner, A. W., & Waltz, J. (1998, November). *What is alexithymia?: Taking the validation of the alexithymia construct beyond self-report measures.* Paper presented at the annual meeting of the Association for Advancement of Behavior Therapy, Washington, DC.

Watson, D., & Clark, L. A. (1991). *The Mood and Anxiety Symptom Questionnaire.* Unpublished manuscript, University of Iowa, Department of Psychology.

Weathers, F. W., Huska, J. A., & Keane, T. M. (1991). *The PTSD Checklist–Civilian version (PCL-C).* (Available from F. W. Weathers, National Center for PTSD, Boston Veterans Affairs Medical Center, 150 S. Huntington Avenue, Boston, MA 02130)

Wells, A. (1994). A multi-dimensional measure of worry: Development and preliminary evaluation of the Anxious Thoughts Inventory. *Anxiety, Stress, and Coping, 6,* 289–299.

Wells, A., & Carter, K. (1999). Preliminary tests of a cognitive model of generalized anxiety disorder. *Behaviour Research and Therapy, 37,* 585–594.

Wells, A., & Carter, K. (2001). Further tests of a cognitive model of generalized anxiety disorder: Metacognitions and worry in GAD, panic disorder, social phobia, depression, and nonpatients. *Behavior Therapy, 32,* 85–102.

Wells, A., & Papageorgiou, C. (1998). Relationships between worry, obsessive–compulsive symptoms, and meta-cognitive beliefs. *Behaviour Research and Therapy, 36,* 899–913.

Westen, D. (1994). Toward an integrative model of affect regulation: Applications to social-psychological research. *Journal of Personality, 62,* 641–667.

Williams, J. B. W., Gibbon, M., First, M. B., Spitzer, R. L., Davies, M., Borus, J., Howes, M. J., Kane, J., Pope, H. G., Rounsaville, B., & Wittchen, H. U. (1992). The Structured Clinical Interview for DSM-III-R (SCID): Multisite test–retest reliability. *Archives of General Psychiatry, 49,* 630–636.

Williams, K. E., Chambless, D. L., & Ahrens, A. (1997). Are emotions frightening?: An extension of the fear of fear construct. *Behaviour Research and Therapy, 35,* 239–248.

Zanarini, M. C., Skodol, A. E., Bender, D., Dolan, R., Sanislow, C., Schaefer, E., Morey, L. C., Grilo, C. M., Shea, M. T., McGashan, T. H., & Gunderson, J. G. (2000). The collaborative longitudinal personality disorder study: Reliability of Axis I and II diagnoses. *Journal of Personality Disorders, 14,* 291–299.

Zung, W. W. K. (1971). A rating instrument for anxiety disorders. *Psychosomatics, 12,* 371–379.

CHAPTER 10

A Meta-Analytic Review
of Cognitive-Behavioral Treatments

ROBERT A. GOULD
STEVEN A. SAFREN
DAVID O'NEILL WASHINGTON
MICHAEL W. OTTO

An accurate review of the outcome literature on cognitive-behavioral treatment (CBT) for generalized anxiety disorder (GAD) faces three immediate challenges. The first is the heterogeneity of interventions that have been applied alone or in combination as the treatment(s) under study. This heterogeneity makes it difficult to form a single standard for CBT; instead, we are best able to describe the *range* of CBT interventions that appear helpful for GAD, and to discuss the magnitude of benefit for each. The second challenge is the heterogeneity of control groups that have been used as the comparison conditions in outcome studies. Not all comparison groups are created equal; a wait-list condition is typically easier to surpass in efficacy than a supportive treatment program or a pill placebo. For these reasons, estimates of the magnitude of treatment gains need to be discussed relative to the standard for comparison.

Finally, in any review, care needs to be taken to ensure that core features of the disorder under treatment—in this case, chronic worry and anxious arousal—are modified by treatment, and that change is not confined to or explained by reductions in co-occurring symptoms (e.g., depressed mood). In the studies of CBT for GAD, many different self-report, clinician-rated, and physiological measures have been utilized.

Measures of anxiety or worry have included the Hamilton Anxiety Rating Scale (Hamilton, 1959), the Fear Questionnaire (Marks & Mathews, 1979), the State–Trait Anxiety Inventory (Spielberger, Gorsuch, & Lushene, 1970), the Zung Self-Rating Anxiety Scale (Zung, 1971), the Covi Scale for Anxiety (Covi & Lipman, 1984), the Fear Survey Schedule (Wolpe & Lang, 1964), the Cognitive–Somatic Anxiety Questionnaire (Schwartz, Davidson, & Goleman, 1978), and the Penn State Worry Questionnaire (Meyer, Miller, Metzger, & Borkovec, 1990). When depressive symptoms are assessed, the Beck Depression Inventory (Beck, Steer, & Garbin, 1988) and the Hamilton Rating Scale for Depression (Hamilton, 1960) have been most commonly used.

Our task in reviewing the literature on the treatment of GAD is made easier by two earlier meta-analytic reviews (Borkovec & Ruscio, 2001; Gould, Otto, Pollack, & Yap, 1997). Meta-analytic reviews have the benefit of providing some of the broadest perspectives on treatment outcome, by helping reviewers to evaluate treatment outcome when every study of adequate design is considered. Also, the focus on effect sizes (ESs) in a meta-analytic review allows greater attention to subtle differences that may arise between active treatments. This is especially important in the literature on CBT for GAD, as most studies include only 15–20 patients per treatment condition, providing only limited power for detecting differences between active treatments. Although these differences are unlikely to attain statistical significance in individual studies, we can use ESs to provide a commentary on the magnitude of these effects across studies.

In addition to global statements about outcome, any review should also provide a perspective on the tolerability of treatments, at least as assessed by the rate of attrition from the trial. This provides a rough metric of whether patients were able or willing to comply with treatment procedures, and thus some suggestion of how well these treatments would be accepted as part of clinical practice, where patients have a choice (nonrandomized) of the type of intervention they will accept. As will be detailed below, acceptability does not appear to be a problem for patients with GAD; dropout rates tend to be relatively low, regardless of the type of treatment provided. Nonetheless, this tentative conclusion, as well as other conclusions discussed below, has to be evaluated relative to the limited number of GAD outcome trials. Interestingly, we have found only three additional studies on GAD that met criteria for inclusion in our meta-analysis since our original 1997 meta-analysis (Laberge, Dugas, & Ladouceur, 2000; Ladouceur et al., 2000; Stanley, Beck, & Glassco, 1996). Despite that fact that GAD has at times been considered the "basic" anxiety disorder (Rapee & Barlow, 1991), investigations of the effectiveness of CBT for this disorder continue to lag behind the advances in CBT for other disorders.

STRATEGIES FOR A META-ANALYTIC REVIEW

We employed methods similar to those detailed in our earlier paper (Gould, Otto, et al., 1997). Briefly, we included only studies utilizing a control group and computed effect sizes relative to the control condition (no treatment, wait list, or psychological placebo) to provide an estimate of the advantage of the active treatment over the control group. Smith and Glass's delta procedures (Glass, McGaw, & Smith, 1981) were used to compute ESs—the difference between the means of the posttreatment control (M_c) and active treatment group (M_t) divided by the standard deviation of the control group (SD_c) at posttreatment:

$$ES = \frac{M_t - M_c}{SD_c}$$

Alternative procedures (see Gould, Otto, et al., 1997) were used when this information was not provided in the research report. Different methods were used if means and standard deviations were not available in the study report. For example, if only a t statistic was reported, the ES was calculated as follows: ES $= t\,(1/n_t + 1/n_c)$. If the results were reported by F score, t was calculated by $t = F$; then the formula for t was applied. Separate procedures were used if only significance levels or the proportions of patients improved or not improved were reported (see procedures by Glass et al., 1981, pp. 128–129). As a rough guideline, Cohen (1988) has estimated that an ES of 0.2 is a small effect, 0.5 is a medium effect, and 0.8 is a large effect.

We categorized studies as "cognitive-behavioral" interventions when cognitive restructuring, situational exposure, imaginal exposure, systematic desensitization, relaxation training (both with and without biofeedback), and/or anxiety management training were utilized. Studies were also required either to employ *Diagnostic and Statistical Manual of Mental Disorders* (DSM-III, DSM-III-R, or DSM-IV) criteria (American Psychiatric Association, 1980, 1987, 1994) for GAD, or clearly to have met those standards had they been applied.

Studies were identified by using four strategies: (1) a CD-ROM PsychLIT (American Psychological Association, 1994) search for the years 1974 (inception of the database) to June 2000; (2) a search of the MEDLINE database (National Library of Medicine, 2000) from 1966 to June 2000; (3) examination of the reference sections of articles located from the first two searches; and (4) inclusions of "in press" articles and unpublished reports if we had knowledge of them from presentations at national conferences prior to October 2000. Our search strategies ultimately produced 16 studies meeting criteria for inclusion; 13 of these studies were from our original 1997 meta-analysis, and 3 others from our search. Four studies were excluded because of a failure to use an adequate control group (e.g., open trials); two for using mixed samples of patients with GAD and with panic disorder; two for reporting data identical to those presented in later-published studies; and one for failing to use DSM criteria for GAD. Two of the studies excluded for inadequate controls were the only unpublished studies uncovered in our search.

When possible, ESs were computed for each dependent variable at posttreatment and at follow-up. If studies employed multiple measures of the severity of anxiety, we calculated a mean ES by averaging across all the dependent measures within a study (see Rosenthal, 1991).

META-ANALYSIS RESULTS

In Table 10.1 we present the ESs for anxiety and depression for each study, along with information regarding the type of control condition employed, sample size, and dropout rates for each experimental group. The ESs in Table 10.1 are for short-term (i.e., less than or equal to 16 weeks) treatment outcome. Statistical comparisons in this meta-analysis are chiefly based on the ES of primary interest—the ES for anxiety severity. Given the limitations of statistical power for some comparisons, 95% confidence intervals (CIs) of the overall obtained ESs are reported for major comparisons in the text of this chapter.

CHARACTERISTICS OF THE SAMPLES IN STUDIES OF CBT FOR GAD

Women constituted an average of 64% of the samples in the studies reviewed. Duration of GAD was reported in 10 of 16 studies, and the mean period for which patients had had GAD was 6 years, 2 months ($SD = 5$ years, 11 months; range = 6 months to 17 years, 1 month). Simple regression analyses revealed that between-study differences in the mean duration of the disorder were not associated with the degree of anxiety reduction achieved ($F = 0.26$, $R = .17$, $df = 9$, $p \approx .65$).

The degree to which researchers assessed comorbid Axis I disorders was variable. Most studies specified that patients with comorbid problems of alcohol or other substance abuse/dependence, psychotic disorders, and suicidality were excluded. Patients with organic brain syndrome, epilepsy, or disabling medical conditions were also typically excluded. Very few researchers required that patients have a relatively "pure" form of GAD with no concurrent Axis I problems. The majority

TABLE 10.1. Mean Posttreatment Effect Sizes (ESs) for Measures of Anxiety and Depression for Cognitive-Behavioral Interventions for Generalized Anxiety Disorder (GAD)

Study
  Treatment group(s)
    Control group
	n	Drop-
		out
		rate
			Tx length	Anxiety
				ES
					Depres-
					sion ES

Barlow et al. (1992)	65		15 weeks		
Relax.		38%		0.77	0.88
CT		24%		0.91	1.13
Relax + CT		8%		0.95	0.95
Wait-list control		50%			
Blowers et al. (1987)	66		10 weeks		
AMT		ND		0.61	NR
Nondir. counseling		ND		0.48	NR
Wait-list control		ND			
Borkovec & Costello (1993)	55		6 weeks		
CBT		ND		0.69	0.71
Applied relax.		ND		0.53	0.43
Nondir. therapy		ND			
Borkovec et al. (1987)	30		6 weeks		
CT + relax.		0%		0.72	0.48
Nondir. therapy + relax.		0%			
Butler et al. (1987)	45		12 weeks		
AMT		0%		0.99	NR
Wait-list control		17%			
Butler et al. (1991)	57		12 weeks		
CBT		0%		0.82	0.98
BT		16%		0.19	0.44
Wait-list control		0%			
Cragan & Deffenbacher (1984)	61		6 weeks		
AMT		5%		1.15	1.16
Relax. self-control		5%		0.62	0.73
Wait-list control		19%			
Laberge et al. (2000)	37		12 weeks		
CBT		11%		0.83	NR
Wait-list control		13%			
Ladouceur et al. (2000)	26		16 weeks		
CBT		0%		1.86	1.91
Wait-list control		0%			
Power et al. (1989)	31		6 weeks		
CBT		16%		1.28	NR
Diazepam		ND		0.42	NR
Pill placebo		ND			

(continued)

TABLE 10.1. *(continued)*

Study Treatment group(s) Control group	*n*	Drop- out rate	Tx length	Anxiety ES	Depres- sion ES
Power et al. (1990)	101		10 weeks		
Diazepam		12%		0.39	0.42
CBT		9%		1.24	0.50
Diazepam + CBT		5%		1.44	0.72
Pill placebo + CBT		14%		0.95	0.41
Pill placebo		14%			
Rice et al. (1993)	45		4 weeks		
Relax. with biofeedback		10%		0.84	NR
Placebo control		ND			
Stanley et al. (1996)	48		14.5 weeks		
CBT		30%		0.48	−0.09
Supportive psychotherapy		35%			
Townsend et al. (1975)	30		4 weeks		
Relax. with biofeedback		7%		−0.17	NR
Nondir. group therapy		47%			
White et al. (1992)	109		6 weeks		
CT		12%		0.80	1.03
BT		15%		0.76	0.91
CBT		16%		0.80	0.89
Subconscious training		0%		0.40	0.35
Wait-list control		0%			
Woodward & Jones (1980)	27		8 weeks		
Cognitive restructuring		0%		0.07	NR
Systematic desensitization		ND		0.59	NR
CBT		ND		0.74	NR
No-treatment control		ND			

Note. AMT, anxiety management training; BT, behavior therapy; CBT, a cognitive–behavioral treatment "package" (i.e., a combination of cognitive and behavioral techniques); CT, cognitive therapy; ND, not determinable; nondir., nondirective; NR, not reported; relax., relaxation; tx = treatment. According to Cohen (1988), 0.2 may be considered a small ES, 0.5 a medium ES, and 0.8 a large ES.

(e.g., Barlow, Rapee, & Brown, 1992; Borkovec & Costello, 1993) allowed patients with comorbid anxiety disorders as long as GAD was the primary disorder. Similarly, the majority of studies allowed patients with depression as long as the depression was secondary to GAD. Rates of comorbid panic disorder (19%; *n* = 7 studies), social phobia (19%; *n* = 7 studies), and major depression (24%; *n* = 5 studies) are unreliable estimates because of the small number of studies reporting these data. Borkovec, Abel, and Newman (1995) found somewhat higher rates of comorbid social phobia (29.1%) for patients with GAD than we found in our sample. Of greater interest, they found that for patients receiving psychotherapy, the presence of comorbid diagnoses declined significantly from pretreament to follow-up. Axis II psychopathology was not used as an exclusionary criterion in any study. None of these studies appeared to have used standardized batteries to assess personality problems. Future research is needed to tease out the relationship between CBT of GAD and Axis II psychopathology.

TREATMENTS AND TREATMENT OUTCOME

CBT interventions for GAD consisted of a number of treatment techniques alone and in combination, including cognitive restructuring, relaxation training, anxiety management training, situational and imaginal exposure, and systematic desensitization. "Anxiety management training" is a specific set of cognitive and behavioral techniques that focuses on patients' fears of being unable to cope with the cause of their worry; it combines relaxation, self-talk, and practice in the use of anxiety-evoking imagery followed by reassuring imagery ("image switching"). Ladouceur and colleagues (2000) used cognitive strategies that specifically targeted intolerance of uncertainty, erroneous beliefs about worry, and cognitive avoidance. Studies that reported using behavior therapy alone ($n = 2$) employed graded exposure, functional analysis of behavior chains, and relaxation training. Studies using relaxation with biofeedback used primarily the same progressive muscle relaxation techniques used in other relaxation studies, along with biofeedback strategies to decrease somatic sensations of anxiety. In total, 16 studies that included 25 treatment interventions utilized cognitive and/or behavioral techniques. Neither the subconscious training intervention (White, Keenan, & Brooks, 1992), the nondirective counseling (Blowers, Cobb, & Mathews, 1987), nor the pill placebo plus CBT intervention (Power et al., 1990) was classified as a CBT technique. The Power and colleagues (1990) intervention was excluded because it was thought to be qualitatively different from a "CBT-alone" condition. Patients receiving a pill placebo plus CBT may have very different expectations for, and attributions about, the effectiveness of treatment than those receiving CBT alone may have. Results from the study also confirmed higher effect sizes for the CBT-alone condition relative to the pill placebo plus CBT at both posttreatment (Day 42) and follow-up (Day 70).

Mean ESs for each CBT condition in each of the treatment studies are presented in Table 10.1. The mean ES for anxiety across all studies was 0.73 (95% CI = 0.58–0.85). Comparison of this effect size to the null hypothesis of no increase in efficacy over the control condition (ES = 0.0) was statistically significant, $t(24) = 10.25$, $p < .0001$. The mean ES for depression was 0.77 (95% CI = 0.64–0.88). Comparison of this ES to the null hypothesis of no increase in efficacy over the control condition (ES = 0.0) was also statistically significant, $t(15) = 9.92$, $p < .0001$. The mean dropout rate was 11.4% ($SD = 10.1$).

The majority of studies employed interventions that combined cognitive and behavioral techniques ($n = 11$ treatment groups), and these interventions had a mean anxiety ES of 0.90. Anxiety management training (utilizing relaxation, cognitive coaching, and use of imagery) was among the next most commonly used strategies ($n = 3$ treatment interventions) and yielded an anxiety ES of 0.91. Both relaxation training alone ($n = 3$ treatment interventions; ES = 0.64) and cognitive therapy alone ($n = 3$ treatment interventions; ES = 0.59) yielded anxiety ESs that were smaller than those of combined cognitive and behavioral therapies. Interventions employing only behavioral techniques, such as graded exposure, functional analysis of behavior chains, and relaxation training ($n = 3$ treatment interventions), yielded similarly modest anxiety ESs (ES = 0.51). Relaxation training with biofeedback ($n = 2$ treatment interventions) had a mean anxiety ES of only 0.34.

Based on our estimates, we can hypothesize that studies comparing a complete CBT package and its component interventions (e.g., relaxation training or cognitive techniques alone) would rarely achieve significant differences between conditions if sample sizes were as small as is typical for this literature (see Borkovec & Matthews, 1988). Although studies to date suggest that there may be an anxiety ES in the range of 0.3 for the difference between full CBT packages and component interventions, ESs in this range require much larger sample sizes to achieve significance than have been included in most studies of CBT for GAD.

COMPARISON TO BENZODIAZEPINE TREATMENT

Two studies compared CBT to medication treatments (Power et al., 1989, 1990). In both cases the medication was the benzodiazepine diazepam, which achieved a mean ES of 0.41 relative to a pill placebo comparison condition. This ES was smaller than the ES for pharmacotherapy studies using benzodiazepines in our previous meta-analysis (ES = 0.70; Gould, Otto, et al., 1997). In the two Power and colleagues studies, CBT achieved large anxiety ESs (mean ES = 1.26) relative to pill placebo. Examination of the ES of the combination of diazepam and CBT in one study (Power et al., 1990) indicated that the combination may have substantial benefit over diazepam alone and a small benefit over CBT alone during acute treatment. However, given evidence for the relatively less successful out-

comes of this combination in the treatment of panic disorder in comparison to CBT alone (Otto, Pollack, & Sabatino, 1996), such combination
treatment strategies should be approached cautiously until additional data
have been accumulated. In addition, benzodiazepines are no longer considered the pharmacological treatment of choice for GAD, with the field
devoting increasing attention to the role of selective serotonin reuptake
inhibitors (SSRIs; Smoller & Pollack, 1996; see also Lydiard & Monnier,
Chapter 14, this volume). We are aware of no published studies comparing CBT with an SSRI in the treatment of GAD.

FACTORS AFFECTING STUDY OUTCOME

We next examined the influence of format and amount of treatment on
outcome. Ten treatment interventions employed a group format, and 15
provided an individual treatment. Statistical analyses revealed no significant differences between studies utilizing group (ES = 0.62) versus individual (ES = 0.83) treatment, t (23) = 1.85, p = .22. Amount of treatment was
operationalized as the product of the number of hours of CBT and the
number of weeks of treatment. For example, a patient receiving 3 hours of
CBT per week for 6 weeks would receive a total of 18 hours of treatment.
The mean number of hours of CBT was 10.1 hours for the 16 studies examined (SD = 3.7; range = 4–16). Simple regression analyses revealed that
studies with greater amounts of treatment were not associated with better
outcome (F = 0.12, R = .05, df = 22, p = .77).

OTHER METHODOLOGICAL ISSUES

Power and Sharp (1995) criticized a number of studies of CBT for panic
disorder because of their failure to control for concurrent psychotropic
medication use (see also Otto, Gould, & McLean, 1996). The authors
questioned whether the positive outcomes seen with CBT would have
been as strong in the absence of concurrent medication. Although controlling for external medication use may improve the internal validity of a
study, it is likely to decrease the external validity of a study, given that
many patients with GAD are on medication at the time that they seek
psychosocial treatment (Borkovec & Whisman, 1996). Nevertheless, we
examined this issue by comparing the ESs of CBT studies that allowed
concurrent medication use (n = 19 treatment interventions) to those that
restricted its use (n = 6 treatment interventions). For purposes of classification, we designated as "allowing use" those studies that did not specify
such use as an exclusion criterion or did not comment on it. The mean

anxiety ES for studies allowing use was 0.70; for those restricting use, it was 0.88. There was no statistical difference between these two conditions, t (24) = 1.55, p = .20. As such, concurrent medication use did not appear to have a positive effect on treatment outcome in these studies.

Another methodological issue concerns the use of independent assessors for the measurement of outcome. Assessors of outcome who are not blind to treatment classification risk biasing the outcome and confounding the interpretation of results. Studies using independent assessors tended to yield a higher mean anxiety ES (ES = 0.77; n = 16) than those that did not (ES = 0.48; n = 9), but these differences were not statistically significant, t (24) = 1.37, p = .18.

LONGER-TERM TREATMENT OUTCOME

Do treatments for GAD maintain their salutary effects over time? In our earlier (Gould, Otto, et al., 1997) meta-analysis, we set a criterion of 6 months as a minimum follow-up period needed to assess long-term outcome. In the present meta-analysis, eight studies provided reliable follow-up data, and these are presented in Table 10.2.

Effect sizes in Table 10.2 are measures of within-group changes in the severity of anxiety and depression from posttreatment to follow-up. ESs were calculated by subtracting the mean of the treatment group at follow-up from the mean of the treatment group at posttreatment and dividing by the standard deviation of the treatment group at posttreatment:

$$\text{ES} = \frac{M_t \text{ (follow-up)} - M_t \text{ (posttreatment)}}{SD_t \text{ (posttreatment)}}$$

The use of this "uncontrolled" ES was necessitated by the practical and ethical difficulties of maintaining patients in control conditions over extended periods of time. With this formula, negative ESs indicate that the treatment group had greater anxiety at follow-up relative to posttreatment, whereas positive values show that the treatment group continued to make gains over time. The mean anxiety ES across 18 treatment interventions was 0.02, suggesting that reductions in anxiety were maintained and very slightly improved at follow-up. Eighty-five percent of patients in these studies were able to complete follow-up measures. Measures of depression severity in the follow-up period were reported in only four studies (8 treatment interventions). The mean depression ES was 0.10, showing continued modest decreases in depression for patients in these studies over time.

TABLE 10.2. Mean 6-Month Follow-up ESs for Measures of Anxiety after Cognitive-Behavioral Interventions for GAD

Study Treatment group(s) Control group	*n*	% sample	Change from post-tx to FU anxiety ES	Change from post-tx to FU depression ES
Barlow et al. (1992)	65	50%		
Relax.			−0.14	ND
CT			−0.14	ND
Relax. + CT			−0.14	ND
Wait-list control				
Borkovec & Costello (1993)	55	94%		
CBT			0.10	NR
Applied relax.			0.25	NR
Nondir. therapy				
Butler et al. (1987)	45	84%		
AMT			0.0	ND
Wait-list control				
Butler et al. (1991)	57	92%		
CBT			0.12	−0.18
BT			0.11	0.14
Wait-list control				
Ladouceur et al. (2000)	26	100%		
CBT			−0.20	−0.44
Wait-list control				
Power et al. (1990)	101	54%		
Diazepam			−0.77	NR
CBT			−0.52	NR
Diazepam + CBT			−0.76	NR
Pill placebo + CBT			−0.66	NR
Pill placebo				
Stanley et al. (1996)	48	100%		
CBT			0.08	0.05
Supportive psychotherapy				
White et al. (1992)	109	85%		
CT			0.34	0.45
BT			0.35	0.39
CBT			0.28	0.15
Subconscious training			0.01	0.20
Wait-list control				

Note. FU, follow-up. For other abbreviations, and for Cohen's (1988) ES guidelines, see Table 10.1.

RETURNING FROM THE FOREST TO THE TREES

Our meta-analysis indicates that on average, combined CBT packages offer outcomes in the range of large ESs based on Cohen's standards (Cohen, 1988, 1994). This magnitude of ES compares well to the those achieved in the treatment of other anxiety disorders with CBT interventions (e.g., Clum, Clum, & Surls, 1993; Gould, Buckminster, Pollack, Otto, & Yap, 1997; Gould, Otto, & Pollack, 1995).

Combined treatment strategies also appear to have a modest advantage (in the range of a small effect size) over single-component treatments. To illustrate this effect, consider the study by Butler, Fennell, Robson, and Gelder (1991) comparing a combined cognitive and behavioral intervention to a more purely behavioral intervention that did not include an explicit cognitive component and to a wait-list condition. The behavior therapy condition included relaxation training, exposures, and planned pleasurable activities. The combined CBT condition included identifying thoughts and generating alternatives, activity scheduling, and planned behavioral assignments, but did not include relaxation training. Significant differences were noted among the three conditions at post-treatment. The general pattern of results was such that both active treatment groups outperformed the wait-list condition, and the combined CBT condition outperformed the behavior therapy condition on several measures.

The Butler and colleagues (1991) study was also noteworthy for illustrating that despite significant improvement, few patients were fully returned to full functioning. Indeed, when we classified the number of patients who scored within the range of scores of nonanxious persons on three of the outcome measures, only 32% of those receiving the CBT and 16% of those receiving the behavior therapy met these criteria for high end-state functioning. Clearly, despite the effectiveness of current treatments, additional advances are required to help more patients make the transition from "improved" to "well."

OTHER RELEVANT STUDIES

Since the publication of our original 1997 meta-analysis, two other important studies have been conducted. These studies are not included in our present meta-analysis but deserve some mention. In a study that did not use a control group, Öst and Breitholtz (2000) compared applied relaxation to cognitive therapy. Thirty-six patients were randomly assigned to either of these conditions and received 12 weekly individual treatment sessions. An uncontrolled, within-group ES analysis (similar to the analysis we did for our follow-up data) yielded ESs of 1.90 for applied relaxation and 2.34 for cognitive therapy. There were no significant differences between these active treatments, given the small sample size. Dropout rates were small for both conditions: 12% for relaxation and 5% for cognitive therapy. The authors reported that the proportions of clinically significant improvement were 53% and 62% for applied relaxation and cognitive therapy, respectively, at posttreatment, and 67% and 56% at 1-year follow-up.

Even more recently, Borkovec, Newman, Pincus, and Lytle (2002) compared cognitive therapy, applied relaxation with self-control desensitization, and CBT in a study with a 2-year follow-up assessment. Seventy-six clients were randomly assigned to one of the three treatment conditions for 14 weekly therapy sessions. Uncontrolled within-group ES analyses produced ESs of 2.20 for cognitive therapy, 1.85 for the relaxation–desensitization treatment, and 1.86 for CBT. These results were largely maintained over a 24-month follow-up period. Taken together, results from the Öst and Breitholtz (2000) and the Borkovec and colleagues (2002) studies support the conclusion of our meta-analysis that CBT approaches yield strong and durable treatment effects. However, it should be noted that ESs from these studies cannot be compared directly to those in our meta-analysis, because they were not derived relative to a control condition.

CLOSING REMARKS

One limitation of meta-analysis should be addressed. First, both for meta-analyses and for review papers, an ES estimate may be inflated because of biases in publication. There may be a tendency for editors and reviewers to publish papers with positive results, whereas studies with negative results may be less likely to emerge in the treatment outcome literature. Thus the true ES of an intervention may be inflated, in that the negative or insignificant ESs may not be included. To account for this, our review did include dissertation abstracts; however, technological and practical limitations do not allow for the inclusion of all unpublished studies. Furthermore, we calculated the fail-safe n value for our meta-analysis based on procedures from Rosenthal and Rosnow (1991). The results indicated that 5,115 unpublished studies with null results would need to exist before one could conclude that our findings were due to sampling bias.

Our meta-analytic review of the GAD treatment outcome literature indicates that CBT tends to offer significant advantages over no treatment, a pill placebo, or a nondirective control. These advantages also appear to be robustly maintained over longer-term follow-up intervals. Moreover, combination treatment strategies—utilizing cognitive restructuring, relaxation training, and at times exposure procedures—appear to have an advantage over single treatment elements, although this advantage is on the order of a small ES. Such small ESs are unlikely to be detected in outcome studies with typically small sample sizes.

Unfortunately, such relatively small sample sizes have been the standard in CBT outcome studies in GAD (as well as many other CBT outcome studies). Consequently, evaluation of treatment effects only in the context of significant differences obtained in a single trial has the potential of obscuring the additive benefit, albeit small, of fuller treatment packages over single-component interventions.

The success of CBT packages for GAD, reflecting large ESs on average, has to be balanced against the reality that these treatments return few patients to "well" status. The clinical and functional significance of treatment gains in these studies needs to be better demonstrated in future studies. Research is also needed to evaluate whether reliable predictors of treatment response can be identified. New treatment interventions tied to better conceptualization of the nature of GAD (see, e.g., Borkovec, Alcaine, & Behar, Chapter 4; MacLeod & Rutherford, Chapter 5; Dugas, Buhr, & Ladouceur, Chapter 6; and Wells, Chapter 7, this volume) hold the potential of providing even larger treatment effects.

REFERENCES

*Denotes study used in this meta-analysis.

American Psychiatric Association. (1980). *Diagnostic and statistical manual of mental disorders* (3rd ed.). Washington, DC: Author.
American Psychiatric Association. (1987). *Diagnostic and statistical manual of mental disorders* (3rd ed., rev.). Washington, DC: Author.
American Psychiatric Association. (1994). *Diagnostic and statistical manual of mental disorders* (4th ed.). Washington, DC: Author.
American Psychological Association. (1994). *PsycLIT database* [CD-ROM]. Washington, DC: Author.
Beck, A. T., Steer, R. A., & Garbin, M. (1988). Psychometric properties of the Beck Depression Inventory: Twenty-five years of evaluation. *Clinical Psychology Review, 8,* 77–100.
*Barlow, D. H., Rapee, R. M., & Brown, T. A. (1992). Behavioral treatment of generalized anxiety disorder. *Behavior Therapy, 23,* 551–570.
*Blowers, C., Cobb, J., & Mathews, A. (1987). generalized anxiety: A controlled treatment study. *Behaviour Research and Therapy, 25,* 493–502.
Borkovec, T. D., Abel, J. L., & Newman, H. (1995). Effects of psychotherapy on comorbid conditions in generalized anxiety disorder. *Journal of Consulting and Clinical Psychology, 63,* 479–483.
*Borkovec, T. D., & Costello, E. (1993). Efficacy of applied relaxation and cognitive-behavioral therapy in the treatment of generalized anxiety disorder. *Journal of Consulting and Clinical Psychology, 61,* 611–619.

Borkovec, T. D., & Mathews, A. M. (1988). Treatment of nonphobic anxiety disorders: A comparison of nondirective, cognitive, and coping desensitization therapy. *Journal of Consulting and Clinical Psychology, 56,* 877–884.

*Borkovec, T. D., Mathews, A. M., Chambers, A., Ebrahimi, S., Lytle, R., & Nelson, R. (1987). The effects of relaxation training with cognitive or nondirective therapy and the role of relaxation-induced anxiety in the treatment of generalized anxiety. *Journal of Consulting and Clinical Psychology, 55,* 883–888.

Borkovec, T. D., Newman, M. G., Pincus, A., & Lytle, R. (2002). A component analysis of cognitive behavioral therapy for generalized anxiety disorder and the role of interpersonal problems. *Journal of Consulting and Clinical Psychology, 70,* 288–298.

Borkovec, T. D., & Ruscio, A. M. (2001). Psychotherapy for generalized anxiety disorder. *Journal of Clinical Psychiatry, 62*(Suppl. 11), 37–42.

Borkovec, T. D., & Whisman, M. A. (1996). Psychosocial treatments for generalized anxiety disorder. In M. Mavissakalian & R. Prien (Eds.), *Long-term treatment of anxiety disorders* (pp. 177–199). Washington, DC: American Psychiatric Association.

*Butler, G., Cullington, G., Hibbert, G., Klimes, I., & Gelder, M. (1987). Anxiety management for persistent generalized anxiety. *British Journal of Psychiatry, 151,* 535–542.

*Butler, G., Fennell, M., Robson, P., & Gelder, M. (1991). Comparison of behavior therapy and cognitive behavior therapy in the treatment of generalized anxiety disorder. *Journal of Consulting and Clinical Psychology, 59,* 167–175.

Clum, G. A., Clum, G. A., & Surls, R. (1993). A meta-analysis for panic disorder. *Journal of Consulting and Clinical Psychology, 61,* 317–326.

Cohen, J. (1988). *Statistical power analysis for the behavioral sciences.* San Diego, CA: Academic Press.

Cohen, J. (1994). The earth is round (*p* < .05). *American Psychologist, 49,* 997–1003.

Covi, L., & Lipman, R. S. (1984). Primary depression or primary anxiety? A possible psychometric approach to diagnose the dilemma. *Clinical Neuropharmacology, 7,* 924–925.

*Cragan, M. K., & Deffenbacher, J. L. (1984). Anxiety management training and relaxation as self-control in the treatment of generalized anxiety in medical outpatients. *Journal of Counseling Psychology, 31,* 123–131.

Glass, G. V., McGaw, B., & Smith, M. L. (1981). *Meta-analysis in social research.* Beverly Hills, CA: Sage.

Gould, R. A., Buckminster, S., Pollack, M. H., Otto, M. W., & Yap, L. (1997). Cognitive-behavioral and pharmacological treatment for social phobia: A meta-analysis. *Clinical Psychology: Science and Practice, 4,* 291–306.

Gould, R. A., Otto, M. W., & Pollack, M. H. (1995). A meta-analysis of treatment outcome for panic disorder. *Clinical Psychology Review, 15,* 819–844.

Gould, R. A., Otto, M. W., Pollack, M. P., & Yap, L. (1997). Cognitive-behavioral and pharmacological treatment of generalized anxiety disorder: A preliminary meta analysis. *Behavior Therapy, 28,* 285–305.

Hamilton, M. (1959). The assessment of anxiety states by rating. *British Journal of Medical Psychology, 32,* 50–55.

Hamilton, M. (1960). A rating scale for depression. *Journal of Neurology, Neurosurgery, and Psychiatry, 23,* 56–62.

*Laberge, M., Dugas, M. J., & Ladouceur, R. (2000). Changes in dysfunctional beliefs before and after a cognitive-behavioural treatment for people with generalized anxiety disorder. *Canadian Journal of Behavioural Science, 32,* 91–96.

*Ladouceur, R., Dugas, M. J., Freeston, M. H., Leger, E., Gagnon, F., & Thibodeau, N.

(2000). Efficacy of a cognitive-behavioral treatment for generalized anxiety disorder: Evaluation in a controlled clinical trial. *Journal of Consulting and Clinical Psychology, 68,* 957–964.

Marks, I. M., & Mathews, A. M. (1979). Brief standard self-rating for phobic patients. *Behaviour Research and Therapy, 17,* 263–267.

Meyer, T. J., Miller, M. L., Metzger, R. L., & Borkovec, T. D. (1990). Development and validation of the Penn State Worry Questionnaire. *Behaviour Research and Therapy, 28,* 487–495.

National Library of Medicine. (2000). *MEDLINE database.* McLean, VA: BRS Information Technologies.

Öst, L. G., & Breitholtz, E. (2000). Applied relaxation vs. cognitive therapy in the treatment of generalized anxiety disorder. *Behaviour Research and Therapy, 38,* 777–790.

Otto, M. W., Gould, R. A., & McLean, R. Y. S. (1996). The effectiveness of cognitive-behavior therapy for panic disorder without concurrent medication treatment: A reply to Power and Sharp. *Journal of Psychopharmacology, 10,* 254–256.

Otto, M. W., Pollack, M. H., & Sabatino, S. (1996). Maintenance of remission following cognitive-behavior therapy for panic disorder: Possible deleterious effects of concurrent medication treatment. *Behavior Therapy, 27,* 473–482.

*Power, K. G., Jerrom, D. W. A., Simpson, R. J., Mitchell, M. J., & Swanson, V. (1989). A controlled comparison of cognitive-behaviour therapy, diazepam and placebo in the management of generalized anxiety. *Behavioural Psychotherapy, 17,* 1–14.

Power, K. G., & Sharp, D. M. (1995). Keep taking the tablets?: Inadequate controls for concurrent psychotropic medication in studies of psychological treatments for panic disorder. *Journal of Psychopharmacology, 9,* 71–72.

*Power, K. G., Simpson, R. J., Swanson, V., Wallace, L. A., Feistner, A. T. C., & Sharp, D. (1990). A controlled comparison of cognitive-behaviour therapy, diazepam, and placebo, alone and in combination, for the treatment of generalized anxiety disorder. *Journal of Anxiety Disorders, 4,* 267–292.

Rapee, R. M., & Barlow, D. H. (Eds.). (1991). *Chronic anxiety: Generalized anxiety disorder and mixed anxiety–depression.* New York: Guilford Press.

*Rice, K. M., Blanchard, E. B., & Purcell, M. (1993). Biofeedback treatments for generalized anxiety disorder: Preliminary results. *Biofeedback and Self-Regulation, 18,* 93–105.

Rosenthal, R. (1991). *Meta-analytic procedures for social research* (rev. ed.). Newbury Park, CA: Sage.

Rosenthal, R., & Rosnow, R. (1991). *Essentials of behavioral research: Methods and data analysis* (2nd ed.). New York: McGraw-Hill.

Schwartz, G. E., Davidson, R. J., & Goleman, D. J. (1978). Patterning of cognitive and somatic processes in the self-regulation of anxiety: Effects of meditation versus exercise. *Psychosomatic Medicine, 40,* 321–328.

Smoller, J. W., & Pollack, M. H. (1996). Pharmacologic approaches to treatment-resistant social phobia and generalized anxiety disorder. In M. Pollack, M. W. Otto, & J. Rosenbaum (Eds.), *Challenges in clinical practice: Pharmacologic and psychosocial strategies* (pp. 141–170). New York: Guilford Press.

Spielberger, C. D., Gorsuch, R. L., & Lushene, R. E. (1970). *State–Trait Anxiety Inventory.* Palo Alto, CA: Consulting Psychologists Press.

*Stanley, M. A., Beck, J. G., & Glassco, J. D. (1996). Treatment of generalized anxiety in older adults: A preliminary comparison of cognitive-behavioral and supportive approaches. *Behavior Therapy, 27,* 565–581.

*Townsend, R. E., House, J. F., & Addario, D. (1975). A comparison of biofeedback-mediated relaxation and group therapy in the treatment of chronic anxiety. *American Journal of Psychiatry, 132,* 598–601.

*White, J., Keenan, M., & Brooks, N. (1992). Stress control: A controlled comparative investigation of large group therapy for generalized anxiety disorder. *Behavioural Psychotherapy, 20,* 97–114.

Wolpe, J., & Lang, P. J. (1964). A fear survey schedule for use in behaviour therapy. *Behaviour Research and Therapy, 2,* 27–30.

*Woodward, R., & Jones, R. B. (1980). Cognitive restructuring treatment: A controlled trial with anxious patients. *Behaviour Research and Therapy, 18,* 401–407.

Zung, W. W. K. (1971). A rating instrument for anxiety disorders. *Psychosomatics, 12,* 371–379.

CHAPTER 11

Cognitive-Behavioral Therapy

ROBERT L. LEAHY

Until recently, the treatment of generalized anxiety disorder (GAD) focused on the use of anxiety management techniques, such as relaxation, activity scheduling, and assertiveness training. Although these primarily behavioral approaches had some efficacy in reducing hyperarousal, the diffuse and general worry that characterizes GAD was not adequately addressed. For example, relaxation training—especially when paired with the presentation of threatening stimuli—has limited value for patients with GAD, since the worries of these individuals are directed at a variety of changing stimuli. Moreover, patients with GAD often do not experience increased arousal during worry, since worry often inhibits emotion (see Borkovec & Hu, 1990; Borkovec, Lyonfields, Wiser, & Diehl, 1993; Wells & Papageorgiou, 1995); this too makes relaxation training alone a treatment of limited relevance. Often, the increased anxious arousal occurs before or after worry.

Increased knowledge of the parameters of worry, a central component of GAD, has increased practitioners' ability to provide a multidimensional treatment approach. As the chapters in this volume illustrate, worry is driven by (1) intolerance of uncertainty (Dugas, Buhr, & Ladouceur, Chapter 6, this volume; Dugas, Gosselin, & Ladouceur, 2001); (2) the belief that worry motivates a person, prepares him or her for events, and prevents negative outcomes (Borkovec, Shadick, & Hopkins, 1991; Wells, Chapter 7, this volume); (3) facilitation of emotional avoidance (Borkovec & Hu, 1990; Borkovec & Inz, 1990; Borkovec et al., 1993; Mennin, Turk, Heimberg, & Carmin, in press); and (4) "incubation" of further worry and emotional arousal as a result of emotional avoidance (Borkovec, Alcaine,

& Behar, Chapter 4, and Wells, Chapter 7, this volume). In the current chapter, I examine how a multicomponent cognitive-behavioral model may address hyperarousal, metacognitive beliefs that sustain worry, emotional and cognitive avoidance, intolerance of uncertainty, and impractical problem solving.

ASSESSMENT

The purposes of clinical assessment are to evaluate possible targets for treatment, establish baselines for various symptoms and behaviors, and to develop a case conceptualization that can guide treatment and anticipate roadblocks that may arise. At the American Institute for Cognitive Therapy, we conduct a rather lengthy evaluation, relying partly on extensive self-report forms that assess depression, anxiety, relationship conflicts, various psychiatric symptoms, emotional processing, and decision making. However, because these are not the focus in the current chapter, I do not focus here on the specifics of these particular evaluations. Several of the measures mentioned in this section are described by Turk, Heimberg, and Mennin in Chapter 9 of this volume.

Comorbid Conditions

Individuals with GAD may often present with other conditions requiring attention. For example, in many cases depression is a consequence of GAD (see Kessler, Walters, & Wittchen, Chapter 2, this volume). Social phobia and other anxiety disorders are also common comorbid Axis I conditions. Clinical experience suggests that avoidant, dependent, and obsessive–compulsive personality disorders are commonly comorbid with GAD as well. A pessimistic outlook, demand for certainty, intolerance of discomfort, low frustration tolerance, and sensitivity to rejection or failure may be common features across the comorbid conditions. Since many of the techniques that are useful with GAD are also useful with these other disorders, the first strategy of treatment might be to focus on these common features, utilizing the interventions and conceptualizations outlined in this chapter. However, when GAD is comorbid with major depression that is accompanied by hopelessness and suicidal ideation, these latter symptoms should be the first focus of treatment.

Physiological Arousal

During the assessment, the clinician should evaluate any signs of excessive arousal, including sweating, motor tension, excessive movement, clenching, sleep disturbance, or startle response. Some of these symptoms can be assessed with the Beck Anxiety Inventory (Beck, Epstein, Brown, &

Steer, 1988; Beck & Steer, 1990). These symptoms may become targets for interventions focusing on reducing general hyperarousal.

Attention and Concentration

Anxiety often interferes with the ability to direct attention to daily life issues, such as work, conversations, or even personal self-care. Inability to remember what one has read, appointments, or work assignments, and "spacing out" during conversations with people, are signs that worry and arousal are interfering. These can be useful targets for change.

Worry

Assessment can also focus on various aspects of worry, such as the extent, content, and metacognitive components of worry and intolerance of uncertainty. Of specific relevance are the Penn State Worry Questionnaire (Meyer, Miller, Metzger, & Borkovec, 1990), the Worry Domains Questionnaire (Tallis, Eysenck, & Mathews, 1992), the Intolerance of Uncertainty Scale (Freeston, Rhéaume, Letarte, Dugas, & Ladouceur, 1994; see also Appendix 6.1 in Dugas et al., Chapter 6, this volume), and the Meta-Cognitions Questionnaire (Cartwright-Hatton & Wells, 1997). Clinicians generally will not utilize these questionnaires at intake; however, once the diagnosis of GAD is considered, one or more of these scales can be helpful in identifying problem areas, helping the patient and therapist develop a cognitive conceptualization of the problem, and targeting metacognitive issues for treatment. Wells's (Chapter 7, this volume) metacognitive model stresses not only schematic vulnerabilities (i.e., the content areas of personal schemata, such as beliefs that the self is defective or unlovable), but also the individual's views of how his or her thinking functions to prevent danger or how this thinking may go out of control. These metacognitive issues include the beliefs that worry protects and prepares the individual, that the individual needs certainty, and that he or she needs to worry about certain content areas (e.g., relationships and money).

Behavioral Deficits and Excesses

Like major depressive disorder, GAD is often characterized by behavioral problems. Assessment should evaluate directly whether the patient is procrastinating or avoiding any activities, is managing time effectively, or is engaging in recurrent off-task behaviors (e.g., watching television, surfing the Web, or other trivial behaviors that interfere with more important behaviors). The therapist should directly raise these issues, since many patients are reluctant to bring up problems that they avoid—often because they utilize cognitive and emotional avoidance to manage their anxiety. Avoided activities may include paying taxes, assuring that one has proper insurance coverage, obtaining adequate medical examinations, planning a healthy diet, exercising, returning phone calls from friends, and completing work assignments.

Cognitive Characteristics

Cognitive assessment should evaluate the patient's typical automatic thoughts, underlying assumptions, and personal and interpersonal schemata. "Automatic thoughts" are thoughts that occur spontaneously and are often associated with negative affect or dysfunctional behavior. Typical categories of automatic thought distortions for patients with GAD are fortune telling (e.g., "I'll fail the exam"), catastrophizing (e.g., "It would be terrible if I got rejected"), mind reading (e.g., "She thinks I'm a loser"), personalizing (e.g., "This only happens to me"), labeling (e.g., "I'm pathetic"), and all-or-nothing thinking (e.g., "Nothing works out for me"). As these thoughts exemplify, many of these patients are depressed precisely because of this pessimistic pattern of thinking.

Other examples of automatic thoughts are "He thinks I'm a loser" (mind reading), "She will leave me" (fortune telling), and "He's always critical" (all-or-nothing thinking). Maladaptive assumptions include "I need a relationship to be happy" and "My value depends on how others see me."

"Underlying assumptions" include many "if–then" rules upon which the patient relies. These include such conditional rules as "If I don't know for sure, then it won't work out," "If I don't have a perfect performance, then I'm a failure," "If people don't like me, then I am a terrible person," and "If I don't know for sure, then I should wait until I do." Conditional strategies or rules for obtaining certainty, perfection, approval, and comfort include the following:

- "I should collect as much information as possible—to be sure."
- "I should wait until I have ruled out all risk."
- "I should wait until I feel ready."
- "I should cover everything, so that my work will be beyond reproach."
- "I need to make up for having waited so long by doing an extraordinary job."
- "I should please everyone."
- "I should avoid any emotional discomfort."

Interpersonal Issues

Many individuals with GAD worry about interpersonal issues. Consequently, assessment of the interpersonal domain should examine relationship conflicts, relationship exits, and problems with assertiveness. For example, one woman with GAD worried about her relationship with her partner, with whom she had frequent arguments. These focused on her concern that he was not attentive enough, that he was losing interest, and that he would leave her. She also had recently experienced a conflict with a friend that appeared to her to mark the end of their relationship. This sensitized her to issues of rejection and abandonment, and activated her mind reading, personalizing, and catastrophic fortune telling.

TREATMENT

Psychoeducation and Therapeutic Contracting

Information on GAD

We provide all patients at the American Institute for Cognitive Therapy with the patient information form for GAD from the book *Treatment Plans and Interventions for Depression and Anxiety Disorders* (Leahy & Holland, 2000). This form is shown in Table 11.1. Patients learn that they have GAD; that this disorder is accompanied by symptoms of arousal, irritability, and worry; and that they may believe that their worries will go out of control, drive them insane, or result in serious illness. It provides the patient with a conceptualization of generalized anxiety, based on his or her probable belief that worry is a form of problem solving and that it may prepare and protect him or her from the worst. This information also states that the patient will be asked to carry out self-help homework assignments, and that cognitive-behavioral therapy has a good chance of reducing the patient's anxiety.

Information on Cognitive-Behavioral Therapy

We also provide each patient with information about cognitive-behavioral therapy. This includes requesting that the patient read David Burns's *The Feeling Good Handbook* (1989). This is an excellent guide for anxious or depressed patients, in that it helps them understand how their thoughts affect their feelings and behavior, and how they can modify their thinking through various cognitive and behavioral interventions. These include identifying the cognitive distortions in various thoughts, examining the degree of belief in and the emotions accompanying each thought, evaluating the evidence for and against the thought, evaluating the costs and benefits of holding the thought, and utilizing the double-standard technique. Examples of cognitive distortions that a patient can track are shown in Table 11.2.

TABLE 11.1. Information for Patients about Generalized Anxiety Disorder

What Is Generalized Anxiety Disorder?

All of us feel anxious at times. We may worry about things that *might* happen. We may have a restless night of sleep. But people with generalized anxiety disorder (or GAD) have physical symptoms that interfere with their normal lives. These problems may include restlessness, fatigue, problems with concentration, irritability, muscle tension, and/or insomnia. In addition, these individuals worry about a variety of events, such as health, financial problems, rejection, and performance, and they find it difficult to control their worry. Many people with GAD feel that their worry is "out of control" and that it will make them sick or make them go insane.

Who Has Generalized Anxiety Disorder?

About 7% of the population will suffer from GAD. Women are twice as likely as men to have this problem. This is a chronic condition, with many people saying that they have been "worriers" all their lives. Most people with GAD have a variety of other problems, including phobias, depression, irritable bowel syndrome, and relationship problems. Many people who have this problem find that they avoid others because of fear of rejection, or that they become overly dependent on others because of their lack of confidence.

What Are the Causes of Generalized Anxiety Disorder?

Only about 30% of the causes of GAD are inherited. There are certain traits that may make people more likely to develop this problem; these include general nervousness, depression, inability to tolerate frustration, and feeling inhibited. People with GAD also report more recent life stresses (such as conflicts with other people, changes in their work, and additional demands placed on them) than those without GAD do. People with GAD may not be as effective in solving problems in everyday life as they could be, or they may have personal conflicts in which they may not be as assertive or effective as they could be.

How Does Thinking Affect Generalized Anxiety Disorder?

People with GAD seem to be worried that bad things are going to happen most of the time. They predict that "terrible" things will happen, even when there is a very low probability of bad things happening. They think that the fact that they feel anxious means that something bad is going to happen—that is, they use their emotions as evidence that there is danger out there somewhere. Many people who worry believe that their excessive worry may keep them from being surprised, or that worrying may prepare them for the worst possible outcome. If you are a chronic worrier, you probably notice yourself saying, "Yes, but what if . . . ?" This "what-iffing" floods you with a range of possibly bad outcomes that you think you have to prepare yourself for. There seems to be no end to the things that you could worry about. In fact, even when things turn out to be OK, you may say to yourself, "Well, that's no guarantee that it couldn't happen in the future!"

In addition to worrying about things that might happen "outside of yourself," you may think that "worrying will make me crazy" or "worrying will make me sick." If you have GAD, you may be locked in a conflict between the fear that worry is uncontrollable and the belief that worry protects you.

(continued)

TABLE 11.1. *(continued)*

How Can Cognitive-Behavioral Therapy Help?

Cognitive-behavioral therapy for GAD can help you identify your beliefs about the costs and benefits of worrying, and show you how to recognize the difference between productive and unproductive worrying. Your therapist will help you carry out experiments in "letting go" of worry and postponing worry. In addition, you will learn how to overcome your avoidance of activities or thoughts about which you worry. Your therapist may also use interventions such as muscle relaxation, biofeedback, breathing exercises, time management techniques, and treatment of insomnia in order to reduce your overall levels of anxious arousal. Other interventions may include addressing your concern that worrying too much may be harmful, assessing your tendency to jump to conclusions that awful things will happen, and helping you learn to distinguish between anxiety and actual facts. Your therapist can teach you to use an extensive self-help form ("Questions to Ask Yourself If You Are Worrying") that can help you get a better perspective on worrying. Finally, since you are worrying throughout the day, your therapist will assist you in limiting worry to "worry time" and will help you keep track of the different themes of worry.

How Effective Is Cognitive-Behavioral Therapy for Generalized Anxiety Disorder?

Given the apparent long course of GAD, it is promising that new forms of treatment are proving to be effective. In some studies, cognitive-behavioral therapy has proven to be more effective than medications in the treatment of GAD. It leads to a reduction of the need to use medications, and in some cases patients continue to improve even more after therapy is completed. About 50% of patients with GAD show significant improvement.

Are Medications Useful?

Many patients with GAD also benefit from the use of medication, which can decrease the feeling of anxiety and apprehension. The value of medication is that it can make you feel less anxious very rapidly. Medication may be an essential part of your treatment, while you learn—in therapy—how to handle your problems more effectively.

What Is Expected of You as a Patient?

Because you may have been a worrier all your life, you may be pessimistic about the chances that anything will help you. It is true that you won't get better overnight, so you will have to work on your worries and anxiety on a regular basis. Your therapist will want you to come to sessions on a weekly basis, to keep track of your worries, to practice relaxation or breathing exercises at home, and to work on managing your schedule so that you are not overburdened. In addition, your therapist will help you identify your worries and help you view things in a more realistic perspective. To do this, you will be asked to write down the things that you are worried about, and to use self-help homework techniques to challenge your negative thinking. You may also be asked to work on solving problems more effectively and on learning how to interact with people more productively.

Note. From Leahy and Holland (2000, pp. 125–126). Copyright 2000 by Robert L. Leahy and Stephen J. Holland. Reprinted by permission of the authors and The Guilford Press.

1. **Mind reading**: You assume that you know what people think without having sufficient evidence of their thoughts. "He thinks I'm a loser."

2. **Fortune telling**: You predict the future negatively: Things will get worse, or there is danger ahead. "I'll fail that exam," or "I won't get the job."

3. **Catastrophizing**: You believe that what has happened or will happen will be so awful and unbearable that you won't be able to stand it. "It would be terrible if I failed."

4. **Labeling**: You assign global negative traits to yourself and others. "I'm undesirable," or "He's a rotten person."

5. **Discounting positives**: You claim that the positive things you or others do are trivial. "That's what wives are supposed to do—so it doesn't count when she's nice to me," or "Those successes were easy, so they don't matter."

6. **Negative filtering**: You focus almost exclusively on the negatives and seldom notice the positives. "Look at all of the people who don't like me."

7. **Overgeneralizing**: You perceive a global pattern of negatives on the basis of a single incident. "This generally happens to me. I seem to fail at a lot of things."

8. **Dichotomous thinking**: You view events or people in all-or-nothing terms. "I get rejected by everyone," or "It was a complete waste of time."

9. **Shoulds**: You interpret events in terms of how things should be, rather than simply focusing on what is. "I should do well. If I don't, then I'm a failure."

10. **Personalizing**: You attribute a disproportionate amount of the blame to yourself for negative events, and you fail to see that certain events are also caused by others. "The marriage ended because I failed."

11. **Blaming**: You focus on the other person as the *source of* your negative feelings, and you refuse to take responsibility for changing yourself. "She's to blame for the way I feel now," or "My parents caused all my problems."

12. **Unfair comparisons**: You interpret events in terms of standards that are unrealistic—for example, you focus primarily on others who do better than you and find yourself inferior in the comparison. "She's more successful than I am," or "Others did better than I did on the test."

13. **Regret orientation**: You focus on the idea that you could have done better in the past, rather than on what you can do better now. "I could have had a better job if I had tried," or "I shouldn't have said that."

14. **What if**: You keep asking a series of questions about "what if" something happens, and you fail to be satisfied with any of the answers. "Yeah, but what if I get anxious?" or "What if I can't catch my breath?"

15. **Emotional reasoning**: You let your feelings guide your interpretation of reality. "I feel depressed; therefore, my marriage is not working out."

16. **Inability to disconfirm**: You reject any evidence or arguments that might contradict your negative thoughts. For example, when you have the thought "I'm unlovable," you reject as *irrelevant* any evidence that people like you. Consequently, your thought cannot be refuted. "That's not the real issue. There are deeper problems. There are other factors."

17. **Judgment focus**: You view yourself, others, and events in terms of evaluations as good–bad or superior–inferior, rather than simply describing, accepting, or understanding. You are continually measuring yourself and others according to arbitrary standards, and finding that you and others fall short. You are focused on the judgments of others as well as your own judgments of yourself. "I didn't perform well in college," or "If I take up tennis, I won't do well," or "Look how successful she is. I'm not successful."

Establishing Goals

After the initial assessment, the therapist can target specific goals for treatment by dividing them into various categories, as in this example:

- *Behavioral*: Increase pleasurable activity; reduce passive rumination.
- *Affective*: Reduce sadness and anxiety; increase sense of pleasure and mastery.
- *Physiological*: Reduce arousal; improve relaxation; and decrease fitful sleep.
- *Cognitive*: Reduce fortune telling, what-iffing, and catastrophizing; increase ability to control worry, see things in perspective, and solve problems.
- *Interpersonal*: Increase assertiveness and ability to reward people; improve communication and listening skills; decrease complaining and withdrawing from others.

The therapist can help the patient set specific and general goals for each of these targets, by including general ratings at baseline and establishing periodic reviews of progress. For example, the patient might rate his or her current assertiveness as 2 on a 10-point scale, and target specific instances of assertiveness—for example, calling a friend, making a request, and asking for a change. These target behaviors can be recorded and compared against baseline to assess progress. The important thing for patients who worry is to have concrete plans for positive change that can stand in contrast to vague negative predictions.

Anxiety Management Techniques

Physiological Arousal and Relaxation

When hyperarousal accompanies generalized anxiety, it can be addressed with a number of standard relaxation techniques, including progressive muscle relaxation, breathing exercises, and meditation. If the patient has found any of these techniques helpful, we urge him or her to utilize them again. Relaxation training is part of general anxiety management and is not used in our program to be "paired" with worries. The patient can practice relaxation on a daily basis at set times.

Sleep Hygiene

Given that both hyperarousal and ruminative thinking can be associated with GAD, both difficulty in getting to sleep and early morning awakening can be problematic; if left untreated, these can increase worry during the waking hours during the day. Research indicates that a frequent contributor to insomnia is mental activity rather than physiological arousal (Espie, 2002; Espie, Inglis, & Harvey, 2001; Harvey, 2002; Harvey, Inglis, & Espie, 2002). We utilize an insomnia handout for patients, instructing them to limit the use of bed to sleep or sex and not to utilize the bed for reading, television viewing, talking on the phone, or ruminating (see Table 11.3). In order to address the mental activity issue, a patient can be asked to do the following:

1. Several hours before bed, make a list of things to do for tomorrow.

2. Write out any worries, and challenge them using the techniques outlined in "Coping Statements for Patients" (see Table 11.4).

3. If you lie in bed for more than 15 minutes, get out of bed and either do something very boring (like reading the business section of the newspaper) or write out your worries, list some rational responses, and list activities to carry out in the future. Return to bed after 15 minutes and "give up going to sleep." The paradoxical nature of "giving up" or "accepting insomnia" is to reduce the intentional force of trying to fall asleep, which often contributes to further insomnia.

4. Try some other behavioral interventions for sleep hygiene, such as regularizing the time of going to bed and getting up, reducing liquids prior to bedtime, setting up a "cooling-down" time prior to bed, and increasing exercise during the day.

Time Management

Many patients with GAD have difficulty managing their time and often feel overwhelmed. This adds to their anxiety and worry. The elements of time management include setting specific goals, prioritizing, scheduling activities, and utilizing self-reward. Some perfectionistic individuals are overwhelmed by tasks because they take on too many responsibilities and they attempt to do a perfect job on each activity. A useful book for such persons is Monica Basco's *Never Good Enough* (2000). Perfectionistic patients can examine the costs and benefits of extremely high standards, consider the evidence that others really care that much, and experiment selectively with reducing the level of their performance. Electronic organizers may be helpful in time scheduling and prioritizing; also, reviewing performance at the end of the day can be reinforcing for patients who may feel that they have not done enough. Periodic stress breaks during the day—such as relaxing for 10 minutes, taking a walk, or reading something light—can serve to decrease the anxious momentum that builds for patients who place high demands on themselves.

Procrastination is a frequent problem for patients with GAD and may augment worry further. Patients can focus on answering the following questions: "Specifically, what goal do you want to accomplish? Describe

TABLE 11.3. Information for Patients about Insomnia

One of the more troubling experiences for depressed and anxious patients is insomnia. Some people experience difficulty falling asleep (onset insomnia or anxiety), while others wake several times during the early morning hours (early-morning insomnia or depression). Usually, as depression and anxiety lift, insomnia decreases and sleep is more restful. However, a number of cognitive-behavioral interventions may assist in the treatment of insomnia.

Before you attempt any interventions, you should record some baseline information about the number of hours per night that you sleep and the number of times that you wake. You can then compare your sleep over the next month or two with the baseline measure.

- **Develop regular sleep times.** Go to bed and get out of bed at about the same time, regardless of how tired you are. Also avoid naps.

- **Use your bed only for sleep and sex.** Insomnia is often the result of increased arousal preceding bedtime and while lying awake in bed. Many who have insomnia use the bed for reading, talking on the phone, and worrying; as a result, the bed is associated with arousal (anxiety). Read or talk on the phone in another room. If you have friends who call late at night, tell them not to call after a specific hour. Avoid anxiety arousal during the hour before bedtime (for instance, avoid arguments and challenging tasks).

- Sleep is often disturbed by **urinary urgency.** Reduce or eliminate liquid intake several hours before bedtime. Avoid all caffeine products, heavy foods, and liquor. If necessary, consult a nutritionist to assist in planning a change in diet.

- **Do not try to fall asleep** – this will only increase your frustration and anxiety. Paradoxically, a very effective way of increasing sleep is to practice giving up trying to fall asleep. You can say to yourself, "I'll give up trying to get to sleep and just concentrate on the relaxing feelings in my body."

- If you are lying awake at night for more than 15 minutes, get up and go in the other room. **Write down your negative automatic thoughts and challenge them.** Typical automatic thoughts are "I'll never get to sleep," "If I don't get enough sleep, I won't be able to function," "I need to get to sleep immediately," and "I'll get sick from not getting enough sleep." The most likely consequence of not getting enough sleep is that you will feel tired and irritable. Although these are uncomfortable inconveniences, they are not catastrophic.

- Your therapist can teach **systematic relaxation and breathing,** which will enhance your restfulness. Try to make your mind go blank. Count backward by threes from 100 or 1,000, as slowly as possible. Visualize a relaxing scene—for example, snow falling on a house in the woods at night.

- Because your disturbed sleep patterns have taken a long time to learn, it may take you a while to unlearn them. **Do not expect immediate results.**

Note. From Leahy and Holland (2000, p. 56). Copyright 2000 by Robert L. Leahy and Stephen J. Holland. Reprinted by permission of the authors and The Guilford Press.

TABLE 11.4. Coping Statements for Patients

Normalize your anxiety:

Anxiety is normal.
Everyone has anxiety.
Anxiety shows that I am alert.
Anxiety may be biologically programmed (this may be the "right response at the wrong time"–there is no danger that I have to escape from).

Take the danger away:

Anxiety is arousal.
I've been through this before, and nothing bad has happened.
Anxiety passes and goes away.

Challenge your negative thoughts:

I'm having false alarms.
I'm not going crazy or losing control.
These sensations are not dangerous.
People can't see my feelings.
I don't need to have 100% control.

Learn from the past:

I've made many negative predictions before that haven't come true.
I have never gone crazy, had a heart attack, or died from my anxiety.
Remember to keep breathing normally–this helps.

Plan acceptance:

I can sit back and watch my arousal.
I can accept that my arousal goes up and down.
I can observe my sensations increasing and decreasing.
I can accept my arousal and examine my negative thoughts.

Note. From Leahy and Holland (2000, p. 91). Copyright 2000 by Robert L. Leahy and Stephen J. Holland. Reprinted by permission of the authors and The Guilford Press.

five steps toward that goal. When would you assign the first step? What are the advantages and disadvantages of taking the first step? Once you do the first step, reward yourself with praise or some pleasant behavior." Procrastination is often the result of beliefs such as "I have to do the entire thing. I can't stand the discomfort. It's too late anyway. I don't like to feel uncomfortable." In such a case, it is helpful to have the patient make discomfort a goal: "Every day, do something that is uncomfortable until you have mastered the ability to experience discomfort without complaining."

Treatment of Worry

Metacognitive Evaluation of the Patient's Personal Theory of Worry

The cognitive-behavioral approach stresses the importance of the patient's personal theory about worry. Patients with GAD often believe that worry has positive functions. Such patients presume that worry will motivate them, give them some control over outcomes, help them anticipate the worst, keep them from being caught by surprise, and assist in problem solving. In addition, these individuals have negative views of worry, including the beliefs that worry is out of control, that it will last forever, that it will cause them to get sick or go crazy, and that it will always be present. Some individuals believe that they have to completely eliminate worry. Several of these beliefs about worry (both negative and positive), and ways of addressing them, are described below. A more detailed description of how these metacognitive beliefs are addressed in cognitive-behavioral therapy is provided by Wells (2000).

BELIEF THAT ONE HAS NO CONTROL OVER WORRY. A common belief for patients who worry is that they have no control over their worry. This is addressed through several interventions: worry time, attentional distraction, and mindfulness training.

Worry Time. When worry time is assigned to the patient, the patient is instructed to worry intensely, and not find any solutions. Any worries that come up outside of worry time should be noted (on a piece of paper) and postponed until the next worry time. The worry time should be set each day for a limited period and should not be conducted while in bed or close to bedtime. Patients often think that this may make matters worse— or that it sounds simply ridiculous—but the therapist should explain that this will help them gain control over worry, limit worry to a specific time, help the patients catalogue typical worries, and help them see that worries are repetitive and therefore finite.

Attentional Distraction. In session, the therapist can demonstrate volitional control by asking the patient to start worrying about something (e.g., an upcoming exam) and then to interrupt the worry by directing attention to objects in the office: "Describe each object that you see in this office." As the patient is distracted from the worry and focuses on the immediate environment, the sense of control is increased.

Mindfulness. Segal, Williams, and Teasdale (2002) have advocated the use of mindfulness training for preventing future depression in patients with recurrent episodes, and Roemer and Orsillo (2002) have indicated that this may be helpful in reducing worry. The rationale behind mindfulness training is that the cognitive style of depressive and worried thinking entails abstract generalizations and attributions beyond the immediate situation, and that "mindfulness" (i.e., being fully present in and aware of the current moment) can counteract such thinking. Although we do not generally use formal mindfulness training for GAD, it can be helpful to have the patient train him- or herself in focusing on the immediate awareness of events, feelings, and thoughts. For example, a man holding a manage-rial post was worried about the performance of his group and predicted dire consequences if things did not shape up. The instruction was to focus on describing the details of the conversation he had had with a colleague and allow himself to experience or feel any emotion that occurred. As he experienced tension and anxiety, he was asked to stand back and observe and describe it without changing it. He observed that his feeling was intense, that he felt it in his arms, that he noticed that his chest was tight-ening, and that this was unpleasant. Staying in the moment—mindfully ob-serving his feelings and his thoughts, without trying to change them—helped him both within the session and over the following week, as he practiced mindfulness, to become less anxious about his anxious thoughts and feelings.

PERCEPTION OF WORRY AS PROBLEM SOLVING. Many patients with GAD believe that worry is problem solving. This belief should be addressed directly. The issue of worry as problem solving is indicated by a patient's re-sponses to the Meta-Cognitions Questionnaire (Cartwright-Hatton & Wells, 1997) and by examining the costs and benefits of worry. The therapist can ask the patient to define "problem solving." Answers to this question may reveal the patient's belief that "worry helps me recog-nize what can go wrong." The therapist can help the patient recognize that identifying possible problems is not the same thing as solving them. Moreover, not all possible problems require solutions. For exam-ple, worrying that there is a possibility of a 90% drop in the stock mar-ket is not the same thing as fixing the problem, nor does it even mean that the problem exists.

ILLUSION THAT WORRY IS A MEANS OF CONTROL. Some patients believe that worry helps them maintain some control over outcomes: "If I worry about it, I'll be able to keep the bad thing from happening." This belief can be chal-lenged by examining the costs and benefits of the belief and the evidence for and against the belief. For example, patients can ask themselves ques-tions such as these:

- "How will worrying that I might have a brain tumor prevent a brain tumor?"
- "How will worrying that people will reject me keep them from re-jecting me?"
- "How do I account for good things that have happened to me, if I didn't worry about them?"
- "When bad things did happen—for example, when my car was hit by someone on the highway—how would worrying have prevented it?"

- "Is it possible that worrying about things makes me actually feel less in control?"
- "Is not having control generally a bad thing or a neutral thing?"

BELIEF THAT WORRY MOTIVATES. Although there is some evidence that worry can motivate some people through the process of defensive pessimism (Norem & Cantor, 1986), most worry is not defensive pessimism. Defensive pessimism is a particular kind of worry—a person's belief that lowering expectations for how well he or she will do (e.g., worry about failing) will motivate him or her to work harder. The question here, in therapy, is whether this particular person is actually working harder or more effectively as a result of worrying. Worrying may lead to interference with attention and concentration, and in some cases to procrastination. The important element is actually mobilizing behavior rather than worrying. For example, a man who was an accountant and worried about being late on filing his own taxes believed that this worry would keep him motivated, but the fact was that his worry led to procrastination. Every time he worried about his taxes and thought of actually taking some action—such as collecting the necessary information—he became anxious and avoided doing anything. A therapist can help such a patient recognize that worry may not motivate. What may motivate the person to solve a problem is identifying possible solutions, reducing the perceived severity of the outcome, and planning small steps forward toward a solution.

Turning Worry into Predictions

WORRY DIARY. The patient is requested to keep a record of his or her worries by writing out each worry, translating it into a prediction, and then reviewing the predictions at the end of the week. The patient first lists each situation that he or she is in when worry begins. For example, "thinking of studying for the exam" is the situation. The worry, "I'm worried about the exam," is translated into "I will get a poor grade on the exam." This is then listed as a prediction to be verified by the next session (or, in this case, 2 weeks later when the grades are posted). The worry diary can be modified to include a more detailed set of questions:

- "What am I predicting?"
- "What degree of belief do I have in this prediction?"
- "What is my emotion and degree of emotion?"
- "What is the evidence for and against this prediction?"
- "What are the worst, best, and most likely outcomes expected?"
- "How would I cope if my worry is accurate?"

Table 11.5 shows an example of a worry diary.

TABLE 11.5. Example of a Worry Diary

Question	Answer
What am I predicting? (Degree of belief, 0–100%)	I'll do poorly on the exam. Belief 75%
Emotions (strength, 0–100%)	Anxious 85% Hopeless 30%
Evidence for and against prediction	*Evidence for:* I didn't study until last night. There's some material I don't know. I'm anxious. Other people know more than I do. *Evidence against:* I have gone to class and done the reading. I'm smart—I get good grades. I have another 2 days to prepare.
Worst, best, and most likely outcome; why is the "most likely" outcome the most likely to occur?	*Worst:* I fail the exam. *Best:* I get an A. *Most likely:* I'll get a B. This is because I do know a lot of the material, and I've been able to cram at the last minute before.
How would you cope if your worry is accurate?	If I did get a poor grade (let's say a C), I still have other grades in that course—the other exams, classroom participation, and the paper.
How would you revise your worry?	I often worry, and things work out OK. I'll study hard now and tomorrow, and when I take the exam I'll probably do OK.

NARROWING THE DOMAIN. The worry diary is helpful in narrowing the issues about which the person is worried. For example, what specific recurring issues (e.g., relationships, achievement, health, etc.) characterize this patient's worry? If the patient is worried primarily about relationship issues, for example, then the therapist can utilize flash cards for self-instruction that identify coping abilities and rational responses. For example, a woman worried that her boyfriend might stop liking her. Her worried predictions, written on one side of an index card, were "He will stop liking me" and "He will break up with me." The rational responses were these: "I talk to him every day. He tells me he likes me. He sees me twice a week. He's affectionate." Coping statements included the following: "I can distract myself from my worries by doing other things. Worrying doesn't help. Even if we broke up, I would be OK. I've gone through breakups before and eventually did OK. I can always get another guy, because I'm attractive and rewarding to be with."

EXAMINING PAST PREDICTIONS OF CATASTROPHES. Worried individuals often treat each new worry as if it were a new phenomenon. For example, the accountant who worried that he had not filed his final return for his own taxes (see above) predicted that he would lose his license and lose his practice. He became engulfed in his current worry and anxiety. It was helpful for him to review past worries and predictions to recognize that his negative predictions almost never came true. These past predictions, over the course of many years, included "I won't graduate from college," "I won't get a girlfriend," "I won't pass the licensing exam," "I won't get a job," and "I won't be able to pay my rent." None of these events had occurred.

Evaluating Cognitive Dimensions of Worries

Many worries are based on cognitive distortions. These include emotional reasoning (e.g., "I'm anxious; therefore something bad will happen"), fortune telling (e.g., "I'll fail the exam"), catastrophizing (e.g., "I'll ruin my life"), negative filter (e.g., "I don't know some of these answers"), discounting the positive (e.g., "Just because I've done well in the past doesn't mean anything"), and labeling (e.g., "I'm an idiot"). Typical cognitive therapy interventions can be utilized to challenge these distortions, including categorizing the distortion (as indicated above), examining the costs and benefits, weighing the evidence for and against, using rational role plays in sessions, and asking the patient to give advice to a friend with the same worries.

Examining the Demand for Certainty

As Dugas and colleagues (Chapter 6, this volume) indicate, much of worry is an attempt to attain certainty in an uncertain world. Because of this excessive demand for certainty, many patients with GAD will continue to engage in worry until they feel certain about an outcome. If they come up with solutions to problems, they will evaluate the solution against the standard of certitude and will reject reasonable solutions because of their demand for certainty. The therapist can evaluate responses on the Intolerance of Uncertainty Scale (Freeston et al., 1994) or can evaluate these needs with the following questions:

- "What are the advantages and disadvantages of demanding certainty?"
- "What is the probability [from 0% to 100%] of each of these outcomes that you are predicting?"
- "Is there anything about which you have absolute certainty?"
- "How do you account for the fact that you are able to tolerate uncertainty in other areas of your life?"
- "Are you assuming that because you have some uncertainty, the outcome will be bad?"
- "What are the best possible outcome, the worst possible outcome, and the most likely outcome?"

Challenging Worries

QUESTIONS PATIENTS CAN ASK THEMSELVES WHEN THEY ARE WORRIED. We (Leahy & Holland, 2000) have developed a self-evaluation form with numerous questions that patients can ask themselves if they are worried. This is shown in Table 11.6. In addition to these questions or challenges to worries, a therapist can ask a patient to examine events along a continuum (i.e., to decastrophize); to examine his or her ability to absorb losses, should they occur; to gain distance from a thought by role-playing both sides of the thought in a session; to use the "point–counterpoint" technique to evaluate underlying assumptions and schemata; to act against a thought; to evaluate how other people who have faced similar problems have handled these situations; to calculate sequential probabilities to examine how unlikely a string of events is to occur; and to develop more adaptive ways of viewing things. Some of these interventions are considered below.

CALCULATING SEQUENTIAL PROBABILITIES. What events trigger or elicit worry? Is it conflict with others, uncertainty about the outcome of events at work, or examining one's appearance in the mirror? These triggers can be a focus for eliciting other automatic thoughts: "What do you think when you have an argument with a friend?" These automatic thoughts can then be used to generate a "vertical descent" (this technique is discussed in more detail below):

"We had an argument . . . "
↓
"I can't stand it when we have an argument. It's terrible . . . "
↓
"We'll never get along . . . "
↓
"Our friendship is over."

Or, in the case of worries about physical ailments, the sequence might be this:

"I have a headache . . . "
↓
"This could be a brain tumor . . . "
↓
"I should have it checked out . . . "
↓
"If I don't, I'll get sick and die."

TABLE 11.6. Questions to Ask Yourself If You Are Worrying: A Self-Help Form for Patients

Specific worry: _____

Questions to ask yourself:	Your response:
Specifically, what are you predicting will happen?	
How likely (0–100%) is it that this will actually happen?	Likelihood:
How negative an outcome are you predicting (from 0% to 100%)?	How negative:
What is the worst outcome?	Worst:
The most likely outcome?	Most likely:
The best outcome?	Best:
Are you predicting catastrophes (awful things) that don't come true? What are some examples of the catastrophes that you are anticipating?	
What is the evidence (for and against) your worry that something really bad is going to happen?	Evidence for: Evidence against:
If you had to divide 100 points between the evidence for and against, how would you divide these points? (For example, is it 50–50? 60–40?)	Rating: Evidence for = Evidence against =
Are you using your emotions (your anxiety) to guide you? Are you saying to yourself, "I feel anxious, so something really bad is going to happen"?	
Is this a reasonable or logical way to make predictions? Why/why not?	
How many times have you been wrong in the past about your worries? What actually happened?	

(continued)

TABLE 11.6. *(continued)*

Questions to ask yourself:	Your response:
What are the costs and benefits to you of worrying about this?	Costs: Benefits:
If you had to divide 100 points between the costs and benefits, how would you divide these points? For example, would it be 50–50? 60–40%	Points: –___ (costs) ___ (benefits) Subtract costs from benefits: ___ – ___ = ___
What evidence do you have from the past that worrying has been helpful to you and hurtful to you?	
Are you able to give up any control in order to be worried less?	
Is there any way that worrying really gives you any control, or do you feel more out of control because you are worrying so much?	
If what you predict happens, what would that mean to you? What would happen next?	
How could you handle the kinds of problems that you are worrying about? What could you do?	
Has anything bad happened to you that you were not worried about? How were you able to handle that?	
Are you usually underestimating your ability to handle problems?	
Consider the thing you are worried about. How do you think you'll feel about this 2 days, 2 weeks, 2 months, and 2 years from now? Why would you feel differently?	
If someone else were facing the events that you are facing, would you encourage that person to worry as much as you? What advice would you give him or her?	

Note. From Leahy and Holland (2000, pp. 130–131). Copyright 2000 by Robert L. Leahy and Stephen J. Holland. Reprinted by permission of the authors and The Guilford Press.

Each element in such a sequence can then be examined for probabilities. In regard to the brain tumor worry, the therapist can ask, "What is the probability that you have a brain tumor?" The patient may say that it is 1%. "What is the probability that you will die from a brain tumor?" The patient may place this at 20%. These subjective probabilities can be examined. The therapist can then continue, "What percentage of people have headaches at some time?" The patient may say 95%. "What percentage of people have brain tumors?" The patient may put this at 1 in 10,000. The sequential probabilities can then be calculated. For the brain tumor, it might be $.05 \times .0001 = .00005$, or $1/200$ of 1%. Even this estimate is quite high.

DISTINGUISHING PRODUCTIVE FROM UNPRODUCTIVE WORRY. Not all worry is irrational and unproductive. Simply telling the patient, "Don't worry, be happy," will appear naive and undermine the credibility of the therapist. Consequently, the therapist can assist the patient in distinguishing productive from unproductive worry by considering such issues as plausibility, possible actions to be engaged in, and current versus possible problems. I examine each of these.

Plausible versus Implausible Worries. Many worries are about events that are highly unlikely and highly implausible. For example, the worry that "The engine in my car will explode on the highway" is highly unlikely. However, the worry that "I might not have given myself enough time to get to my destination" is plausible. The patient can distribute his or her worries along a continuum, or divide them into categories of plausible versus implausible or likely versus unlikely.

Action versus Fantasy. Another dimension of significance is whether the worry concerns a fantasy or an action that can be taken. For example, the fantasy that the car's engine will explode is simply a catastrophic prediction. An action statement would be "Is there a reasonable action to take?" In this case, even though the worry is implausible, the reasonable action to take is to check the coolant and the oil. The therapist should encourage the patient to translate fantasies into actions to be taken.

Current versus Possible Problems. As Dugas and colleagues (Chapter 6, this volume) make clear, worries can be divided into current versus possible problems. A current problem might be car maintenance. Here the patient can be guided by standard or conventional standards: "How often do you check the oil?" The action to be taken is for the current problem—in this case, checking the oil. Possible problems are generally "what-if" thoughts about potential bad outcomes, usually with remote possibilities. In this case, the image of the car's engine blowing up can be used for an imaginal exposure exercise—for example, repeating the image of the car explosion for 10 minutes. Reducing the anxiety in response to the image by habitu- ating to "possible problems" can also be accompanied by having the pa- tient repeat for 10 minutes, "It's always possible that the engine in my car could blow up on the highway." We have found it useful for the patient to practice repeating what-ifs in imaginal exposure whenever they arise dur- ing the day. For example, if the patient has a what-if worry about his or her car crashing off the side of a bridge, the exercise will be to repeat the statement "It is always possible that my car could crash." Repeating the feared thought, especially if it is accompanied by a visual image, prevents the patient from using worry as a "coping" or "problem-solving" strategy and demonstrates to the patient that the thought or image becomes less evocative with exposure.

EXAMINING FEARS UNDERLYING WORRIES. As Borkovec and colleagues (Chapter 4, this volume) note, worries may maintain a focus on relatively superficial concerns that are abstract or linguistic. In order to access the fear struc- ture underlying the initial worry, it is helpful to examine the sequential implications of worries, via the techniques of vertical descent and expo- sure to feared fantasy.

Vertical Descent. A patient is often focused on how problems may be averted, and therefore avoids thinking through the worst possible out- come. The therapist may utilize the vertical descent procedure to get at the underlying most feared outcome (Burns, 1989). "Vertical descent" re- fers to a sequence of statements by the patient about the outcomes or meanings of different negative thoughts, and the therapist's questioning of those statements. For example, the accountant who worried that he hadn't filed his own taxes (a fact) gave the following responses to the ther- apist's repeated questions, "What might happen next?":

"The IRS will fine me and attach penalties . . . "
↓
"I'll be charged with tax evasion . . . "
↓
"I will go to prison . . . "
↓
"My life will be ruined . . . "
[Therapist: "What does it look like to think your life is ruined?"]
↓
"I will become a homeless person. No one will want to talk to me. I'll die."

Exposure to Feared Fantasy. Because worries are abstract and linguistic, they prevent access to the emotionally laden images and thoughts that constitute the fear structure. Worries about finances may be linked, through vertical descent, to images of being incarcerated. Worries about relationship conflict may eventually be linked to images of being alone in a deserted room. The cognitive-behavioral approach to these concerns is first to help the patient access these "feared fantasies" through vertical descent and imagery induction, and then to practice exposure, as explained below.

The patient described above was utilizing worry in order to prevent himself from having the feared fantasy images of going to prison and ending up on the street as a homeless person. These were catastrophic, fortune-telling thoughts for the patient, with very low probabilities of occurrence. However, the worry prevented him from having these images and kept him in a worrisome and avoidant style—he worried about how he might have violated the law, and he avoided doing his own taxes. The therapist evoked the catastrophic image of ending up in prison in order to elicit the emotional component:

THERAPIST: Describe the visual image of yourself in prison.

PATIENT: I see myself in a cell with a toilet in the corner. I am all alone and depressed as hell.

THERAPIST: What happens next?

PATIENT: What do you mean?

THERAPIST: Describe your day in the prison.

PATIENT: I guess I would want to do some reading. Maybe I'd read some novels.

THERAPIST: What authors?

PATIENT: I don't know. Probably crime novels (*laughs*).

THERAPIST: Then what happens?

PATIENT: I guess I go to lunch.

THERAPIST: Whom do you talk to?

PATIENT: Other prisoners. I guess we talk about sports or things going on in the prison. I've never thought it through.

The therapist can also have the patient write out the feared fantasy in detail. (For example, in this case, the feared fantasy included the images of being arrested for tax evasion, being taken to jail, going to court, ending up in prison, sitting in his cell, and talking with other prisoners.) The therapist then can assign reading this narrative aloud (or silently) for 20 minutes each day, in order for the patient to habituate to these feared images. During the reading of these narratives in the therapy session, the therapist should note whether the patient responds with intense emotion or with emotional numbing to these images, which are often referred to as "hot spots" (see Grey, Holmes, & Brewin, 2001) in the treatment of post-traumatic stress disorder. For example, the accountant expressed intense emotion with the image of a trial; he imagined being humiliated in front of friends and family members. His automatic thoughts were "Everyone will think I'm a crook. They'll never want to talk with me again." Other hot spots included imagining being in the cell and thinking, "I'll never get out." These hot spots then became the focus of questioning via standard cognitive therapy techniques: "What is the likelihood that you would be arrested for being late on taxes? What evidence do you have for and against this? Could you contact a tax lawyer or the IRS (anonymously) and find out how things can be rectified? What is your prediction? Have you ever heard of anyone going to jail for being late on taxes? Could you find out from the IRS or a tax lawyer how many people are late filing taxes?" The therapist also engaged in role plays to get the patient to challenge these negative feared fantasies:

THERAPIST: (*As negative voice*) You are going to go to prison for the rest of your life for being late on taxes!

PATIENT: (*As rational responder*) That's absurd. The IRS only attaches penalties and interest for lateness. If they arrested everyone who is late on taxes, then a third of the people in the United States would be in jail.

THERAPIST: (*As negative voice*) But you can't be absolutely sure. They might make an example of you.

PATIENT: You can't be sure of anything. But I have never heard of this happening, so it makes no sense to worry about it happening to me.

DEVELOPING POSITIVE NARRATIVES AND IMAGES. Since patients have been avoiding their negative feared fantasies through worry and telling themselves stories about how things can go wrong, it will be useful to develop positive narratives of outcomes that are neutral or positive. In the foregoing case, the therapist requested the patient to write out a story in detail about a positive outcome. This was the patient's positive narrative:

> I get all of my tax information together for the previous 2 years and have another accountant go over them with me. I then call the tax attorney and find out that all you have to do is file a late return. I find out that almost all the taxes had been paid through withholding and that there is a small penalty with interest attached. I then make a payment arrangement with the IRS and pay off the small debt. I learn to get my taxes done on time in the future.

The therapist then turned the positive narrative into a series of problem-solving behaviors, with assigned times: "When will you call the tax lawyer? When will you get the tax information together? Specifically, what information will you gather, and when will this be gathered?" As the patient engaged in this proactive behavior—acting against his anxiety—he would reevaluate the catastrophic or negative predictions. For example, after the patient talked with the tax attorney, the prediction that "I will go to jail" was reevaluated and the patient gave it a rating of 10%, as opposed to his previous 50% rating.

Worry and Personal Schemata

CORE BELIEFS ABOUT SELF/OTHERS AND WORRY. The patient's worry is often related to one or more core beliefs about self and others. A man who worked as an investment broker worried about not producing a high enough profit for his investors; a woman worried about losing her looks and consequently being abandoned by her husband; and a compulsive woman worried that she would not be viewed as conscientious by her colleagues at work. The core schemata for these respective people were not being superior (the investment broker), being unlovable (the woman worried about her looks), and not having self-control and conscientiousness (the compulsive worker). As such, it may be helpful for a patient to identify what he or she does *not* worry about. For example, the investment broker did not worry about whether people liked him; the worried woman did not worry about money; and the compulsive worker did not worry about getting sick from too much work.

WORRY AS A CONDITIONAL RULE OF ADAPTATION. Individuals may worry because they believe that it helps them achieve their desired goals. The investment broker compulsively checked his monitor in his office, watching stocks go up and down. His assumption was that "If I worry and check, I'll be able to catch something before it goes down too much." The worried wife claimed that her worry allowed her to identify any physical flaws so that she could either correct them or hide them, and that this would prevent her from being humiliated. The compulsive worker believed that her worries about all the details would assure that she would not make mistakes. In each case, these people believed that worrying prevented them from being exposed to their schematic fears of being ordinary, abandoned, or irresponsible.

WORRY'S REINFORCEMENT OF THE PERSONAL SCHEMA. Just as worry may be utilized to prevent a schematic threat from arising, the reliance on worry may reinforce the personal schema. Guidano and Liotti (1983) have referred to this as the "protective belt." Thus coping strategies at a more peripheral level (such as worry and avoidance) may prevent the individual from examining the validity of more core schematic issues. For example, the investment broker had not examined whether he needed to be special and superior; the worried wife had not examined whether she was lovable or if she needed someone to love her; and the compulsive worker had not examined any evidence that she might be irresponsible (or, if she were, how this would be so terrible).

MODIFICATION OF THE SCHEMA. Having considered how reliance on worry protects a patient from examining a core schema, the therapist and patient can examine how the schema can be modified so that it does not require "protection." In the case of the investment broker, he was able to consider the value of doing things for other people that did not require his being superior—in this case, volunteering to be a "Big Brother" to a poor child. The broker and his therapist also examined how his parents would literally require him to achieve something before they would give him any love or reward. He was taught that his self-esteem was entirely contingent on achievement. The therapist was able to assist him in challenging this contingent worthiness by role-playing himself with a good parent. He played the good parent providing unconditional love and respect to himself (played by the therapist).

　　The worried wife focused on being more attractive than all other women in order to be special to her husband. The therapist asked her to consider an episode from the book *The Little Prince* (Saint-Exupery, 1943/2000). A fox meets the Little Prince and states that, with time, they will become special to each other. He will be the only fox for the boy, and the boy will be the only boy for the fox. In becoming special to one another, they will begin to view each other with the heart, not just the mind. After relating this story, the therapist asked the patient to rate her teenage daughter on a scale of 1–10 on attractiveness. She was hesitant. She indicated that she could not be objective about her daughter, since she loved her. The therapist noted that this was the same issue she had with her husband—they could not be objective, since they loved each other. The patient was able to understand that being special to her husband meant that he would never be objective about her appearance, since he would see her through a schema of love.

CONCLUSION

Patients presenting with GAD often describe themselves as having always worried. Many of these people believe that there are advantages to worry—such as preparing for events, preventing disaster, and solving problems. They also typically believe that their worry is out of control. The cognitive-behavioral model described here attempts to target the meta-cognitive aspects of worry, as well as to help patients with increased arousal, sleep problems, and difficulties with time management. Structured self-help assignments, together with in-session challenges to dysfunctional demands for certainty and reassurance, are essential components of this approach. Moreover, highlighting how worry is related to core beliefs and personal schemata—such as schemata related to defectiveness, overresponsibility, or abandonment—can increase the effectiveness of the cognitive interventions described here.

REFERENCES

Basco, M. R. (2000). *Never good enough: How to use perfectionism to your advantage without ruining your life.* Carmichael, CA: Touchstone Books.

Beck, A. T., & Freeman, A. M. (1990). *Cognitive therapy of personality disorders.* New York: Guilford Press.

Beck, A.T., Epstein, N., Brown, G., & Steer, R. A. (1988). An inventory for measuring clinical anxiety: Psychometric properties. *Journal of Consulting and Clinical Psychology, 56,* 893–897.

Beck, A. T., & Steer, R. A. (1990). *Beck Anxiety Inventory manual.* San Antonio, TX: Psychological Corporation.

Borkovec, T. D., & Hu, S. (1990). The effect of worry on cardiovascular response to phobic imagery. *Behaviour Research and Therapy, 28,* 69–73.

Borkovec, T. D., & Inz, J. (1990). The nature of worry in generalized anxiety disorder: A predominance of thought activity. *Behaviour Research and Therapy, 28,* 153–158.

Borkovec, T. D., Lyonfields, J. D., Wiser, S. L., & Diehl, L. (1993). The role of worrisome thinking in the suppression of cardiovascular response to phobic imagery. *Behaviour Research and Therapy, 31,* 321–324.

Borkovec, T. D., Shadick, R. N., & Hopkins, M. (1991). The nature of normal and pathological worry. In R. M. Rapee & D. H. Barlow (Eds.), *Chronic anxiety: Generalized anxiety disorder and mixed anxiety–depression* (pp. 29–51). New York: Guilford Press.

Burns, D. D. (1989). *The feeling good handbook: Using the new mood therapy in everyday life.* New York: William Morrow.

Cartwright-Hatton, S., & Wells, A. (1997). Beliefs about worry and intrusions: The Meta-Cognitions Questionnaire and its correlates. *Journal of Anxiety Disorders, 11,* 279–296.

Dugas, M. J., Gosselin, P., & Ladouceur, R. (2001). Intolerance of uncertainty and worry: Investigating specificity in a nonclinical sample. *Cognitive Therapy and Research, 25,* 13–22.

Espie, C. A. (2002). Insomnia: Conceptual issues in the development, persistence, and treatment of sleep disorder in adults. *Annual Review of Psychology, 53,* 215–243.

Espie, C. A., Inglis, S. J., & Harvey, L. (2001). Predicting clinically significant response to cognitive behavior therapy for chronic insomnia in general medical practice: Analyses of outcome data at 12 months posttreatment. *Journal of Consulting and Clinical Psychology, 69,* 58–66.

Freeston, M. H., Rhéaume, J., Letarte, H., Dugas, M. J., & Ladouceur, R. (1994). Why do people worry? *Personality and Individual Differences, 17,* 791–802.

Grey, N., Holmes, E., & Brewin, C. R. (2001). Peritraumatic emotional "hot spots" in memory. *Behavioural and Cognitive Psychotherapy, 29*, 367–372.

Guidano, V. F., & Liotti, G. (1983). *Cognitive processes and the emotional disorders*. New York: Guilford Press.

Harvey, A. G. (2002). A cognitive model of insomnia. *Behaviour Research and Therapy, 40*, 869–893.

Harvey, L., Inglis, S. J., & Espie, C. A. (2002). Insomniacs' reported use of CBT components and relationship to long-term clinical outcome. *Behaviour Research and Therapy, 40*, 75–83.

Leahy, R. L., & Holland, S. J. (2000). *Treatment plans and interventions for depression and anxiety disorders*. New York: Guilford Press.

Mennin, D. S., Turk, C. L., Heimberg, R. G., & Carmin, C. N. (in press). Focusing on the regulation of emotion: A new direction for conceptualizing and treating generalized anxiety disorder. In M. A. Reinecke & D. A. Clark (Eds.), *Cognitive therapy over the lifespan: Theory, research and practice*. New York: Guilford Press.

Meyer, T. J., Miller, M. L., Metzger, R. L., & Borkovec, T. D. (1990). Development and validation of the Penn State Worry Questionnaire. *Behaviour Research and Therapy, 28*, 487–495.

Norem, J. K., & Cantor, N. (1986). Defensive pessimism: Harnessing anxiety as motivation. *Journal of Personality and Social Psychology, 51*, 1208–1217.

Roemer, L., & Orsillo, S. (2002) Expanding our conceptualization of and treatment for generalized anxiety disorder: Integrating mindfulness/acceptance-based approaches with existing cognitive-behavioral models. *Clinical Psychology: Science and Practice, 9*, 54–68.

Saint-Exupéry, A. de. (2000). *The little prince* (R. Howard, Trans.). Fort Washington, PA: Harvest Books. (Original work published 1943)

Segal, Z. V., Williams, M. J. G., & Teasdale, J. D. (2002). *Mindfulness-based cognitive therapy for depression: A new approach to preventing relapse*. New York: Guilford Press.

Tallis, F., Eysenck, M. W., & Mathews, A. (1992). A questionnaire for the measurement of nonpathological worry. *Personality and Individual Differences, 13*, 161–168.

Wells, A. (2000). *Emotional disorders and metacognition: Innovative cognitive therapy*. New York: Wiley.

Wells, A., & Papageorgiou, C. (1995). Worry and the incubation of intrusive images following stress. *Behaviour Research and Therapy, 33*, 579–583.

CHAPTER 12

Supportive–Expressive Psychodynamic Therapy

PAUL CRITS-CHRISTOPH
MARY BETH CONNOLLY GIBBONS
KATHERINE CRITS-CHRISTOPH

In this chapter, we present a description of a standardized, interpersonally oriented psychodynamic psychotherapy treatment model for generalized anxiety disorder (GAD). The background for the approach, including reasons for the development of a psychodynamic treatment of GAD plus empirical evidence supporting an interpersonally oriented psychodynamic theoretical model of GAD, is first briefly reviewed. This is followed by a description of the essential features of the clinical treatment model. The results of an initial study implementing the treatment model are then presented, and we conclude with recommendations regarding future research and clinical applications of the model. Further details about the treatment method and results of our evaluation of the approach are presented elsewhere (Crits-Christoph, Connolly, Azarian, Crits-Christoph, & Shappell, 1996; Crits-Christoph, Crits-Christoph, Wolf-Palacio, Fichter, & Rudick, 1995).

BACKGROUND

There are five major reasons why we embarked on the development of an interpersonally oriented psychodynamic treatment of GAD. The first is that GAD is a relatively prevalent disorder that involves significant degrees of impairment (see Kessler, Walters, & Wittchen, Chapter 2, this volume). Thus, for public health reasons, it is important to develop and test treatments for this disorder. The second reason is that existing treatments for GAD have been insufficient. Although there has been some success with medication and cognitive-behavioral treatments for GAD, there are clear limitations to these approaches. In their review of cognitive-behavioral treatments for GAD, Chambless and Gillis (1993) indicate that clinically significant change occurs in only about 50% of patients. In regard to medications, benzodiazepines are the most widely used treatments for GAD and, until recently, the only medications with U.S. Food and Drug Administration (FDA) approval for the treatment of GAD in the United States. However, studies have revealed a number of concerns about benzodiazepine treatment of GAD, including (1) inadequate improvement in a significant minority of patients (about 30%) (Greenblatt, Shader, & Abernethy, 1983a); (2) less effect on the core GAD symptom of worry (Rickels et al., 1982); (3) a variety of side effects, including attentional, psychomotor, cognitive, and memory-impairing effects, as well as possible teratogenic risk in female patients of childbearing years (who constitute a majority of the population with GAD); (4) the potential for abuse, with associated physical dependence, withdrawal, and effects on coping and stress response capabilities (Greenblatt, Shader, & Abernethy, 1983b; Rickels, Schweizer, & Lucki, 1987; Woods, Katz, & Winger, 1992); and (5) documented high relapse rates (e.g., Rickels et al., 1987). More recently, venlafaxine has been approved by the FDA for the treatment of GAD, but the magnitude of the treatment effect relative to placebo appears modest (Davidson, Dupont, Hedges, & Haskins, 1999), with little information available regarding relapse rates.

The third reason for developing a psychodynamic approach to GAD is that the psychodynamic perspective remains relatively common among practicing psychotherapists (Jensen, Bergin, & Greaves, 1990). To the extent that a treatment approach acceptable to these clinicians can be developed and is shown to produce effects at least equal to those of medication and cognitive-behavioral treatments, a larger number of providers can implement effective treatment of patients with GAD, rather than having to refer these patients to physicians or cognitive-behavioral clinicians.

The fourth reason for the development of a psychodynamic approach to GAD is that there has been a long-standing interest in the theory and treatment of anxiety from a psychodynamic perspective. Many writers from this perspective, including Freud, Sullivan, Fairbairn, Klein, and Kohut, have proposed ideas about the etiology and treatment of anxiety (see Zerbe, 1990, for a review). Of course, it is an important question as to whether the chronic anxiety problems ("anxiety neurosis") described by these theorists is the same as GAD. It is not unreasonable to assume that some aspects of GAD fit well with psychodynamic conceptualizations of chronic anxiety.

Freud's writing about anxiety are potentially confusing, since over time he offered two theories of anxiety. His earlier writings (before 1926) suggested that anxiety is the consequence of repressed or nondischarged sexual impulses. The emergence of the warded-off, unacceptable sexual feelings in psychoanalytic treatment brings the anxiety out in the open to be channeled in a more productive direction, including appropriate expression of sexuality. In Freud's second theory of anxiety, the "signal" theory (see Compton, 1972), a small amount of anxiety from a perceived danger "signals" the ego to be alert to the threat. In order to keep the threat out of consciousness so that it does not become overly traumatic, defenses are activated. However, if the defenses fail, a full anxiety attack will occur. Within this model, treatment focuses on insight about the perceived danger, so that the patient can see that the danger is not as great as he or she imagines. Interestingly, this idea is similar to aspects of modern cognitive-behavioral approaches to the treatment of anxiety disorders. For example, the cognitive-behavioral treatment of panic disorder involves educating (and sometimes demonstrating) to the patient that the danger from panic symptoms is not what the patient imagines (e.g., that the panic symptoms are those of a heart attack). Similarly, exposure-based treatments of anxiety disorders probably involve a cognitive component of demonstrating to the patient that reality is not as dangerous as what the patient imagined.

Psychodynamic writers subsequent to Freud proposed a number of modified or alternative explanations for chronic anxiety. Perhaps the greatest modification involved a shift away from a focus on sexual impulses as the cause of anxiety and toward the impact of human relations on psychological growth. For example, Horney (1950) suggested that in the developing child, relationships that hinder psychological growth (e.g., relations with caretakers who are dominating, overprotective, over-exacting, indifferent, etc.) lead to a lack of confidence in self and others. In the face of this lack of confidence, the child feels isolated and helpless, and views the world as potentially hostile; all this leaves the child with a "basic anxiety." As part of efforts to cope with this anxiety, the child becomes extremely clinging, rebellious, or distant from others, often being pulled in several of these directions at once. In an effort to escape from the resultant feelings (inferior, lost, anxious, and conflicted), the individual creates an idealized self-image that he or she attempts to achieve in life. The ideal self, however, can never be achieved, and these failures led to self-hate and neurotic conflict.

A purely interpersonal perspective on anxiety was proposed by Sullivan (1953), who postulated that anxiety is often a result of anticipated disapproval from the primary caregiver earlier in life. In treatment, the therapist provides a climate of security that provides a context for patients to gradually develop their own security operations over time. This concept of therapeutic security is similar to the notion of the therapeutic alli-

ance that is a major component of the supportive–expressive (SE) treatment described in this chapter. The interpersonal perspective was further
articulated by Fromm-Reichmann (1955), who emphasized the anxiety-
producing role of distorted views of other people. In this model, there is
a hypothesized reciprocal relationship between anxiety and distorted
thoughts about people, with anxiety leading to distorted thoughts about
others, and distorted thoughts producing further anxiety. This pattern is
first generated from early relational experiences.

From the object relations school, Fairbairn (1952) emphasized the
role of separation conflict originating in infancy. A conflict develops between the child's feelings of dependency on the primary caregiver and a
fear of being engulfed and loss of identity, with both sides of the conflict
generating anxiety. In contrast, Klein (1975a, 1975b) linked anxiety to the
infant's experience and subsequent fear of not being able to evoke the primary caregiver when needed. Since the primary caregiver cannot be
evoked when needed, a sense of being persecuted by others develops.
Moreover, there is a lack of confidence in the ability to sustain or repair
relationships. These internalized representations of self and others are
carried over and activated later in life, with consequential impacts on relationships with other people. This object relations view is incorporated
into our SE therapy for GAD in regard to the meaning of separation from
the therapist at treatment termination. It is hypothesized that the impending termination of the relationship with the therapist activates relationship themes involving attachment and loss.

Although psychodynamic writers of varying perspectives ranging
from classical psychoanalysis to object relations to self psychology have offered theories on chronic anxiety, our SE treatment model is more closely
aligned with the interpersonal view. This brings us to the final, and perhaps most compelling, justification for development of an interpersonally
oriented psychodynamic therapy for GAD: the emerging empirical literature that highlights the central role of interpersonal factors in the etiology
and/or maintenance of GAD.

The first study to suggest a link between interpersonal factors and
GAD was reported by Borkovec, Robinson, Pruzinsky, and DePree (1983),
who showed that worry (the central feature of GAD) was associated with
high levels of interpersonal concerns. Further indirect evidence for this
connection was apparent in the data reported by Brown and Barlow
(1992) regarding the high level of comorbidity between GAD and social
phobia—the latter being fundamentally a disorder involving anxiety about
interpersonal situations.

The possible origins of the interpersonal issues in GAD have been explored in several studies. Lichtenstein and Cassidy (1991) reported a study
in which people with GAD were asked to recall memories of the nature of
attachment to primary caregivers in childhood. Significantly more inse-

cure attachment to primary caregivers was found in the subjects with GAD than in those without GAD. In particular, the subjects with GAD reported greater enmeshment (overinvolvement with parents) and role reversal (i.e., taking on parental responsibilities as children), as well as greater preoccupying anger and oscillating feelings toward their caregivers. Furthermore, the subjects with GAD felt more rejected as children by their primary caregivers than did the subjects without GAD.

A second, related area of relevant research on GAD concerns the incidence of past traumatic events. Borkovec (1994) reported that subjects meeting criteria for GAD were found to have a significantly greater frequency of past traumatic events than subjects without GAD had. Moreover, subjects meeting all the diagnostic criteria for GAD reported more frequent traumatic events than subjects meeting only some of these criteria. Further analysis of data from this study (Molina, Roemer, Borkovec, & Posa, 1992) indicated that subjects with GAD more often experienced traumas related to emotional events involving friends or family, or physical/sexual assault, than did subjects without GAD.

Interesting data on the content of current worries in patients and subjects with GAD have been presented by Borkovec (1994). Nonanxious subjects worry about serious traumatic events (e.g., death/illness/injury) more often than do treatment-seeking patients and non-treatment-seeking subjects with GAD. A speculation from these data is that the subjects/ patients with GAD avoid thinking about those past events that are most traumatic (Borkovec, 1994). Consistent with this hypothesis, Roemer, Borkovec, Posa, and Lyonfields (1991) report that worrying appears to distract subjects with GAD from more disturbing emotional contents ("Worrying about most of the things I worry about is a way to distract myself from worrying about even more emotional things, things that I don't want to think about"). Translated into psychodynamic terms, worrying appears to serve a defensive function for people with GAD.

THEORETICAL MODEL OF GAD

Drawing upon the above-described empirical research on interpersonal factors, our theoretical model of GAD hypothesizes that a set of dangerous or traumatic experiences leads to a set of basic wishes/desires, expectations, beliefs, and feelings about oneself and other people. The wishes/ desires typically involve obtaining love, security, stability, or protection from others, and are connected to fears that others may disappoint, abandon, abuse, reject, or criticize. The fears connected to these desires/ beliefs are so strong and troubling that the person with GAD would prefer not to think about the desires, feelings, or relevant present or past events that have contributed to the fears. In psychodynamic terminology, defensive mechanisms are activated that lead the patient with GAD to become overly concerned ("worried") with certain current events in his or her life as a way of avoiding thinking about the more basic, important emotional issues and desires. It is important to emphasize that our model also deviates from a classical psychoanalytic one, in that it does not restrict the development of GAD to early childhood events. Such traumas and relationship issues can occur at any phase of life. However, a sustained period of insecure attachment during childhood is more likely to generate rather powerful expectations about others as one moves into early adulthood.

Although largely out of conscious awareness, the troubling feelings and desires remain apparent in repetitive, maladaptive relationship patterns. A central part of this model is that the relationship patterns are cyclical; this means that they end up recreating the same sort of perceived circumstances that originally generated the fear. For example, people with GAD may have a desire to be close to others, but because of the expectation that others will abuse or abandon them (which would make them feel out of control or in danger), they become very controlling (or distant) in a relationship, which ends up sabotaging the relationship—recreating the abandonment (or perceived abuse) that they have come to expect from others. Alternatively, they may seek out someone who tolerates their controllingness, leading to a somewhat stable, but not satisfying or intimate, ongoing relationship that still contains the expectation that others are dangerous. The SE model operationalizes such a cyclical maladaptive relationship pattern in terms of the "core conflictual relationship theme" (CCRT). The CCRT is the maladaptive pattern, originating in prior relationships, that is evident in current interpersonal interactions. Three components constitute the CCRT: (1) the wish or desire, (2) the perceived or expected response from the other person, and (3) the response of the self. As treatment develops, therapists formulate a CCRT for each patient and use this formulation to guide interventions.

The anxiety in GAD, which is the response-of-self component of the CCRT, is hypothesized to consist of multiple components. The most basic anxiety is the fear of not obtaining what one needs in relationships and life. This fear in itself can generate ongoing worry. However, as mentioned, much of the worry component of GAD is assumed to be a defensive response (constantly thinking about relatively less important issues as a way of avoiding thinking about emotionally troubling events or concerns). The somatic symptoms of GAD can also be a defensive response (i.e., focusing on bodily symptoms as a way of avoiding emotions), as well as simply part of the physiology of the fear response. It is acknowledged that life presents difficult or traumatic experiences that may add "realistic" anxiety to the mix of fears and defenses being brought from past relationships into current relationships.

Anxiety as the CCRT response of self feeds back to maintain the CCRT pattern. An example will help clarify how this can occur. A CCRT commonly found in some patients with GAD is as follows:

Wish: To be taken care of
Response from other: Does not protect or nurture
Response of self: Fear of losing the relationship; anxiety

The patient with this CCRT engages in a number of possible strategies to reduce the anxiety. For example, the patient becomes controlling toward the other person to prevent loss of the relationship. Consequently, the other person becomes less protective/nurturing, and instead responds with either anger or increased distance. In the patient's mind, the response of the other person "validates" the patient's fear of losing the relationship. In addition, the patient does not achieve fulfillment of his or her need to be taken care of. The need therefore remains active and in search of fulfillment, propagating the pattern. However, this wish/need, or any other CCRT wish/need, is not seen as a drive that is discharged when met. Gratification of the wish/need can reduce its immediate potency, but the wish/need generally remains ongoing.

The SE model does not presuppose that one specific CCRT is evident in all patients with GAD. This is because the traumas and relationship problems that are part of the origins of GAD occur in multiple forms and at various levels of severity. These different environmental inputs are modified by other aspects of a person's past and current social world and temperament. The fact that expectations and feelings about others may change in the context of current, relatively positive relationships provides the opportunity for psychotherapy—a relationship with a caring and insightful therapist—to change these patterns.

Although human beings certainly have wishes and desires that are not interpersonal in nature, the wishes/desires that are inherent within CCRT patterns, and therefore implicated in the sequential pattern that ends in anxiety, are generally interpersonal (e.g., wishes for closeness, independence, nurturance, etc.). Research on CCRT patterns in psychotherapy indicates that multiple wishes and multiple CCRTs are commonly found, although one CCRT predominates across most of the interactions with other people described by patients in therapy (Connolly et al., 1996). Most interpersonal wishes that are part of CCRT formulations are not problematic or inappropriate in themselves. However, some patients (particularly those with more severe psychological disturbances) do express inappropriate wishes, such as the wish to hurt someone else. In many such cases, the inappropriate wish is derived from an underlying CCRT that contains an appropriate wish. For example, a patient may have the underlying wish to be close to other people that is connected to the expectation that others will take advantage of him or her. In response to the fear that others will take advantage of him or her, the patient displays the wish to hurt others.

TREATMENT MODEL

The SE model of treatment for GAD is an adaptation of Luborsky's (1984) general SE manual. The "supportive" component of SE treatment consists of efforts to bolster the patient's self-esteem and adaptive abilities. The therapist accomplishes this in part through enhancing or maintaining a positive therapeutic alliance, which is seen as a major curative factor in its own right. Other aspects of the treatment process (e.g., the regular sessions, consistent boundaries in the therapeutic contract and relationship) also provide supportive structure. The "expressive," or "exploratory," component of SE treatment is the process of expressing thoughts and feelings during treatment in order to gain insight about the underlying factors that play a role in maladaptive interpersonal patterns. Although most of the techniques in our adaptation of SE treatment for GAD are derived from the general manual (Luborsky, 1984), there are some modifications and additions to tailor the treatment to GAD. Thus our goal is not to propose a totally new treatment; however, the greater level of specificity provided in our adaptation allows for implementation of SE treatment in a research context where there is a need for standardization of treatment, so that studies can be replicated. For further details of the basic elements of the general SE approach to treatment, including historical influences on the development of the SE model, the reader is referred to Luborsky (1984). Here we present information on the selection of patients suitable for our approach, the treatment format, and the setting of treatment goals. In subsequent sections, we describe the basic theory of core interventions for change, as well as techniques and other technical issues.

Selection of Patients for Treatment

The treatment is designed for patients who present with a principal *Diagnostic and Statistical Manual of Mental Disorders*, fourth edition (DSM-IV) diagnosis of GAD. Because of the high rates of comorbidity of other Axis I conditions (particularly major depressive disorder) with GAD, the presence of other disorders is not a reason for exclusion, but GAD should be primary. However, patients with any current or past history of schizophrenic disorders, bipolar disorders, or Axis II Cluster A personality disorders (schizoid, schizotypal, or paranoid) are excluded, as are patients with alcohol or other substance dependence. In a clinical context, as opposed to a research study, patients with any of these other disorders do not have to be excluded, provided that they receive additional concurrent treatment targeting the comorbid disorder(s).

Treatment Format

SE treatment for GAD is administered in weekly individual psychotherapy (50-minute sessions). Basic treatment is for 16 sessions, but this is followed by monthly booster sessions for 3 months. In a research context, diagnostic evaluation occurs independently before assignment to a therapist. In a clinical context, assessment sessions (presumably 1 or 2) would occur before the initiation of the 16-session treatment.

Treatment Goals

Once a patient has begun therapy, one of the first tasks is the setting of goals. The therapist begins treatment, after introductions, by asking a general question (e.g., "Can you tell me what's going on?") in order to understand the patient's chief complaints. The intent of this inquiry phase is to elicit relevant material to assist in formulating goals. If possible, preliminary goals are set at the end of the first session, but often a second session is needed to obtain more information or to establish more of a therapeutic alliance before setting goals.

Typical patient goals include symptom reduction, improvements in self-esteem, and/or interpersonal changes. Sometimes patients with GAD focus solely on their symptoms, in which case the therapist needs to encourage exploration of the interpersonal domain. Specifically, the therapist obtains information about relationship themes by asking the patient directly for descriptions of interactions with other people (see "Techniques," below, for the elicitation of relationship episodes). If no interpersonal goals can be formulated, SE therapy may still achieve some success with a patient, based upon the supportive elements of treatment. It is rare, however, that a therapist is unable to introduce some interpersonal goals as part of the treatment.

Once the therapist has a good sense of possible goals, these goals are reviewed with the patient; the patient's own language is used as much as possible. Because the treatment is brief, goals have to be appropriate for a short-term treatment (e.g., major comprehensive personality change would not be an appropriate goal). Examples of interpersonal goals would include "reducing the number of arguments with my spouse" or "setting limits with my boss." A good goal is one that is interpersonal, clearly articulated, and achievable within the time frame of brief therapy. A less helpful goal is one that is vague or based upon a fantasy (i.e., achieving some unlikely success in life). If less appropriate goals are suggested by a patient, the therapist attempts to clarify/refine the goal or to make it clear that certain goals cannot be achieved within the brief time frame of therapy, so other goals needs to be set.

As treatment advances, the therapist periodically refers to the goals as a way of monitoring progress and setting new goals. If new goals are added during treatment, they have to be appropriate for the amount of time remaining. Essential to our model is that the therapist attempts, if possible, to add a goal (if it is not one of the originally agreed-upon goals) relating to greater mastery over the patient's CCRT.

THEORY OF CHANGE

We hypothesize that a number of factors contribute to psychotherapeutic changes for patients receiving SE treatment for GAD. The relative salience of each of these factors may vary from patient to patient as a function of a patient's unique interpersonal patterns and characterological style. These factors naturally interact and overlap. We discuss each factor as a separate category, acknowledging that the division of these therapeutic change factors into separate categories is somewhat arbitrary.

The theory of change for the generic model of SE treatment is described by Luborsky (1984, Ch. 2). Three main psychological changes are specified: (1) an increase in self-understanding of the CCRT, which leads to mastery over the impairing relationship conflicts, including understanding of the relation between symptoms and the CCRT; (2) an increased feeling that the therapist is an ally working collaboratively with the patient to change the self-defeating relationship patterns; and (3) an internalization of the helpful therapist and the tools of therapy, which will ensure that the treatment gains are maintained. A full description of each of these factors is provided by Luborsky, including an account of the patient's and therapist's roles in bringing about these changes. Below, we discuss each of these factors as they relate to SE psychotherapy for GAD. We further expand upon each factor through a review of the empirical literature. We also discuss concepts specific to our work with patients who have GAD.

Change in the CCRT

The primary determinant of successful treatment is hypothesized to be change in the patient's CCRT. In a naturalistic sample of outpatients receiving dynamically oriented psychotherapy, changes in the pervasiveness of the CCRT wish, response-of-other, and response-of-self components have been shown to significantly predict improvements in symptomatology and general functioning (Crits-Christoph & Luborsky, 1990). In this investigation, changes in the pervasiveness of CCRT components were relatively small in magnitude, indicating that even small changes in the CCRT pattern could affect symptom course. Of note is that this study did not examine the causal sequence of change in CCRT pervasiveness and symptom change. It could be that symptom changes lead to changes in core patterns, or that a third variable may result in both symptomatic and core pattern changes. However, this empirical evidence is consistent with the hypothesis that changes in the pervasiveness of the CCRT are an important part of the therapeutic process.

Within our dynamic framework, we see changes in psychiatric symptoms as important, but not as constituting the sole definition of therapeutic change. We see changes in the CCRT as a necessary part of successful psychotherapy. This is not to say that symptom relief is not an important part of psychotherapeutic change; indeed, it is likely to be very important from the patient's perspective. Rather, we would hypothesize that symptom change in the absence of substantial CCRT change would result in higher rates of relapse and recurrence of GAD symptoms following treatment.

Our focus on brief therapy, where the time limits may not allow for complete changes in relationship patterns, is supported by the empirical evidence suggesting that even small changes in CCRT pervasiveness can influence symptom course. Our model does not suggest that interpersonal conflicts are completely explored and resolved in a brief course of therapy. Rather, our theory is that maladaptive interpersonal patterns, although rooted in earlier interpersonal experiences, are triggered by relationships and events throughout the patient's lifespan. The goal of a brief course of psychotherapy is to help the patient identify the underlying CCRT, understand the current developmental or relationship manifestations of the pattern, explore the maladaptive coping responses that are currently hindering successful life adjustment, and work through new expectations of self and others. This process begins during the brief treatment and, if the patient has successfully learned the tools of self-exploration, continues to influence the patient's exploration of new relationship experiences following treatment. We hypothesize that the maintenance of treatment gains and the prevention of future relapses and recurrences are associated with the degree to which the patient continues to utilize the tools of psychotherapy.

A successful psychotherapy is expected to demonstrate a variety of changes to the CCRT. The primary goals are to move the patient toward a less self-defeating response of self and to help the patient develop more adaptive coping responses. A successful treatment might also result in less rigid projection of perceived responses from others into new relationship experiences. Although the patient's wish may not change substantially in a brief treatment, a modification of the wish in certain interpersonal contexts might be achieved. Furthermore, the patient may demonstrate changes in the CCRT by choosing new, more adaptive relationships that allow for appropriate expression of the CCRT wish.

Both increases in self-understanding and the development of a positive therapeutic alliance are hypothesized to contribute to change in the CCRT across psychotherapy. "Self-understanding," traditionally referred to as "insight" in the psychoanalytic literature, is a complex construct that encompasses various aspects of the therapeutic change process. Changes in self-understanding include the uncovering of feelings or patterns that are largely out of the patient's awareness. Complete repression of a traumatic event, with sudden emergence during treatment, is probably rare. More typical is the case where a patient has access to traumatic memories and the corresponding feelings, but engages in a variety of defenses (such as the worrying typical of patients with GAD) to avoid thinking about painful feelings. A therapist implementing the SE model uses interpretation of these defenses and resistances in order to help the patient learn to confront fears and interpersonal conflicts directly, instead of engaging in processes to avoid the painful feelings.

A cognitive, or general intellectual, understanding about one's own relationship conflicts is also an important aspect of self-understanding. Although purely cognitive learning may appear superficial, we feel that such learning is a necessary part of therapeutic change. However, patients are not likely to learn from interpretations that provide intellectual information regarding their dynamic conflicts before defenses and resistances have been lowered. Such a premature interpretation is likely to result in increased anxiety and further activation of the defenses. Thus the first step is to lower defenses/resistances. Next, cognitive learning of CCRT patterns can occur. After the defenses have been lowered and emotions connected to the conflictual themes have been accessed, emotional insight can then occur. Such emotional insight provides the opportunity to move beyond intellectualized insight. With emotional insight, the patient experiences the power of the CCRT pattern in his or her life. When this happens, the patient achieves greater certainty about the significance of the CCRT, thereby increasing motivation to master the theme and/or generate new behaviors. In fact, because patients with GAD engage in excessive worrying, there is a danger in remaining at only a cognitive level of self-understanding: The patients may simply incorporate the cognitive information into their worry systems (e.g., "I'm worried about needing too much from my spouse").

Self-understanding can also be thought of as a skill rather than only an outcome. One goal of our brief dynamic therapy is for patients to learn the skill of self-exploration. As described earlier, we see the acquisition of this skill as important in carrying on the work of therapy after treatment termination.

The therapist's interpretations of the CCRT pattern are the main techniques used to encourage self-exploration and increase self-understanding (see "Techniques," below). Research studies have found that the accuracy of therapists' interpretations relative to the CCRT pattern is associated with treatment outcome (Crits-Christoph, Cooper, & Luborsky, 1988) and the development of a positive therapeutic alliance (Crits-Christoph, Barber, & Kurcias, 1993). These studies were performed by having independent judges, who were unaware of treatment outcome and the quality of the therapeutic alliance for each patient, formulate CCRT patterns from relationship episodes extracted from transcripts of therapy sessions. Another set of judges identified therapist interpretations in transcripts of sessions. These interpretations were then extracted from the transcripts, and a different set of independent judges (also unaware of outcome and alliance) rated the extent to which each therapist interpretation mentioned each component of the patient's CCRT pattern. Based upon these results, our model of SE treatment for GAD places heavy emphasis on accurate formulation and interpretation of the CCRT throughout treatment.

Therapeutic Alliance

The second curative factor described by Luborsky (1984) in the general SE manual is an increased sense of a joint struggle with the therapist to overcome the symptoms and problems. We see the development of a positive therapeutic alliance as an important change factor for multiple reasons. First, the therapeutic alliance has consistently been found to be a robust predictor of psychotherapy outcome (Horvath & Symonds, 1991). Second, the therapeutic alliance is an important change factor because it relates to our formulation of the dynamic issues typical of patients with GAD. We hypothesize that patients with GAD have insecure or conflicted attachment patterns. The experience of a positive therapeutic relationship may provide a corrective emotional experience for the patients and therefore may be fundamental to effective treatment of GAD. Some patients with GAD may experience guilt that they have done something wrong to another that fuels their anxiety reaction. A positive therapeutic alliance with the therapist can provide a safe environment that helps ease the feelings of guilt and decrease anxiety.

A positive therapeutic alliance may further provide an environment in which the patient feels safe enough to approach his or her fears. The safe context of a positive therapeutic alliance may allow patients to lower their defenses and to access fears they do not normally think about. For patients who may be more aware of their fears, the positive alliance may allow them to explore fears that they are reluctant to disclose to others because of possible negative reactions. These patients may be more likely to disclose difficult issues to significant people in their lives once they have had success disclosing and exploring these issues with their therapists. In addition, the safe relationship with the therapist may encourage a patient to approach feared interpersonal situations. This process is not simply one of desensitization. Rather, the therapy works to change the patient's internal representations of others and their expected responses.

A positive therapeutic alliance not only provides the safety for the patient's explorations of fears, but also supports the patient in trying new behaviors. As described by object relations theorists in the concept of separation–individuation, we assume that patients wish to become independent and try new things, but that a secure positive attachment must first be present. Alternatively, the therapist must be careful not to undermine treatment by activating a patient's fears of engulfment and loss of identity.

Finally, a positive therapeutic alliance provides the necessary context in which interpretive interventions are most likely to be effective. A positive therapeutic alliance should convey the sense that the patient and therapist are working collaboratively to explore the patient's conflicts, rather than a sense that the therapist is coming up with explanations for the patient's conflicts that may be heard as critical. The alliance sets the stage for other therapeutic change mechanisms.

New Behaviors

The psychodynamic perspective focuses on the patient's gaining self-understanding of maladaptive relationship patterns, in order to give him or her the opportunity to grow in a more positive direction. However, we also acknowledge the need for patients to engage successfully in new behaviors. For patients with GAD, as well as any patients suffering from anxiety disorders, the adoption of new, more adaptive behaviors is particularly important. As progress is made in lowering defenses and understanding the CCRT patterns, the therapist's role is to encourage new more adaptive responses on the part of the patient. For example, after the patient comes to see how his or her needs and wishes tend not to be satisfied because of the "vicious cycle" that occurs with a CCRT pattern, the therapist can encourage the patient to ask directly for what he or she wants from others.

Comparison with Cognitive-Behavioral Therapy

In order to further understand the theoretical model for our SE treatment for GAD, it is instructive to compare our approach to cognitive-behavioral therapy—the treatment that has received the most attention in the empirical literature. As psychodynamic therapy has become more focal and briefer (as in the model described here), and as cognitive-behavioral therapy has been modified over the years to place more emphasis on schemata, or core beliefs, the degree of similarity between these two major modalities of treatment has increased. Despite the focus in our theory of change on "beliefs" about others and the self, as well as the encouraging of new behaviors, it is important to point out where differences remain. Some of these differences are mostly a matter of relative emphasis, and some are clear theoretical divergences.

Although the cognitive model of anxiety (Beck & Emery with Greenberg, 1985) has a major focus on the concept of the schema, which seems quite similar to the notion of the CCRT, the CCRT model specifically defines important schemata as interpersonal in nature, rather than simply beliefs about the self or the world in general. Note that the cognitive model does not exclude interpersonal schemata, but it does not emphasize them to the extent that the SE model does. More recently, some cognitive-behavioral models (e.g., Safran & Segal, 1990) have begun to have a more explicit interpersonal focus.

The CCRT model also specifies the interpersonal pattern in terms of three sequential components: the wish, the response from other, and the response of self. In particular, the wish component is a major difference between the SE model and the cognitive model. The notion that the wish drives the whole sequence is distinctively a psychodynamic one.

The SE model also places greater emphasis on self-understanding and working through as the major elements in the change process, whereas cognitive-behavioral therapy emphasizes the identification of automatic thoughts, homework, exposure, and evaluating evidence for a belief. However, both treatments contain elements of all these processes, and the differences are more a matter of emphasis or terminology. In the SE model, however, at least some of the material (i.e., aspects of the CCRT pattern) are thought to be less accessible to the patient, at least initially in therapy; the cognitive model assumes that material can be fairly easily accessed with some probing.

One clear difference between SE therapy and cognitive-behavioral therapy relates to the theory of defenses. Whereas the cognitive model would describe the concept of defenses as simply another set of beliefs, the psychodynamic model would add that defenses are motivated by anxiety. This distinction has implications for how a therapist formulates the pathway for progress over the course of psychotherapy. If a patient is seen as having pathological defenses that obscure the issues or lead to avoidance of anxiety and important interpersonal issues connected to the anxiety, the psychodynamic therapist will probably want to address such defenses as a preliminary step.

Because of the importance of defenses and the theory that some important material is not readily available to consciousness, the SE model, compared to the cognitive model, places more emphasis on the need to develop material over the course of treatment. This leads to a treatment process that is less structured than the cognitive-behavioral therapy process, even in a brief, focal SE treatment like our treatment for GAD.

TECHNIQUES

The reader is referred to the generic manual for SE treatment (Luborsky, 1984, Chs. 5–9) for a discussion of the major techniques of SE psychotherapy. Here we discuss the techniques that are most applicable to brief SE therapy and that should be emphasized in the treatment of GAD. In addition, our experience with providing a time-limited 16-session SE treatment for GAD has helped us map out the details for applying brief SE therapy in greater detail than was originally provided in the section on time-limited SE therapy in Luborsky's (1984) generic manual. We describe the predominant techniques used in each of 4 phases of treatment.

Early Phase

Sessions 1–5 constitute the early phase of treatment. During this phase, the therapist and patient work together to set initial goals. The most important task of this phase is to build a positive therapeutic alliance with the patient. The therapist uses supportive interventions as described by Luborsky (1984, Ch. 6) to build trust and a positive bond with the patient. For example, conveying support for the patient's wish to achieve treatment goals helps to build the alliance. Along these lines, the therapist might say, "When you started treatment, one of your goals was to reduce your anxiety. We can see that we're working together to achieve that." The therapist can also explicitly mention when progress has been made toward goals: "You noticed, in what you just said, that you are feeling less anxious since you started treatment. You are making progress with your goal." Simply encouraging a "we bond" by using the word "we" in referring to the work of therapy helps to build a sense of a team working together. Another supportive technique to build the alliance involves making positive comments on the patient's strengths and areas of competence, as well as encouraging positive steps in the patient's life: "I see you are helping yourself to feel better by finding ways to manage your problems at your job."

In addition to supportive techniques, during the early phase of treatment, the therapist further attempts to formulate and interpret a preliminary CCRT during this phase. The patient is encouraged to share descriptions of his or her interactions with other people, so that the therapist can obtain the material needed for formulating the CCRT. These descriptions of interactions with other people are termed "relationship episodes" in SE therapy. The therapist uses techniques to help the patient describe his or her interactions with other people, as described by Mark and Faude (1995). Because of the time limits of SE treatment for GAD, it cannot be assumed that once the resistances are lifted the relevant material will naturally flow, so the therapist has to be active in drawing out interpersonal material. A patient, for example, may make a general statement such as "My girlfriend is annoying." The therapist may begin by asking, "What would be an example of that?" Once the patient begins recounting a specific example, the therapist asks questions to ensure that a detailed and complete narrative account of the specific interaction is obtained (e.g., "Do you recall what you said to her?", "How did she respond to you?", "What happened next?", "What was it that you were angry about?"). Mark and Faude recommend reviewing tapes of sessions with a supervisor as the best way to teach therapists to develop ways to help patients describe interpersonal interactions.

Once a patient has described in detail several accounts of his or her interactions with other people, the therapist begins to formulate a CCRT by identifying the most common wishes, responses from the other person, and responses of the self across the multiple interactions that the patient has described. Although most patients discuss such relationship episodes from both the recent and distant (i.e., childhood/adolescence) past, the predominance of material is generally from ongoing relationships or recently occurring interactions with other people.

Some patients, particularly those with an additional Axis II diagnosis, may develop negative transferential issues with the therapist during the early phase of treatment. In such a case, the therapist should continue to try to build a positive alliance by empathizing with the patient's feelings as much as possible. The therapist should try to manage the personality issues in order to keep the patient engaged in treatment, but should try to focus the treatment on the anxiety and worry problems. Axis II defenses should be addressed in an empathic way, while maintaining the goal of exploring the CCRT feelings and issues. This treatment is not recommended for patients with severe Axis II disorders, such as borderline personality disorder.

Middle Phase

Sessions 6–11 are defined as the middle phase of treatment. The goal of the therapist during this phase is to refine the CCRT formulation, using information from the patient's narratives. During this phase, in the context of a positive therapeutic alliance, the patient feels safer, the defenses have been lowered, and the patient begins to recall and discuss more memories and experiences. The therapist uses this phase to "work through" the CCRT by relating the CCRT pattern to earlier relationships

and by helping the patient see the pervasiveness of the patterns across relationships in the patient's life, including the relationship with the therapist. In brief SE therapy, most of the focus is upon current or relatively recent relationships, not early childhood. Thus "working through" consists
of identifying and discussing how the CCRT pattern is evident repeatedly
within a single current relationship (i.e., many interactions with a current
person in the patient's life are colored by the CCRT themes), as well as
across a number of current/recent relationships. The therapist makes interpretations such as "We can see how you are again getting yourself in
the same situation—where you want to be close to someone, but then you
expect that they will reject you, and you consequently become anxious."

Unlike in many psychodynamic therapies, in SE therapy the therapist
does not pursue interpretations of the therapeutic relationship as the central technique with all patients. The therapist interprets a CCRT pattern
applied by the patient to the therapeutic relationship as just another (although sometimes vivid) example of how the pattern comes out in multiple relationships. The therapist also addresses the CCRT in the therapeutic relationship if treatment is not progressing because the CCRT with the
therapist has created an impasse (e.g., the patient expects to be take care
of and is therefore not working actively in therapy). Research suggests that
within brief SE therapy, about 60% of patients display an explicit CCRT
pattern with the therapist (Connolly et al., 1996). Furthermore, among all
therapist interpretations (which reflect only 4% of all therapist statements) in brief SE therapy, only about 7% directly address the patient–
therapist relationship (Connolly, Crits-Christoph, Shappell, Barber, &
Luborsky, 1998).

Sometimes new patient material emerges in the middle of the 16-ses-
sion treatment, leaving the therapist feeling unsure of which therapeutic
direction to take. For example, it is not uncommon for a patient with
GAD to introduce a past trauma, including past abuse, about halfway
through treatment. We feel that in most such cases the traumatic episode
can be explored with the patient and used to achieve further understanding of the patient's symptoms, defenses, and interpersonal conflicts. Although some psychoanalytic theorists feel that is countertherapeutic to
explore such material in a brief treatment, we feel that such exploration
can be helpful in unfolding and learning about the CCRT. However, if the
patient begins to deteriorate during the exploration of traumatic experiences, the patient can be referred for additional treatment.

Termination Phase

Sessions 12–16 are considered the termination phase and play a central
role in brief SE therapy for GAD. Mann's (1973) brief therapy makes the
termination issues the primary focus throughout brief treatment. We be-

lieve that termination exploration is critical, but do not include it as the primary focus across the entire length of treatment. Luborsky (1984) describes the termination phase as characterized by a resurgence of symptoms, resulting from the activation of the patient's CCRT in anticipation of the loss of the therapist. The patient may experience the realistic loss of an important person (the therapist) in his or her life, but further experiences the fear of not obtaining, for example, CCRT wishes for support, nuturance, love, or closeness. Thus a patient may begin to experience that the therapist is "like other people" (in that the therapist is abandoning the patient, not caring, being arbitrary, etc.). The therapist links the upcoming termination to the CCRT pattern as a way of illustrating once again the pervasiveness of the pattern. Moreover, the activation and working through of the CCRT at termination become an opportunity to illustrate to the patient that there are alternatives to the feared negative outcomes that are connected to the patient's CCRT.

We suggest that the therapist begin work on termination no later than Session 14, but preferably as early as Session 12. In the absence of references to termination on the patient's part, the therapist may collude with the patient to avoid discussion of painful feelings regarding termination, and may instead explore other topics that seem more pressing. We have found that termination issues often explode in the last sessions if left undiscussed. Both patient and therapist may be left with the sense that there is not enough time to deal with the feelings and issues that emerge. Supervision can be helpful in training therapists to address termination issues early enough and to be less apprehensive about their own termination feelings.

In brief SE treatment, the therapist's goal is to have the patient complete treatment with a good understanding of his or her CCRT, although intellectual understanding is not the only ingredient of successful treatment. During the termination phase, the therapist should provide a clear and succinct summary to the patient regarding what has been learned about the CCRT. The therapist should further encourage the patient to express an understanding of the CCRT in his or her own words.

Booster Phase

We designed a final phase of treatment, called the "booster phase," on an experimental basis as part of our research project. Based on our positive experience, we recommend the use of booster sessions as part of the clinical treatment package. Three monthly booster sessions are scheduled following the 16 acute-phase sessions. The goals of the booster phase are to monitor gains and reinforce the changes that the patient has made; to encourage and support the patient to do the work of therapy on his or her own (i.e., internalization of the treatment tasks); and to help the patient explore relapses in terms of the CCRT and the loss of the therapist. The patient should be referred for further treatment if a serious relapse occurs during the booster phase.

Some psychodynamic therapists are concerned that booster sessions "water down" the termination process. However, we find that the 16th session is still experienced by the patient as the end of the regular therapy. Thus we feel that the positive aspects of the booster sessions far outweigh the potential interference with the termination process. We do recommend that booster sessions not be scheduled more frequently than once a month.

GAD-Specific Technical Issues

There are a number of technical issues specific to SE treatment for GAD, beyond the modifications related to the 16-session format. The general SE manual advises therapists to adjust the relative number of supportive versus expressive (exploratory) techniques, depending on the degree of patient pathology. For patients with GAD, we recommend a moderate number of supportive techniques to build a positive alliance and create a safe environment for the exploration of painful memories and feelings. Although the larger goal of treatment is to reduce anxiety symptoms, some amount of anxiety is helpful to the therapeutic process by providing the motivation to the patient for working actively in the therapy. Therefore, the therapist does not attempt to support the patient to the extent that all anxiety is relieved within sessions.

Several points regarding the interpretation of the CCRT are salient to the treatment of GAD. A patient with GAD often experiences a primitive wish (such as the wish to feel safe) early in the treatment process, while the patient is overwhelmed by the symptoms and feelings of hopelessness. The therapist's goal is to help bring this wish to the surface in the context of the alliance. The therapist may make the interpretation that the patient's wishes are unfulfilled in other relationships and may explore whether such wishes are fulfilled in the therapeutic relationship. As the primitive wishes are brought into consciousness and gratified in the alliance, the patient is motivated to move on to more mature wishes. The therapist helps to focus the therapeutic explorations on these more mature CCRT wishes in the patient's current relationships.

The therapist also works to link the CCRT wishes to the anxiety symptoms (one of the responses of self). Initially, the therapist should establish the link between the wishes and the feelings of anxiety. After the link is established, the therapist should help the patient to explore those responses of self that are self-defeating and that perpetuate the cyclical maladaptive pattern. For example, a patient may wish to be close to others but may distance him- or herself in response to perceived rejections from others. In such a case, the therapist helps to link the patient's response of self to the wishes and perceived responses of others, pointing out the self-defeating nature of the response. The focus on the response of self helps to lay the groundwork for developing new, more adaptive responses of self as therapy progresses.

Resistance and Defenses

The generic SE manual by Luborsky (1984) does not provide much discussion about defenses and resistances. We have borrowed from Mark and Faude (1997), who elaborate on how defenses and resistances should be handled within the SE model. For patients with GAD, we see worry as a common defense used to avoid exploration of more painful experiences and feelings. However, we do not recommend interpretation or confrontation of this defense or other defenses as the primary intervention strategy of this treatment approach. Unlike Davanloo (1980), we do not attempt to analyze and confront defenses routinely. Rather, defenses and resistances are explored to the extent that they influence or hinder the understanding of the CCRT.

We recommend a variety of techniques to deal with defenses in SE treatment. The therapist can (1) encourage the patient to explore reality, rather than arguing with the patient; (2) use questions to explore relationship experiences, rather than stating truths; and (3) consider sidestepping the patient's defenses when the therapist feels it is more important to support the patient.

It is important that the therapist be aware of resistances and defenses as he or she attempts to formulate the CCRT. It is possible that the manifest response of self may disguise an underlying wish. For example, the response of self may be a defense to the underlying wish. If it is not helpful to interpret the underlying defense, the therapist may explore the less threatening wish.

Past Traumas

Past traumas are frequent in patients with GAD. Within our treatment model, the therapist does not specifically search for past traumas. Such experiences will often be brought up by the patient if they are relevant to the relationship issues being discussed. The therapist should provide empathy for the patient's traumatic experience. When relevant, the therapist should explore with the patient how the trauma might have exacerbated the CCRT. Furthermore, the therapist can help the patient explore what he or she would have wanted in regard to the trauma. For example, the patient may have wanted to express anger or elicit help.

EMPIRICAL EVIDENCE FOR THE APPROACH

We have conducted two studies of SE treatment for GAD. The first was a single-group trial. The main results of this study have been published elsewhere (Crits-Christoph et al., 1996) and are briefly summarized here. Follow-up data from this first study that have not been previously reported are presented here as well. A second study comparing SE therapy to supportive therapy alone for GAD is currently being completed, and the results are not yet available.

The first study had several goals. Because this was our first investigation of the treatment model, one goal was to refine the treatment approach for patients with GAD. Aspects of the treatment described in this chapter have emerged from this first systematic experience of treating patients with GAD. A second goal was to objectively evaluate therapists' performance in applying the SE treatment protocol for GAD. For this purpose, audiotapes of treatment sessions were rated for competence and adherence to the SE approach. A third goal of the pilot study was to obtain preliminary efficacy data. Although this was not a controlled study, these preliminary data would help justify continuing with further research efforts to establish the efficacy of the treatment. Below we describe the study sample, followed by the results of analyses of efficacy and treatment fidelity data.

Sample Characteristics

The sample consisted of 26 patients, 23 of whom completed at least 12 of the required 16 sessions. All 26 patients were evaluated after 16 weeks, regardless of whether they had dropped out earlier. Patients met DSM-IV diagnostic criteria for GAD, with 65% also receiving a concurrent Axis I diagnosis and 42% a concurrent Axis II diagnosis at intake. The average age was 44 years; 62% were female; 8% were members of an ethnic minority group; 73% were married, 15% were single, and 12% were divorced. Five highly (10 years) experienced psychotherapists (four with PhDs and one with an MSW) participated in the study.

Pre–Post Changes

Outcome data for a number of efficacy measures are given in Table 12.1. Statistically significant changes across 16 weeks of treatment were apparent for all outcome measures. In particular, scores on the Beck and Hamilton measures of anxiety symptoms were markedly reduced. Importantly, the effects of treatment were broader than changes in anxiety symptoms, with relatively large decreases found on the Inventory of Interpersonal Problems and the Hamilton and Beck depression scales.

TABLE 12.1. Baseline, Termination (Week 16), and Follow-Up Mean (*SD*) Outcomes for Patients with GAD Treated with SE Therapy

Measure	Intake (n = 26)	Termination (n = 26)	6-month follow-up (n = 21)	12-month follow-up (n = 23)
HAM-A	15.8 (5.6)	7.9 (6.1)**		
HAM-D	10.6 (4.1)	5.9 (4.1)**		
BAI	21.5 (7.1)	7.4 (8.1)**	6.7 (5.9)	7.9 (7.4)
BDI	16.0 (7.8)	7.5 (7.0)**	8.0 (6.3)	8.4 (8.6)
WORRY	53.3 (6.4)	47.2 (7.8)**	47.2 (7.8)	44.4 (8.4)*
IIP	1.24 (0.55)	1.10 (0.62)*	1.04 (0.62)	1.01 (0.64)

Note. Intake and termination data are taken from Crits-Christoph et al. (1996). HAM-A, Hamilton Anxiety Rating Scale (Hamilton, 1959); HAM-D, Hamilton Rating Scale for Depression (17-item) (Hamilton, 1960); BAI, Beck Anxiety Inventory (Beck, Epstein, Brown, & Steer, 1988); BDI, Beck Depression Inventory (Beck, Steer, & Garbin, 1988); WORRY, Penn State Worry Questionnaire (Meyer et al., 1990); IIP, Inventory of Interpersonal Problems (Horowitz et al., 1988). The p values for termination are from paired t tests comparing baseline to termination. The p values for follow-up are from paired t tests comparing termination to each follow-up assessment.
*p < .05;**p < .001.

At termination, 79% of patients no longer qualified for a diagnosis of GAD.

Follow-Up Data

We conducted follow-up assessments at 6 and 12 months after termination. Only self-report measures were gathered at follow-up, with 21 patients available for the 6-month assessment and 23 available for the 12-month assessment. These data are also presented in Table 12.1. In general, there were no significant changes from termination to either follow-up assessment, indicating that patients maintained their gains. The exception was a significant reduction (t = 2.3, p = .03) in worry (the central feature of GAD) from termination to the 12-month follow-up. This is particularly important, because worry changed the least from baseline to termination. All variables changed significantly (p < .05) from baseline to each follow-up visit, with the exception of the IIP, which justed missed significance (p = .057) in the comparison of baseline with 12-month follow-up.

Treatment Fidelity and Discriminability

Independent judges provided ratings of adherence and competence on a 45-item general SE scale (Barber & Crits-Christoph, 1996) modified for

GAD. Each item is rated on a 1–7 scale for both frequency of each technique (adherence) and quality of implementation (competence). The scale produces summary mean scores for adherence and competence for both the supportive and expressive aspects of SE therapy. Ratings were made from audiotapes of one session drawn from all 26 patients receiving SE treatment. As a comparison, ratings were also made for one session of 23 patients receiving cognitive therapy for GAD or other anxiety problems.

The mean summary competence score for SE treatment was 4.0 and for cognitive therapy was 3.1 (Cohen's d effect size = 1.7, t = 5.3, $p <$ .00001). Competence in supportive techniques demonstrated a smaller effect (effect size = 0.70, t = 2.4, p .02), while competence in the delivery of expressive techniques evidenced a larger effect (effect size = 1.9, t = 5.9, p .00001). These data indicate that SE therapy for GAD can be adequately implemented according to our protocol and can be readily discriminated from another psychotherapy.

SUMMARY AND FUTURE DIRECTIONS

We have developed a treatment for GAD that is sensible, given what is known about the interpersonal factors that may contribute to the development of this disorder. The treatment model can be successfully implemented by trained psychotherapists. Moreover, our preliminary outcome data are encouraging, and we await the results of our controlled evaluation.

Despite these promising indicators, several potential limitations of our approach need to be acknowledged. It is clear that GAD is a chronic disorder with disturbances in cognitive, interpersonal, and somatic domains. The ultimate answer to the treatment of the disorder may lie with a treatment package that can address these multiple components. Thus many patients may require medication in addition to a psychotherapy that addresses interpersonal issues. Furthermore, it may be necessary to combine the teaching of specific coping skills (e.g., relaxation training) with an interpersonally oriented psychotherapy.

The potential integration of other treatment approaches into SE therapy for GAD is part of our long-term research plan. Although we initially need to document efficacy through controlled studies of SE therapy, future studies will turn to ways to enhance outcome through combinations with medication or other psychotherapies. Another potential future direction is the identification of patients who respond or do not respond to SE treatment for GAD. If such predictors can be identified, alternative treatment can be tried with patients who do not respond to SE therapy.

REFERENCES

Barber, J. P., & Crits-Christoph, P. (1996). Development of an adherence/competence scale for dynamic therapy: Preliminary findings. *Psychotherapy Research, 6,* 81–94.

Beck, A. T., & Emery, G., with Greenberg, R. (1985). *Anxiety disorders and phobias: A cognitive perspective.* New York: Basic Books.

Beck, A. T., Epstein, N., Brown, G., & Steer, R. A. (1988). An inventory for measuring clinical anxiety: Psychometric properties. *Journal of Consulting and Clinical Psychology, 56,* 893–897.

Beck, A. T., Steer, R. A., & Garbin, M. G. (1988). Psychometric properties of the Beck Depression Inventory: Twenty-five years later. *Clinical Psychology Review, 8,* 77–100.

Borkovec, T. D. (1994). The nature, function, and origins of worry. In G. C. L. Davey & F. Tallis (Eds.), *Worrying: Perspectives on theory, assessment, and treatment* (pp. 5–33). New York: Wiley.

Borkovec, T. D., Robinson, E., Pruzinsky, T., & DePree, J. A. (1983). Preliminary exploration of worry: Some characteristics and processes. *Behaviour Research and Therapy, 21,* 9–16.

Brown, T. A., & Barlow, D. H. (1992). Comorbidity among anxiety disorders: Implications for treatment and DSM-IV. *Journal of Consulting and Clinical Psychology, 60,* 835–844.

Chambless, D. L., & Gillis, M. M. (1993). Cognitive therapy of anxiety disorders. *Journal of Consulting and Clinical Psychology, 61,* 248–260.

Compton, A. (1972). A study of the psychoanalytic theory of anxiety: I. The development of Freud's theory of anxiety. *Journal of the American Psychoanalytic Association, 20,* 3–44.

Connolly, M. B., Crits-Christoph, P., Demorest, A., Azarian, K., Muenz, L., & Chittams, J. (1996). The varieties of transference patterns in psychotherapy. *Journal of Consulting and Clinical Psychology, 64,* 1213–1221.

Connolly, M. B., Crits-Christoph, P., Shappell, S., Barber, J. P., & Luborsky, L. (1998). Therapist interventions in early sessions of brief supportive–expressive psychotherapy for depression. *Journal of Psychotherapy Practice and Research, 7,* 290–300.

Crits-Christoph, P., Barber, J., & Kurcias, J. (1993). The accuracy of therapists' interpretations and the development of the therapeutic alliance. *Psychotherapy Research, 3,* 25–35.

Crits-Christoph, P., Connolly, M. B., Azarian, K., Crits-Christoph, K., & Shappell, S. (1996). An open trial of brief supportive–expressive psychotherapy in the treatment of generalized anxiety disorder. *Psychotherapy, 33,* 418–430.

Crits-Christoph, P., Cooper, A., & Luborsky, L. (1988). The accuracy of therapists' interpretations and the outcome of psychotherapy. *Journal of Consulting and Clinical Psychology, 56,* 490–495.

Crits-Christoph, P., Crits-Christoph, K., Wolf-Palacio, D., Fichter, M., & Rudick, D. (1995). Supportive-expressive dynamic psychotherapy for generalized anxiety disorder. In J. P. Barber & P. Crits-Christoph (Eds.), *Dynamic therapies for psychiatric disorders: Axis I* (pp. 43–83). New York: Basic Books.

Crits-Christoph, P., & Luborsky, L. (1990). The changes in CCRT pervasiveness during psychotherapy. In L. Luborsky & P. Crits-Christoph (Eds.), *Understanding transference: The CCRT method* (pp. 133–146). New York: Basic Books.

Davanloo, H. (Ed.). (1980). *Short-term dynamic psychotherapy.* New York: Aronson.

Davidson, J. R. T., Dupont, R. L., Hedges, D., & Haskins, J. T. (1999). Efficacy, safety, and tolerability of venlafaxine extended release and buspirone in outpatients with generalized anxiety disorder. *Journal of Clinical Psychiatry, 60*, 528–535.

Fairbairn, W. R. D. (1952). *An object-relations theory of the personality*. New York: Basic Books.

Fromm-Reichmann, F. (1955). Psychiatric aspects of anxiety. In C. M. Thompson, M. Mazer, & E. Witenberg (Eds.), *An outline of psychoanalysis* (pp. 113–133). New York: Modern Library.

Greenblatt, D. J., Shader, R. I., & Abernethy, D. R. (1983a). Current status of benzodiazepines: I. *New England Journal of Medicine, 309*, 354–358.

Greenblatt, D. J., Shader, R. I., & Abernethy, D. R. (1983b). Current status of benzodiazepines: II. *New England Journal of Medicine, 309*, 410–416.

Hamilton, M. A. (1959). The assessment of anxiety status by rating. *British Journal of Medical Psychology, 32*, 50–55.

Hamilton, M. A. (1960). A rating scale for depression. *Journal of Neurology, Neurosurgery and Psychiatry, 23*, 56–62.

Horney, K. (1950). *Neurosis and human growth: The struggle toward self-realization*. New York: Norton.

Horowitz, L. M., Rosenberg, S. E., Baer, B. A, Ureno, G., & Villasenor, V. S. (1988). Inventory of Interpersonal Problems: Psychometric properties and clinical applications. *Journal of Consulting and Clinical Psychology, 56*, 885–892.

Horvath, A. O., & Symonds, B. D. (1991). Relation between working alliance and outcome in psychotherapy: A meta-analysis. *Journal of Counseling Psychology, 38*, 139–149.

Jensen, J. P., Bergin, A. E., & Greaves, D. W. (1990). The meaning of eclecticism: New survey and analysis of components. *Professional Psychology: Research and Practice, 21*, 124–130.

Klein, M. (1975a). *Envy and gratitude and other works 1946–1963*. New York: Delacorte Press/Seymour Lawrence.

Klein, M. (1975b). *Love, guilt, and reparation and other works 1921–1945*. New York: Delacorte Press/Seymour Lawrence.

Lichtenstein, J., & Cassidy, J. (1991, April). *The Inventory of Adult Attachment (INVAA): Validation of a new measure*. Paper presented at the biennial meeting of the Society for Research in Child Development, Seattle, WA.

Luborsky, L. (1984). *Principles of psychoanalytic psychotherapy: A manual for supportive–expressive treatment*. New York: Basic Books.

Mann, J. (1973). *Time-limited psychotherapy*. Cambridge, MA: Harvard University Press.

Mannuzza, S., Fyer, A. J., Martin, M. S., Gallops, M. S., Endicott, J., Gorman, J., Liebowitz, M. R., & Klein, F. (1989). Reliability of anxiety assessment: I. Diagnostic agreement. *Archives of General Psychiatry, 46*, 1093–1101.

Mark, D., & Faude, J. (1995). Supportive-expressive therapy of cocaine abuse. In J. P. Barber & P. Crits-Christoph (Eds.), *Dynamic therapies for psychiatric disorders: Axis I* (pp. 294–331). New York: Basic Books.

Mark, D., & Faude, J. (1997). *Psychotherapy of cocaine addiction: Entering the interpersonal world of the cocaine addict*. Northvale, NJ: Aronson.

Meyer, T. J., Miller, M. L., Metzger, R. L., & Borkovec, T. D. (1990). Development and validation of the Penn State Worry Questionnaire. *Behaviour Research and Therapy, 28*, 487–495.

Molina, S., Roemer, L., Borkovec, M., & Posa, S. (1992, November). *Generalized anxiety disorder in an analogue population: Types of past trauma*. Paper presented at the annual meeting of the Association for Advancement of Behavior Therapy, Boston.

Rickels, K., Wiseman, K., Norstad, N., Singer, M., Stoltz, D., Brown, A., & Danton, J. (1982). Buspirone and diazepam in anxiety: A controlled study. *Journal of Clinical Psychiatry, 43*, 81–86.

Rickels, K., Schweizer, E., & Lucki, I. (1987). Benzodiazepine side effects. In R. E. Hales & A. J. Frances (Eds.), *American Psychiatric Association annual review* (Vol. 6, pp. 781–801). Washington, DC: American Psychiatric Press.

Roemer, L., Borkovec, M., Posa, S., & Lyonfields, J. (1991, November). *Generalized anxiety disorder in an analogue population: The role of past trauma*. Paper presented at the annual meeting of the Association for Advancement of Behavior Therapy, New York.

Safran, J. D., & Segal, Z. V. (1990). *Interpersonal process in cognitive therapy*. New York: Basic Books.

Sullivan, H. S. (1953). *The interpersonal theory of psychiatry*. New York: Norton.

Woods, J. H., Katz, J. L., & Winger, G. (1992). Benzodiazepines: Use, abuse, and consequences. *Pharmacology Review, 44*, 151–347.

Zerbe, K. J. (1990). Through the storm: Psychoanalytic theory in the psychotherapy of the anxiety disorders. *Bulletin of the Menninger Clinic, 54*, 171–183.

CHAPTER 13

Integrative Psychotherapy

MICHELLE G. NEWMAN
LOUIS G. CASTONGUAY
THOMAS D. BORKOVEC
CHRISTINE MOLNAR

Psychotherapy integration has become a dominant movement (Castonguay, Reid, Halperin, & Goldfried, 2003). Convinced that "pure-form" orientations have neither provided a satisfactory understanding of psychopathology nor resulted in sufficiently effective treatments for the majority of their clients, many psychotherapists have integrated constructs and methods belonging to diverse approaches. In fact, "eclectic/integrative therapy" is the most frequent self-identified orientation among clinicians (Mahoney, 1991).

Although a number of innovative treatments have emerged from within the integration movement (see Norcross & Goldfried, 1992; Stricker & Gold, 1993), integrative therapists have failed to devote considerable attention to research (Castonguay & Goldfried, 1994). There is currently, no convincing empirical evidence that integration has fulfilled its promise to provide treatments that are more effective than traditional, "pure-form" approaches. The goal of this chapter is to present an integrative treatment for generalized anxiety disorder (GAD).

Our integrative therapy is based on an interesting convergence of ideas and research findings. Thomas Borkovec had conducted experimental trials on CBT for GAD for over 12 years. Toward the end of this period, several significant findings emerged. First, Cassidy (1995) found that clients with GAD reported greater role-reversed and enmeshed relationships with their primary caregivers in childhood than did matched nonanxious controls. Shortly thereafter, Pincus and Borkovec (1994) found that clients with GAD also had more interpersonal problems, especially in being overly nurturing and intrusive in their relationships with others. Finally, interpersonal dimensions that remained untreated by cognitive-behavioral therapy (CBT) predicted outcome at follow-up (Borkovec, Newman, Pincus, & Lytle, 2002). After many years of focusing on the intrapersonal anxiety process of clients with GAD, Borkovec concluded that it would be necessary to address their interpersonal problems as well if further increments in therapeutic efficacy were to be accomplished. Thus he envisioned an additive therapy investigation that would contrast CBT with and without therapeutic interventions focused on interpersonal functioning.

Independently of Borkovec's research and insights, Michelle Newman and Louis Castonguay arrived at similar conclusions with regard to the effectiveness of CBT. Having graduated from the State University of New York at Stony Brook, they were fully trained in cognitive and behavioral techniques. However, their backgrounds combined with additional training in humanistic, psychodynamic, and interpersonal therapies convinced them that several important dimensions of human functioning were not explicitly or systematically addressed in the CBT literature. Furthermore, repeated clinical observations led them to conclude that successful CBT often required more than the skilled application of learning-based techniques prescribed in treatment manuals. Their own process and outcome research also led them to believe that CBT could be improved by addressing (differently and more frequently) clients' interpersonal difficulties, exploring developmental events at the core of clients' view of self and others, deepening clients' emotional experience, and attending more adequately to the complexity of the therapeutic relationship (including alliance ruptures). Thus the arrival of Newman and Castonguay at Penn State provided an exciting opportunity for collaboration in mutual efforts to improve the effectiveness of CBT.

This chapter begins with a description of the conceptual and empirical bases of the integrative treatment. The general structure of the treatment protocol (within the current investigation) and the therapeutic rationale provided to clients are then presented. Also described are the techniques that were added to CBT to address two specific factors involved in the etiology and/or maintenance of GAD: interpersonal problems and emotional avoidance. Preliminary process and outcome data are then briefly reviewed.

THEORETICAL AND EMPIRICAL BASES
FOR AN INTEGRATIVE THERAPY FOR GAD

To date, CBT has demonstrated strong efficacy for GAD. Studies suggest that it is superior to no treatment, analytic psychotherapy, pill placebo, nondirective therapy, and placebo therapy (Borkovec & Ruscio, 2001).

Furthermore, CBT has the largest effect sizes when compared to other therapy and control conditions, and improvement is maintained for up to 1 year following treatment termination (Borkovec & Ruscio, 2001). Moreover, CBT is associated with maintenance of gains or further improvements during the follow-up period (Borkovec & Newman, 1998; Borkovec & Ruscio, 2001).

Despite its therapeutic value, there is room for improvement in CBT for GAD. Replicated findings show that at best, it leads only to an average of 50% of clients achieving high end-state functioning. One interpretation of this finding is that some clients need to receive more sessions of CBT to benefit fully from this intervention. To test this hypothesis, Borkovec and colleagues (2002) conducted a trial that substantially increased client contact time from a prior study (Borkovec & Costello, 1993). Despite almost twice as much contact time, however, the rate of high end-state functioning was not improved.

A second hypothesis is that CBT has failed to address important factors in the etiology and/or maintenance of GAD. Guided by this hypothesis our research group (Newman, Castonguay, & Borkovec, 1999a) examined theoretical criticisms of CBT, as well as applied and basic research, and determined that the addition of techniques designed to address interpersonal problems and to facilitate emotional deepening might improve the effectiveness of CBT for GAD.

INTERPERSONAL AND EMOTIONAL PROBLEMS

Several authors with a cognitive-behavioral orientation have criticized CBT for overlooking the importance of the client's interpersonal reality (e.g., Coyne & Gotlib, 1983; Goldfried & Castonguay, 1993; Goldfried & Davison, 1994; Robins & Hayes, 1993). For these authors, CBT has placed too much of an emphasis on appraisals of self in relationships, and has devoted insufficient attention to clients' potential contributions to their own interpersonal difficulties.

Summarizing these critiques, Robins and Hayes (1993) have suggested that the traditional view of clients' cognitions has failed to consider fully that clients' constructions of past and current relationship (e.g., scripts for how to behave with others, expectancies about reactions of others) are at the core of clients' views of self. Although they argue that such constructions often determine clients' actions toward others, they also assert that interpersonal behaviors can become habitual over time and therefore deserve to be addressed on their own, in addition to the cognitions themselves.

Moving beyond the critiques of models underlying CBT, several CBT therapists have incorporated constructs and intervention methods developed in humanistic, psychodynamic, and interpersonal traditions. Guidano and Liotti (1983), for example, note the influence of early attachment on an individual's view of self and patterns of interpersonal relating. In addition such techniques as examination of past and present interpersonal behaviors, use of the client–therapist relationship, and examination of the clients' impact on others have become an intrinsic part of the theoretical framework and intervention focus in CBT for personality disorders (Beck, Freeman, Davis, & Associates, 2003). Furthermore, the role of an early invalidating environment, is central to Linehan's (1993) dialectical behavior therapy for borderline personality disorder.

Writing specifically about anxiety disorders, Barlow (2002) has advised clinicians to consider the interpersonal context within which clients' difficulties are maintained, as well as comorbid personality disorders. Chorpita and Barlow (1998) have also highlighted the contribution of attachment patterns to specific vulnerabilities (i.e., cognitions of uncontrollability and unpredictability) that may be at the core of anxiety.

Jeremy Safran (Safran & Segal, 1990) has offered a particularly insightful integration of complex interpersonal issues within a CBT perspective. Guided by the work of such therapists as Sullivan, Kiesler, and Bowlby, he has argued that individuals construct internal models of relationships based on their early relationships with caregivers. These models, labeled by Safran as "interpersonal schemata," determine perceptions of others and guide clients' interpersonal behaviors in ways that typically confirm and reinforce these schemata.

The integrative treatment presented in this chapter has been informed by Safran's model of interpersonal schema. This model provides a comprehensive and coherent integration of cognitive, interpersonal, and emotional issues. It is important to note, however, that our integrative treatment is considerably different from the approach described by Safran. Whereas several techniques described in Safran and Segal's (1990) approach have been incorporated into the present integrative treatment, (e.g., procedures to deal with alliance ruptures), others have been added or modified to better address the needs of clients with GAD. In addition, whereas Safran and Segal's (1990) protocol focuses simultaneously on cognitive, interpersonal, and affective dimensions, this is not the case in the present treatment. For empirical and theoretical reasons described later, our treatment provides CBT and non-CBT techniques in two distinct therapeutic segments. The non-CBT techniques are labeled "interpersonal/emotional processing" (I/EP), because they are specifically designed to address interpersonal problems and to facilitate emotional deepening. Within a session lasting 2 "standard therapy hours" (i.e., 1 hour and 50 minutes), therapists consecutively conduct 55 minutes of CBT and 55 minutes of I/EP.

Based on the theoretical and clinical contributions described above, as well as the research findings presented below, we have identified four types of difficulties that are important targets for GAD treatment and that have not been systematically addressed by traditional CBT. These difficulties include (1) current interpersonal relationship patterns, (2) origins of current relationship problems, and (3) interpersonal difficulties that may emerge in the therapeutic relationship, (4) avoidance of emotion. These issues are briefly described here to highlight their importance in our conceptualization of GAD and to present empirical support for their therapeutic value. The ways in which each of these dimensions is addressed in the clinical context of our research program are described later in this chapter.

The Role of Current Interpersonal Problems in GAD

Evidence clearly demonstrates that interpersonal difficulties are associated with GAD. For example, clients with GAD worry more often about interpersonal issues than about any other topic (Roemer, Molina, & Borkovec, 1997). In addition, the most common comorbid Axis I diagnosis among persons with GAD is social phobia (Barlow, 2002), and nearly 50% of clients with GAD have one or more personality disorders (Sanderson, Wetzler, Beck, & Betz, 1994), which by definition involve maladaptive and enduring ways of relating to others. Moreover, persons with GAD report more interpersonal distress and rigidity than nonanxious controls, and they score significantly higher than clinical norms on most Inventory of Interpersonal Problems Circumplex Scales (Alden, Wiggins, & Pincus, 1990; Pincus & Borkovec, 1994). These findings suggest that relationship problems may contribute to the development or maintenance of GAD.

There is also evidence that interpersonal problems are not sufficiently addressed within CBT approaches. Research by Castonguay, Hayes, Goldfried, and DeRubeis (1995) found that CBT therapists emphasized intrapersonal issues (e.g., links between thoughts and emotions) more than interpersonal issues (e.g., relationship patterns of clients). They also found that CBT therapists focused more on the impact others had on clients than on the clients' potential contributions to their own interpersonal difficulties. Other studies showed that a focus on interpersonal issues was positively related to clients' improvement in psychodynamic therapy, but not in CBT (Castonguay et al., 1998; Kerr, Goldfried, Hayes, Castonguay, & Goldsamt, 1992).

In an attempt to understand how cognitive therapists deal with interpersonal issues, Hayes, Castonguay, and Goldfried (1996) discriminated between a focus on clients' cognitions about others and an effort to promote change in clients' patterns of interacting with others. Although cognitive therapists focused more frequently on clients' cognitions about others, such a focus was *negatively* related to outcome. While therapists' direct attention to real interpersonal difficulties of the client was significantly less frequent, it was related to positive change at the end of treatment.

These studies suggest that CBT therapists focus less on interpersonal issues than on intrapersonal issues, and that the way they typically focus on interpersonal issues is not effective. These studies further suggest that CBT therapists may improve their effectiveness by considering the ways with which interpersonal issues are dealt within psychodynamic and interpersonal therapies.

A recent study demonstrates the limitations of CBT in dealing with interpersonal problems in GAD. Borkovec and colleagues (2002) found that most interpersonal problems assessed were minimally responsive to CBT, and that the degree of remaining interpersonal problems was predictive of failure to maintain follow-up gains. This study is in line with previous evidence showing that Axis II comorbidity predicts poorer response to CBT (e.g., Durham, Allan, & Hackett, 1997; Hofmann, Newman, Becker, Taylor, & Roth, 1995). Such evidence points to the necessity of using therapy techniques to address interpersonal problems, including clients' maladaptive ways of relating to others.

Developmental Origin of Interpersonal Problems

CBT researchers have acknowledged the potential role of early attachment patterns in the development of anxiety (Chorpita & Barlow, 1998). Similarly, CBT conceptualizations have been influenced by the work of Bowlby (1982), who theorized that diffuse anxiety is the typical consequence of some forms of insecure attachment. For example, Safran and others (e.g., Guidano & Liotti, 1983), have suggested that childhood patterns of attachment shape individuals' core views of self, as well as their recurrent ways of interacting with others.

Despite acknowledging the importance of attachment, evidence from controlled trials suggests that CBT therapists focus less on clients' past and less on their relationship with early caregivers than do psychodynamic therapists (Goldfried, Castonguay, Hayes, Drozd, & Shapiro, 1997; Jones & Pulos, 1993). Nonetheless, a focus on developmental issues has been found to be positively related to outcome in CBT (Hayes et al., 1996; Jones & Pulos, 1993).

Developmental difficulties may be especially relevant to GAD. Basic research shows that persons with GAD report greater unresolved feelings of anger toward and vulnerability surrounding their primary caregivers than do persons without GAD (Cassidy, 1995). Thus our integrative therapy explores developmental origins of clients' current interpersonal difficulties and their potential links with current problems.

Clients' Interpersonal Problems and the Therapeutic Relationship

Respected CBT therapists have recognized that clients' interpersonal problems are frequently manifested in the therapeutic relationship (Beck et al., 2003; Goldfried, 1980). For example, Goldfried (1980) notes that therapeutic interactions may create a rich context in which therapists can observe and change clients' maladaptive interpersonal behavior.

Despite potential usefulness of the therapeutic relationship, research suggests that CBT therapists do not pay much attention to issues emerging between themselves and their clients, at least when they follow manualized treatments (Castonguay et al., 1995; Goldfried et al., 1997; Jones & Pulos, 1993). Interestingly, however, Jones and Pulos (1993) found that although CBT therapists did not spend much time focusing on "transferential" issues, clients benefited from it when they did.

Another issue that has not received a lot of attention in CBT is maintenance of the therapeutic relationship. Although CBT therapists establish and maintain a good working alliance (Raue & Goldfried, 1994), they pay less attention to the ways they can adversely affect relationships with clients (Goldfried & Castonguay, 1993). For example, Jones and Pulos (1993) found that although CBT therapists were more approving and reassuring than psychodynamic therapists, they were also more tactless, condescending, and patronizing to clients. In addition, when compared with psychodynamic therapists, CBT therapists' own emotional reactions more frequently intruded on the therapeutic process. In another study, Castonguay, Goldfried, Wiser, Raue, and Hayes (1996) found that techniques used in cognitive therapy to address alliance ruptures seemed to exacerbate relationship problems and interfere with clients' improvement. Later in this chapter, we describe techniques developed by humanistic and interpersonal therapists to resolve alliance problems. A preliminary study suggested that the integration of these techniques within traditional cognitive therapy increased treatment effectiveness for depression (Castonguay et al., In Press).

Emotional Deepening

In traditional CBT, emotion has been frequently viewed as an epiphenomenon to be controlled, rather than as something to be experienced (Mahoney, 1980). Indeed, studies show striking differences between CBT and other approaches in the manner in which affective experiences are handled. Whereas psychodynamic and interpersonal therapies view evocation of affect as essential to therapeutic change, traditional CBT tends to promote control or suppression of the full range of negative affect (Jones & Pulos, 1993; Wiser & Goldfried, 1993).

Ironically, a focus on affective control in CBT overlooks the theoretical importance placed on affective arousal by CBT experts (Beck, 1976; Foa & Kozak, 1986; Rachman, 1980). Furthermore, a number of studies have found a positive relationship between level of affective experiencing and clients' improvement in CBT (e.g., Castonguay et al., 1996; Foa, Riggs, Massie, & Yarczower, 1995; Jones & Pulos, 1993). Experimental research also supports the value of emotional processing to an individual's well-being and health (e.g., Pennebaker & Traue, 1993).

The failure of CBT to elicit and deepen emotional experience may be particularly consequential in the treatment of GAD. As shown by Borkovec, Alcaine, and Behar (Chapter 4, this volume), basic research suggests that the function of worrisome thinking may be one of avoidance of painful emotions. In fact, persons with GAD report that a major reason for their worry is to avoid thinking about more troublesome emotional experiences. As with any type of fear-motivated avoidance, worry may thus persist via negative reinforcement—it becomes a habit constantly reinforced by its ability to prevent the person from feeling worse (at least in the short term). Without deliberate exposure to feared emotions, opportunities for extinction of fear are precluded; as a consequence, worry is much more likely to persist (as the only way, albeit inefficient and costly, to reduce emotional pain). Thus the incorporation of experiential techniques designed to facilitate emotional processing may directly address a major underlying mechanism maintaining GAD symptomatology.

The importance of emotional processing to therapeutic change is highlighted by Safran and Segal (1990) who suggest that interpersonal schemata are coded, at least in part, in affective or expressive/motor form. Thus it is important to work with clients in an "emotionally alive fashion." Similarly, Foa and Kozak's (1986) neobehavioristic theory of emotional processing, originally developed to explain underlying mechanisms of action of exposure for fears, can be extended to explain the usefulness of therapy for interpersonal issues. For example, Safran and Greenberg (1991) note that interpersonal schemata are most amenable to modification by exposure to corrective experiences when related emotions are activated. Furthermore, experiencing emotions increases clients' awareness of needs about which they were previously unaware (Greenberg & Safran, 1987) and can guide them in choosing new behaviors to meet these needs, as well as behaviors to abandon.

In order to facilitate emotional processing, the present integrative treatment makes use of various techniques that help clients increase their awareness, experience, and expression of interpersonally relevant primary emotions. These techniques are aimed at creating an affective context to facilitate the assessment and challenge of clients' core perceptions of self and others.

STRUCTURE AND RATIONALE OF INTEGRATIVE THERAPY FOR GAD

As mentioned earlier, each session of the integrative treatment is composed of two separated components: a CBT segment of 55 minutes, followed by an Interpersonal/Emotional processing (I/EP) segment of 55 minutes. The decision to divide these components in this manner was based on empirical and theoretical considerations. The primary goal of our research is to determine whether the efficacy of CBT can be improved for GAD (Newman, Castonguay, Borkovec, & Schut, 1999b). Methodologically, the most appropriate strategy to test this question is an additive design (Borkovec & Castonguay, 1998). Thus we are currently comparing CBT + I/EP to a treatment protocol of the same length that is composed of a CBT segment and a supportive listening (SL) segment (the SL segment controls for time in therapy and common factors such as the therapeutic relationship). If CBT + I/EP leads to greater improvement than CBT + SL, it will provide evidence that the I/EP techniques add a therapeutic benefit above and beyond CBT.

The CBT component of the integrative protocol has been previously tested by Borkovec and Costello (1993) and Borkovec, Newman, Pincus, and Lytle (2002). Because CBT treatments are fully described elsewhere in this book, the rest of this chapter is devoted to the I/EP techniques (see also Borkovec & Newman, 1998, and Newman, 2000a, for additional information on our approach to CBT).

Although I/EP involves techniques not typically associated with CBT, it rests on a conceptualization that is perfectly compatible with CBT. In both the CBT and the I/EP segments of treatment, maladaptive symptoms of GAD are viewed as arising from overlearning of bad habits. The bad habits addressed in CBT are associated with clients' searching for threats in their environment and trying to control them via worrying. In I/EP, clients are told that they have overlearned the bad habit of avoiding painful emotion. Furthermore, they may be so busy trying to avoid what they fear from others that they fail to actively pursue their interpersonal needs. Ironically, although avoidance of emotion and some maladaptive relationship patterns may be motivated by a desire to anticipate and avoid danger, clients often create situations that are more likely to lead to negative outcomes. In particular, their approach to protecting themselves from the negative reactions of others has been to avoid letting others know who they are and what they feel. However, rather than making them more likeable, this approach makes them hard to connect with, and they may appear cold and uninterested in others.

The solution in both of these therapy segments is to replace maladaptive habits with new, more adaptive habits. The techniques used in the two segments, however, are substantively different. Whereas in the CBT segment therapists apply techniques that make use of the clients' current strengths (e.g., ability to analyze situations cognitively and critically, desire to control their negative responses to situations and to feel less anxious), in the I/EP segment therapists attempt to address clients' deficits (e.g., inability to get in touch with and process emotion, discomfort with interpersonal vulnerability and spontaneity).

Much of I/EP involves attempting to expose clients to feared emotions, to feared critical feedback about their impact on others, and to their fear of being vulnerable to other people by showing who they really are. Clients are encouraged to try things that may help them confront their immediate fears and to become aware of how their avoidance of negative emotions in the short term comes at a great cost in terms of a restricted lifestyle in which their needs are not met in the long term. Furthermore, we attempt to help them shift their attentional focus away from anticipating danger and toward openness, spontaneity, and vulnerability to others, as well as toward more empathic attention to the needs of others.

Thus our conceptualization is consistent with most CBT models. What is added in I/EP is the recognition of dangers (painful affect, interpersonal fears) as well as learned habits to cope with these threats (avoidance of emotion, maladaptive ways of relating with others) that have not been typically identified in traditional CBT. In addition, many I/EP techniques are based on mechanisms of change underlying most CBT procedures for anxiety: exposure, modeling, and skills training. Furthermore, the target of intervention in I/EP is based on a functional analysis. Indeed, therapists always specify interpersonal behaviors that should be changed or acquired, interpersonal situations within which such behaviors take place or fail to take place, short- and long-term impacts of such behaviors, and the functions the behaviors have served in clients' lives. Therapists gather this evidence from their emotional responses to clients, from clients' self-reports, and from clients' in-session behavior and emotional responses.

SPECIFIC I/EP TECHNIQUES

I/EP techniques can be classified into two major categories: addressing problematic relationship patterns and facilitating emotional deepening.

Addressing Problematic Relationship Patterns

Exploring Past and Current Relationships

Early in I/EP, clients are asked about people with whom they have had intimate relationships, familial links, and important friendships. Therapists avoid focusing on developmental issues until they have fully explored current interpersonal problems, especially if these problems are manifested in the therapeutic relationship. This is based on our observation that clients with GAD often talk about the past to avoid talking about their immediate feelings. It is easy indeed for these clients to engage in storytelling about what happened in their lives, and quite difficult for them to be "present-focused" and in touch with feelings in the here and now of the therapy session. Such an intellectual description, in effect, may serve the same role that worry plays. By "remaining in their heads," such clients avoid experiencing painful emotion.

On the other hand, clients will frequently draw a connection between their current affective experience (with the therapist or a current significant person) and an earlier moment in their lives when therapists facilitate the exploration of feelings associated with a current interpersonal event. Such an emotionally immediate connection (especially when a client makes it, rather than having it pointed out by a therapist) can become a powerful way to understand why patterns of relating with others may have been realistic and functional in the past but have become archaic and maladaptive.

Once a therapist has gathered general information about a client's interpersonal relationships (which takes one or two sessions), the therapist chooses a person who seems important to the client and explores in more depth the client's relationship with this individual. Because persons with GAD are more apt to focus on a description of the other individual than to describe the relationship, the manner in which the therapist asks the client about the relationship is important. Even a directive such as "Tell me about your relationship with John" tends not to elicit the relevant information from GAD individuals. In our experience, if asked about the general state of any one relationship, a person with GAD may either deny difficulties or blame current relationship problems on the other person.

This point is illustrated by the case of Clark, a 55-year-old professor. When Clark started treatment, he was in the midst of intense conflict with his ex-wife and was estranged from his two children. Clark initially represented himself as a victim of his ex-wife and children, and he attempted to illustrate this point by describing instances where they had treated him badly. In one of these scenarios, he reported that his son and daughter had ignored him. He had visited them to celebrate the combination of his daughter's graduation and Father's Day, and to attend a reception hosted by his ex-wife for his daughter.

Rather than accept Clark's characterization that he was blameless in his problems with his children, the therapist asked him to talk about a specific interaction that took place during this visit, in which he was left feeling as though he did not really get what he wanted or needed. The therapist instructed him to do this in a blow-by-blow manner (i.e., "What did you do, and then what did he do, and then what did you do?"). To guide

Clark in responding to this request (and to redirect him when he wandered off topic), the therapist used a chart that we have developed to explore the interpersonal situations (see Figure 13.1).

After Clark had described an interaction with his son, the therapist asked him what emotion he felt and he replied that he had felt angry. Then the therapist asked what he needed or wanted from his son and what he was afraid might happen. As demonstrated in the following vignette, the therapist then tried to determine whether Clark did something or failed to do something that decreased the probability of getting his needs met.

CLARK: I decided that I wanted to have lunch with my son for Father's Day, so I called him up to find out whether he was free.

THERAPIST: When exactly did you make this phone call?

CLARK: When I got into town.

THERAPIST: So tell me exactly what you said to him when you called him.

CLARK: I said that I thought it would be fun if we had lunch on Saturday. Then he said, "Mom already planned a special Father's Day lunch with Grandpa, so I can't make it, but I would like to stop by before then to give you your Father's Day gift."

THERAPIST: And what did you say to that?

CLARK: I said, "Well I really wanted to have lunch, but I guess that would be better than nothing."

THERAPIST: Then what happened?

CLARK: We said goodbye. However, I thought about what happened over and over until he stopped by, and the more I thought about it, the an-

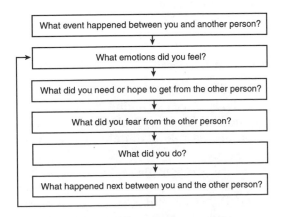

FIGURE 13.1. I/EP interpersonal exploration chart.

grier I got. I mean, I'm his father, so don't I deserve to be honored on Father's Day?

THERAPIST: When was the next time you spoke with him?

CLARK: When he came by to give me my Fathers Day gift later that day, but by that time I really didn't want to see him. When he handed the gift to me, I said, "Why don't you get the hell out of here and go figure out who your father really is!" Then I called my daughter to tell her I would not attend her graduation reception, because I would not get to spend the kind of time with her that I had expected.

Clark told the therapist that his role as father was not being acknowledged adequately, since he had received the same invitation to his daughter's graduation reception that everyone else had. Even though his daughter reminded him that she was hoping she could see him at her reception, this was not good enough. In the end he felt dishonored and discounted.

The therapist's goal was to help Clark to become aware of his role in these problematic interactions. In this instance, the therapist noted how he had waited until the last minute to invite his son to lunch, and how some of his angry behaviors toward his children served to push them away from him. As noted earlier, such problematic behaviors are often a result of clients' misguided attempts to avoid what they fear. However, some attempts to avoid a feared reaction may actually evoke that reaction. Specifically, Clark feared that his children would not value him. Because of this fear, he made plans with his children at the last minute and did not communicate directly to them how important it was for him to see them. His behavior contributed to his children's unavailability, which he interpreted as evidence that they did not value him. He then pushed his children away even further by yelling at his son and refusing to attend his daughter's graduation. Interpersonal events such as these are what the therapist hopes to target in I/EP.

Teaching Clients Alternative Ways to Handle Interpersonal Interactions

Once identified, problematic relationship patterns become the target of direct intervention. Thus, after examining the ways in which clients have created or exacerbated an interpersonal problem, therapists and clients work on (most typically via role plays) alternative ways of relating with others.

Of course, such skills training interventions are consistent with a CBT model. However, social skills' training has never been part of Borkovec's CBT protocol for GAD, because the goal of this protocol was to directly target GAD symptomatology (i.e., worrisome thinking and muscular tension). On the other hand, social skills interventions are perfectly in line with the I/EP focus on interpersonal issues, as well as with it's emphasis on learning as the basis of both the etiology and treatment of GAD.

Social skills training targets a deficit frequently observed in individuals suffering from GAD. In our experience, when asked to generate specific ways that they could have handled their relationship problems differently, persons with GAD often come up with extreme, "all-or-none" solutions (e.g., "I could either yell at him, or I could say nothing"). Most likely because of a fear of being vulnerable, clients often do not even consider the option of talking to others in a way that would help them understand what the clients are feeling.

In doing role plays, therapists first encourage clients to play themselves and to attempt to recapture what they said as well as how they said it. Once therapists have a sense of what the clients did, they assume the clients' role and ask the clients to assume the role of the person with whom they were interacting. Clients, who are playing the role of the other, are asked to imagine how they would have been impacted in the interaction, as if in the other person's shoes. Such a reverse role play often elucidates for clients the impact they had on the other person. We have found it important to emphasize that clients pay attention to the impact that therapists (who are playing the role of the client) have on them, rather than to use the role play as an opportunity to feel vindicated and understood by their therapists.

In the following role play, the therapist attempted to make Mindy (a college student with GAD) aware of her impact on her friend Ellen. In particular, Mindy realized that even though she was not meeting Ellen's needs, she nonetheless expected Ellen to meet her needs:

MINDY: Ellen told me she thought I went home too often. When she said this I laughed and said, "Thanks for your opinion!"

THERAPIST: What did you feel?

MINDY: Criticized.

THERAPIST: Sounds like your friends wish they could see you more often.

MINDY: I don't feel like they are hearing me, though.

THERAPIST: I wonder how well you are hearing them. They are saying they enjoy your friendship, yet you feel like you are not being heard.

MINDY: I'm often told I'm sensitive. But I feel condemned by them. I just feel like ending the friendship.

THERAPIST: Let's do a role play where I am you and you are Ellen. Try to imagine what she was feeling.

MINDY: OK. (*As Ellen*) You go home too often and spend too much time with John [Mindy's boyfriend]. I feel like I am second best to John.

THERAPIST: (*As Mindy*) Thanks for your opinion!

MINDY: (as Ellen) I guess I really miss spending time with you. I am going to graduate soon, and we won't have as many chances to spend time together.

THERAPIST: How did you feel as Ellen?

MINDY: I don't like being Ellen.

THERAPIST: What does Ellen need from you?

MINDY: She wants to spend more time with me. But I don't want to spend time with her if she is going to be critical of me and condemn me.

THERAPIST: Do you think your response to her got you what you needed?

MINDY: I guess not.

THERAPIST: How did it feel as Ellen to hear your response?

MINDY: Bad. I didn't feel like Mindy cared about what I wanted.

THERAPIST: Seems like your friends have needs they are not getting met, and that if you consider their needs, maybe you will get more of what you want.

Once maladaptive relationship patterns have been identified, and clients have learned to respond in ways that can have a better impact, homework is assigned so that clients can apply new responses outside of therapy. As is commonly done in CBT, I/EP therapists always follow up to determine whether clients did the assignment and how it went. For Mindy, the homework was to listen actively to others in order to understand better what they needed from her.

At one point, Mindy noted that whenever her boyfriend, John, was not attending fully to her, she interpreted his silence as meaning that he was going to leave her. Her fear initially prevented her from realizing that there could be an alternative explanation. The therapist set up a role play in which Mindy played the role of John. In this role, Mindy recreated a recent episode in which she talked at length about events in her life, and while she was talking, she expected John to be totally attentive to her feelings. However, the role play helped her realize that she did not give John much space to talk about himself—that his silence was actually the price she had to pay for her to have "the stage," and that she was "guilty" of what she accused him of (i.e., not being attentive to the other's needs). As highlighted by the following transcript, she then tried to be more attentive to John:

MINDY: I told John how excited I was about us getting engaged and moving close to my family when we graduate, and he didn't say anything. He hasn't been professing his love to me like he did when we first started dating.

THERAPIST: How did you respond to his silence?

MINDY: At first I was scared, but then I thought about how I don't always hear people. So I tried to understand his feelings and to talk to him about them.

THERAPIST: What did you say?

MINDY: I said, "Don't you want to get engaged any more? How come you don't tell me how much you love me any more?" He said he wanted to get engaged, but it was hard for him to think about living so far away from his parents. He said, "Imagine how you would feel if you had to live far away from your family," and then I realized that it would be hard for John to live hundreds of miles away from his own family when I got to live so close to mine.

THERAPIST: Sounds like it was important for John that you understand where he was coming from.

MINDY: Yeah. I want to hear him. He may leave me if he doesn't feel supported by me.

Communicating directly and less defensively allowed Mindy to develop empathy for John and to understand further how her focus on self was actually increasing the likelihood that John would not feel understood in the relationship. Interestingly, the relief that Mindy experienced after directly asking John what he was feeling negatively reinforced her more adaptive behavior of trying to understand his needs. Such negative reinforcement made it likely that she would engage in this behavior with others, thereby increasing the probability of having her own needs met in relationships.

Making Use of the Client–Therapist Relationship

The interpersonal component of I/EP is founded on the idea that clients' maladaptive patterns of relating are often repeated in the therapeutic relationship. This is consistent with Safran and Segal's (1990) suggestion that successful therapy often requires therapists to be "hooked" into clients' maladaptive ways of relating to others (i.e., to be pulled by clients into behaving consistently with the clients' expectations). Thus, in I/EP therapists try to identify when and how they have been participating in clients' interpersonal schemata. Once therapists identify that they have been hooked, they need to act in ways that oppose clients' expectations of them, thereby disconfirming clients' cognitive–interpersonal schemata. The goal is to help clients gain awareness of their maladaptive ways of relating and any rigid construals of interpersonal relationships that may underlie these patterns. Such awareness helps them identify their contribution to their interpersonal difficulties, as well as the needs that motivated their behaviors (e.g., what they were trying to gain or were afraid to lose as a result of the interaction). Once the needs are identified, concrete behavioral strategies can teach clients better ways to satisfy them.

It is often difficult for I/EP therapists to recognize when they have been hooked in a way that enables clients' interpersonal or emotional avoidance. Among the indicators that therapists have been hooked are therapists' impression that therapy isn't going anywhere, that they feel emotionally detached from certain clients, and the sense that they are persistently frustrated or feeling helpless with the clients. To deal with such issues, therapists make notes after each session about things they may have done, intentionally or unintentionally, to contribute to clients' enactment of interpersonal and/or emotional avoidance. In addition, therapists attempt to adopt the attitude of a participant-observer (Sullivan, 1953). By taking some distance from the interaction, they can identify markers as they are unfolding. Therapists have reported, for example, allowing clients to provide irrelevant background information, to tell long tangential stories, to change the topic, and to provide only abstract descriptions of events and/or feelings. Another example is a therapist and client becoming engaged in an analysis of why something happened, why the client had a particular feeling, or why another person acted a certain way. The focus on "why" is an indication that the client is avoiding being emotionally present.

Although clients' ways of relating can pull therapists into patterns of avoidance, therapists have their own vulnerabilities with regard to being hooked. For example, the impulse to try to make clients feel better quickly, rather than to help them stay with painful emotions. Other issues have included therapists' discomfort with clients' anger when it is directed at them, or bringing humor into the room when clients are talking about a difficult experience. It is important for therapists to identify and change negative ways that they may act on those issues.

As a means to identify clients' maladaptive interaction patterns that may be manifested in the therapeutic relationship, and to determine quickly when they may have been hooked, therapists continually check in on their own emotions, with particular awareness of how the clients' behaviors would affect them if they had a friendship with the clients rather than a therapeutic relationship. By doing this, therapists become more sensitive to clients' behaviors that might be ignored or excused in the therapy context, but that may be creating problems for the clients outside therapy. Checking in on their feelings requires therapists to take a step back from the ongoing interaction and to adopt the attitude of a participant-observer (Sullivan, 1953).

Once therapists become aware of clients' negative impact, they are encouraged to address this issue in an open and nondefensive manner, thereby modeling the communication style that clients are encouraged to use. A helpful way of presenting the information can be "I feel _____ when you do _____ (e.g., "I feel pushed away, when you don't answer my questions"). After providing feedback, therapists invite clients to talk about their affective responses to such feedback (e.g., "How do you feel about what I just said to you?"). Clients' ability and willingness (or lack thereof) to examine their own emotional responses following such feedback (e.g., being hurt or angry), as well as their behavioral responses to these emotions (e.g., changing the subject), provide unique opportunities for therapists to observe clients' openness to their affective experiences. These moments in therapy also inform therapists about clients' ability and willingness to accept and respond positively to others' self-disclosure—and, reciprocally, to allow themselves to be open and vulnerable with another person.

One common client reaction to therapists' feedback is to explain how doing what they did helps them (e.g., "I changed the subject because talking about my emotions made me uncomfortable"). Clients often seem to feel that if they provide a reason for their behavior, the behavior becomes acceptable. However, the actual reason for their behavior may be to avoid painful emotion. Furthermore, justification does not mitigate the negative impact of the behavior. When clients do express an emotion (which may require repeated but gentle invitations), therapists' immediate task is to empathize with and validate their affective experiences. Therapists are then asked to share their own reactions to clients' self-disclosures (e.g., "Of course you would want to avoid a topic that made you uncomfortable. However, not answering my question also has an impact on me and makes me feel as though what I am asking for, isn't important"). Therapists are also encouraged to observe whether clients' responses to their openness help them feel understood by clients.

In addition to paying attention to the therapeutic relationship, therapists try to facilitate links between interaction patterns observed in the session and patterns in clients' past or current relationships outside the session. However, therapists try not to make such connections until they have fully processed any negative feelings that may have emerged in the therapeutic relationship. As illustrated in the following example, when clients and therapists are open to their own experience (and that of each other) during the session, the exploration of the here-and-now situation and of outside (past and present) relationships can have a synergistic and beneficial impact.

To return to the case of Mindy, it became apparent that she sometimes felt the same negative emotions toward the therapist that she had been feeling with her friends. The following segment occurred immediately after the therapist asked Mindy how she felt.

MINDY: I don't like this hour as much, because you hear about my bad qualities—like how I don't like to be with my friends because I feel anxious, and like they are being critical of me.

THERAPIST: I feel like I know more about who you are when you share more with me, instead of saying "Mmm-hmm" to everything I say. That sounds like you are saying, "I'm not bad. I'm not bad." I don't feel like I know you at all or what you are feeling when you are always the good student.

MINDY: I would form negative opinions of someone who told me about their bad qualities.

THERAPIST: Close your eyes and try to get in touch with what you are feeling in your body about sharing bad parts of yourself with me.

MINDY: My fists are clenched. I don't like this. I'm scared I'll find out more bad things about myself.

THERAPIST: What have you found out about yourself?

MINDY: I need control. I don't like being with my friends. I'm angry. I don't want this to be me!

THERAPIST: It is hard to be with others when you can't control what they will do and how they will see you. It seems like how you feel with your friends is similar to how you feel with me, wanting to be viewed positively by me.

MINDY: (*Speaking in a very distant way*) There could be elements of that that would be applicable.

THERAPIST: Check your body.

MINDY: I'm afraid. I'm surprised you don't know me, because I feel with you like I feel with my friends, so maybe they don't know me either. I tried to figure out how to be more vulnerable with people and hear them, but it's like getting on a horse that I fell off of, only the horse is much taller now.

THERAPIST: It's a struggle to let yourself be vulnerable.

MINDY: I've been hurt when I've let myself be vulnerable. I feel sad, and I need to put the suit on [Mindy's way of describing her false self].

THERAPIST: It seems hard for you to allow all of what you feel.

MINDY: I keep my feelings to myself, but I still have them. When I was younger, I had a best friend, Rick. I told him I liked a guy in my school, and he told the guy how I felt. I didn't think my friend would betray my secret.

THERAPIST: (*Pulling up a chair*) Tell Rick how you feel.

MINDY: (*Speaking to the empty chair*) It's your fault that I turned into the suit person. I mean, I know it isn't fair to blame you for all of it.

THERAPIST: Slow down—stay with what you are feeling.

MINDY: I feel empty. (*Mindy relaxes her muscles, becomes visibly sad, and begins to cry freely.*)

THERAPIST: It's nice to meet you, Mindy [referring to the fact that Mindy has revealed her "true self"].

MINDY: Really?

THERAPIST: Yes, it is really nice to meet you.

MINDY: How do I fix it?

THERAPIST: Feel it and let it teach you what you want.

(*Mindy sits with sadness.*)

THERAPIST: When threat is all you pay attention to, relief is all you can ever have, but you can feel even more when you are not trying to escape. What did you find out today about yourself?

MINDY: I want to be myself with my friends instead of avoiding them. I'm ready for whatever they say to me.

THERAPIST: You learned about who you were when you took a risk with me.

Another aspect of the therapeutic relationship that is targeted in I/EP has to do with alliance ruptures. In line with Safran's model, the emergence of therapeutic ruptures in I/EP is viewed as an opportunity to disconfirm clients' maladaptive interpersonal schemata and to help them gain more realistic perceptions of themselves and others, as well as more adaptive ways of behaving. Using markers developed by Safran, Crocker, McMain, and Murray (1990), therapists are trained to identify such ruptures. These markers include clients' overt expressions of dissatisfaction; indirect expressions of hostility (e.g., sarcasm, passive–aggressive behavior); disagreement about the goals or tasks of therapy; overly compliant behavior; evasive behavior (e.g., constant confusion, skipping from topic to topic, never really answering a direct question, arriving late); and self-esteem-boosting maneuvers (e.g., self-justifying or self-aggrandizing).

One type of alliance rupture frequently observed with clients who have GAD happens when they begin to address questions posed by therapists but then move to a totally different topic. Another type occurs when clients suggest that before therapists can understand their answers, they must first give therapists some background information. These behaviors can be in-session manifestations of an overlearned pattern of avoidance. Such noncompliance is often a response to therapists' attempts to facilitate emotionally immediate exploration of significant interpersonal issues related to the therapeutic relationship or a significant outside relationship.

Although we recognize that alliance ruptures can be the result, at least in part, of clients' avoidance patterns, I/EP therapists are trained not to focus on possible avoidance behavior as they begin addressing such ruptures. This is based on research evidence (Castonguay et al., 1996; Piper et al., 1999) suggesting that assigning responsibility for alliance ruptures to clients may actually exacerbate them. Instead, therapists use techniques that are consistent with strategies used in humanistic and interpersonal therapies. These techniques involve three steps (Castonguay et al., in press).

First, a therapist explicitly communicates that he or she has noticed the client's negative reaction and invites the client to talk about it (e.g., "I have a sense that you aren't as engaged as you have been in other sessions. Is that how you are feeling?"). The second step is to reflect back the client's perception and emotions, and then to invite the client to express additional emotions and thoughts about unhelpful or invalidating events that have taken place in the treatment. This step continues until the therapist has the sense that the client feels understood.

The third step is accomplished by using the technique of "disarming" (Burns, 1989). Using this technique, the therapist finds some truth in the client's reaction, even when the reaction may seem unreasonable. The assumption underlying this technique is that even when a treatment obstacle seems related to the client's difficulties (such as the overlearned coping device of emotional avoidance), it is always the case that the therapist has contributed in some fashion to the lack of synchrony between the two participants. The therapist's openness to his or her experiences and recognition of his or her own contribution to a relationship problem often facilitate the client and therapist to step out of an unproductive process (Castonguay, 1996).

In a situation where a client has been evasive, for example, the therapist may say something like this: "I am sorry that my questions don't seem relevant to you. I realize now that I haven't always clearly explained the rationale of my approach to you." To clients who frequently change the topic, even after repeated attempts by therapists to refocus their attention to a specific issue, therapists might say something such as this: "I am afraid that I have been pressuring you to talk about something that might not be important to you, or that you might not be ready to talk about now."

The positive impact of Burns's disarming technique is consistent with Carl Rogers's (1961) observation that openness of one person frequently leads to openness by another. It is our experience that therapists' explicit and nondefensive recognition of their contribution to alliance problems is often followed by clients' recognition of their own role (e.g., "I appreciate your saying that. I guess I did feel some pressure, but I think I avoid talking about these things, even though I should talk about them").

It is also important to note that not addressing an alliance rupture is a frequent manifestation of being hooked. Following the steps described above is a difficult task, since it frequently involves inviting a client to talk about negative feelings toward the therapy and/or the therapist him- or herself. However, avoiding alliance ruptures is likely to be another way for therapists to mimic how other people in clients' lives may respond to them. In contrast, actively addressing and resolving problems in the therapeutic relationship is likely to provide clients with are important corrective experiences (Safran & Segal, 1990). In particular, it shows clients how being open and vulnerable about their emotions can be a way to get closer to another person. Contrary to the habit of avoidance typically used by GAD individuals, such vulnerability (and exposure to fear) can actually, and paradoxically, be the best strategy for them to have their worries decrease and get their interpersonal needs met.

Facilitating Emotional Deepening

An important element of I/EP is the facilitation of emotional experience. Emotional awareness and deepening are used to facilitate exposure to previously avoided affect and, conversely, to achieve the extinction of a learned (i.e., negatively reinforced) habit of cognitive avoidance (i.e., worry). The use of emotional processing techniques is also based on Greenberg and Safran's view that emotion provides information about a person's needs.

Thus therapists are asked to track markers of emotionality. Examples include changes in voice quality, the sound of tears in the voice, and a slowing or quickening of conversational pace. When such markers are noted, clients are encouraged to stay with their emotions and to allow themselves to fully experience them. Therapists also need to pay attention to moments of emotional disruption or disengagement. When clients stop emoting and/or being attentive to their affective experience, therapists invite them to focus on their immediate experience (e.g., "What just happened? You were allowing yourself to cry, and you quickly moved away from your feeling").

Our clinical observation matches basic science findings that clients with GAD are incredibly avoidant of, and uncomfortable with, their emotions. One common problem is that when asked what they are feeling, clients describe what they are thinking. Thus an early step in therapy may be to teach the difference between thoughts/observations and feelings. Our therapists use the phrase "You are going into your head" as a way to help clients notice when they are moving away from their affective experience and are instead focused on thoughts. We sometimes find that even requiring clients to put words to their affective experience can move them away from the initial feeling. Therefore, therapists will at times tell clients to stay with their current feelings.

We have also observed that the emotion most commonly described by clients with GAD is frustration or anger. In part, we believe this is because frustration and anger are the emotions that make these clients feel least vulnerable to others. I/EP therapists therefore explore the possibility that beneath the frustration, clients also experience other feelings. This is illustrated in the following segment, where Marie described running into her friend Gail, who said she felt bad for Fran (one of Marie's ex-roommates):

THERAPIST: How did you respond?

MARIE: I laughed and told her I have problems of my own. It's not my problem that Fran lacks social skills and nobody wants to room with her.

THERAPIST: How did you feel?

MARIE: I was pissed that Gail wasn't supportive of me.

THERAPIST: Let's slow this down, so you have a chance to feel that anger. What did you want from Gail?

MARIE: I wanted sympathy. I wanted support.

THERAPIST: What did you fear?

MARIE: Conflict. I didn't want to get upset. I mean, the whole world has been ganging up on me. University housing messed up again, and I have to move out for a second time. And she feels bad for Fran? What about me?

THERAPIST: Try to slow down.

MARIE: I feel like if I get it all off my chest, then I'll feel relief.

THERAPIST: You don't allow your feelings to sink in when you talk about this so quickly. Often anger isn't the first emotion, but it covers up another emotion. Do you think there was a feeling underneath the anger?

MARIE: (*Speaking while laughing*) Maybe hurt was under the anger. I'm angry at the world. (*Smiling*) I needed someone to understand me.

THERAPIST: There is that smile again, but this doesn't really make you happy. Could you have responded in a different way to Gail? How about, "Gail, I've been through a lot with all of this moving. I feel like I need support and understanding about what it has been like to go through all of this."

MARIE: I kind of want her to mysteriously know what I need without my having to ask, and to ask if I am OK.

THERAPIST: What stopped you from asking for what you want?

MARIE: I feel bad, as if I'll hurt someone and they won't like me. I'm scared

I'll be alone if I ask for what I need. I feel sad because I want to be allowed to feel what I'm feeling. (*Marie goes off on a tangent.*)

THERAPIST: I feel a little lost, like I'm running to keep up.

MARIE: I don't want to slow down. I can get hurt and do damage. If I bring up feelings from the past it will hurt me twice.

THERAPIST: I feel like there is an urgency right now.

MARIE: I felt like there was an urgency with Gail.

THERAPIST: I can't absorb what you say when you talk so quickly. You're telling me you are scared and angry, but I don't feel like you are connected to those feelings.

MARIE: I'm afraid if I let my feelings in that they won't go away.

In addition to general markers of underlying emotionality, I/EP therapists pay attention to markers of what humanistic therapists label "internal conflicts," "unfinished business," and "problematic reactions" (Greenberg, Rice, & Elliott, 1996; Greenberg & Safran, 1987). In each of these instances, experiential techniques are employed to help clients to get in touch with, own, and deepen previously unprocessed emotions.

Markers for internal conflicts are usually expressions by clients that they are "of two minds" about something (e.g., "A part of me wants to leave my husband, but another part of me can't imagine life without him"). Once a client has acknowledged an internal conflict, a therapist asks the client to take part in a two-chair exercise wherein the client distinguishes the two parts of the self—as though they were two separate people—and then embodies each one separately. It can often be helpful for the client to label each of the parts.

One of our clients, Sara, experienced a persistent conflict between the facade that she felt she needed to show others and her true feelings, which she felt she should discount. She labeled the facade "outside Sara" and her needs and wishes "inside Sara." The therapist placed two chairs facing one-another and had Sara first take the role of "outside Sara" and talk about her feelings to "inside Sara." After a time, the therapist had her switch chairs and roles, this time being "inside Sara" telling "outside Sara" how she felt. She was then asked to switch roles multiple times. Eventually she realized that she spent a great deal of time trying to repress "inside Sara." Nonetheless, her true feelings often leaked out eventually. She also realized that "outside Sara" sometimes operated on avoidance of fear. Therefore, she worked on finding a better balance between showing the side of her that she believed others wanted to see and allowing her own needs to come through.

Unfinished business refers to a client's unresolved feelings toward another person (who may still be alive or may have passed away). The primary intervention to deal with this is an empty-chair exercise (Greenberg et al., 1996). In this exercise, the client expresses his or her feelings toward the other person, who is imagined sitting across from the client in an empty chair. Interestingly, unresolved feelings are not always negative. We have often found that clients with GAD regret never having told someone how much they value them. One client had a father who was terminally ill. After much exploration, she realized that she was trying to show her father through her actions how important he was to her, but had never expressed what she felt. The therapist recognized that it was important for this client to process what her father meant to her. She was asked to imagine her father in the empty chair and to tell him how she felt about him. She spent several sessions getting in touch with her feelings and eventually told her father how she felt, which brought them closer together.

Markers for a problematic reaction include clients' surprise, confusion, or ambivalence about a particular reaction of theirs. When such markers are observed, clients are asked to close their eyes and imagine themselves back in the situation that evoked the reaction. It is helpful for clients to play the scene in slow motion, to vividly imagine every aspect of the scene, and to describe in detail the events and their feelings during the situation. The key is to help clients pay attention to every internal cue as they repeatedly describe the situation. By reexperiencing fine-grained details and their reactions to them, clients can express and own the emotions that first surprised them. Clients will frequently gain access to previously implicit emotions as a result of this technique, appropriately called "systematic evocative unfolding" (Greenberg et al., 1996). This technique is also used when clients do not seem to know what they felt in a particular instance.

As has been noted throughout this chapter, clients with GAD find emotional processing difficult, particularly the expression of vulnerable emotion in front of another person (i.e., the therapist). The expression of feeling provides a safe corrective experience, and is an important step in overcoming fear of vulnerability with others. Ultimately, however, such exposure will be of limited benefit if clients do not also change their habitual avoidance of emotion outside therapy. Because of their fear of emotions, clients with GAD may agree to be "pushed" toward emotionality during sessions, only to remain avoidant of their feelings between sessions. Homework is therefore assigned to encourage clients to focus on and stay with emotions outside of therapy. Because of a tendency to interpret instructions with an "all-or-none attitude" (e.g., "Either I shove my emotions aside, or I express whatever I happen to feel all the time"), clients are also told that the goal is to help them achieve a better balance between emotional expression and lack of expression. It is further emphasized that the goal of becoming aware of their feelings is not necessarily to stimulate emotional/cathartic expression. Clients are reminded that their emotions are above everything else aspects of themselves that they need to accept, and that rather than attempting to avoid their feelings, they should see emotions as an important source of information for what they need in their lives. Once they have accepted their emotions, whether or not they act on them depends on the long-term costs and benefits of doing so.

RESEARCH

As noted earlier in this chapter, our integrative treatment (i.e., CBT + I/EP) is currently being compared to a control condition (i.e., CBT + SL) (Newman et al., 1999) to determine whether the addition of I/EP techniques can improve the efficacy of CBT, which is currently the only empirically supported therapy for GAD. Although it is too early to present the results of the study in progress, we have conducted a preliminary investigation of the integrative treatment (Newman et al., 1999). The first goal was to determine whether it would be possible to train therapists to conduct a treatment that required 55 minutes of CBT followed by 55 minutes of I/EP. The second goal was to conduct a preliminary examination, albeit limited, of the efficacy of the integrative treatment.

Eighteen individuals meeting *Diagnostic and Statistical Manual of Mental Disorders*, fourth edition (American Psychiatric Association, 1994) criteria for GAD received 15 sessions of CBT + I/EP. Three experienced therapists, two of them with a primarily psychodynamic background and the other originally trained in CBT, conducted the therapy. Therapists (one female and two males) were trained by Newman, Borkovec, and Castonguay and followed two treatment manuals, one for I/EP and one for CBT. They also received weekly individual supervision (by Newman and Borkovec) and group supervision (provided by Newman, Castonguay, and Borkovec).

Systematic adherence and quality checks revealed no major breaks in the treatment protocol and competent delivery of treatment (Newman et al., 1999). The two segments also did not differ in quality of alliance and credibility of the therapy (Borkovec, Newman, & Castonguay, 1998). Furthermore, analysis of outcome data suggested, although tentatively, that the integrative treatment can lead to greater therapeutic change then CBT. Indeed, the within-group effect sizes on commonly used anxiety outcome measures for CBT + I/EP compared favorably with those for a comprehensive CBT package (Borkovec et al., 2002) at posttreatment (2.87 vs. 2.16) and 1 year follow-up (2.74 vs. 1.93).

Although preliminary, these results suggest that I/EP techniques can be added to CBT, even if these techniques have been derived from different theoretical orientations. These results are also promising with regard to the possibility of improving the efficacy of CBT for GAD. Of course, more definitive conclusions, especially with respect to outcome, must await the results of the current clinical trial.

CONCLUSION

As CBT therapists, we are aware of the therapeutic impact of CBT. However, we also recognize that CBT (like any other approach) has its weaknesses. Findings on the role of interpersonal, developmental, and emotional processing difficulties in the development and maintenance of GAD; on the clinical and conceptual limitations of CBT; and on the treatment process strongly suggest that the addition of I/EP techniques may be helpful to CBT for GAD. The addition of these techniques is also consistent with recent conceptual developments in CBT.

One may argue that because we conduct CBT and I/EP as distinct segments separated in time, we are not really doing integrative therapy. However, a number of treatments involving the sequential or concurrent use of different approaches have been described in the integrative literature (Glass, Victor, & Arnkoff, 1993). The key here is that although our therapy protocol uses techniques derived from divergent theoretical orientations, it is nonetheless based on a coherent theoretical framework. As described elsewhere, it represents a perfect example of one of the current trends in psychotherapy integration—that is, the improvement of effective therapies (in this case, CBT) by the assimilation of constructs and methods of other orientations (Castonguay et al., 2003). Furthermore, the use of different approaches (simultaneously or in succession) with the same patient has been recommended as relevant for future research on psychotherapy integration (Elkin, 1991). Whether the therapy would be improved by flexibly combining the techniques in one 2-hour block is, of course, an empirical question. However, given how difficult it is to keep therapists and clients focused on emotional processing and negative interpersonal patterns in I/EP, it would be even more difficult for therapists and clients not to get hooked into avoiding addressing these issues, without a specific block of time allotted for the delivery of these techniques. Furthermore, given how difficult it is for Clients with GAD to get in touch with and process emotions, anything less than a full therapy hour devoted to this process might diminish the efficacy of this intervention.

Finally, we would like to end this chapter by acknowledging that some psychotherapy approaches may have a lower direct cost than the ones that we have described (e.g., Newman, 1999; Newman, Consoli, & Taylor, 1997, 1999; Newman, Kenardy, Herman, & Taylor, 1997). However we would argue that although this integrative treatment requires more time than typical CBT protocols, it is likely to be more cost-effective. As demonstrated by Newman (2000b), individuals with anxiety disorders who do not respond to CBT end up requiring a considerable amount of costly medical and psychological care. The present integrative protocol is specifically aimed at addressing factors that are predictive of nonresponse to CBT. As our research program progresses, we hope to show that the use of a more comprehensive treatment such as this one will, in the long run, be effective for a larger number of individuals by adequately addressing a larger number of variables involved in the etiology and maintenance of GAD (Newman, 2000b).

ACKNOWLEDGMENT

Preparation of this chapter was supported in part by National Institute of Mental Health Research Grant No. MH-58593.

REFERENCES

Alden, L. E., Wiggins, J. S., & Pincus, A. L. (1990). Construction of circumplex scales for the Inventory of Interpersonal Problems. *Journal of Personality Assessment, 55*, 521–536.

American Psychiatric Association. (1994). *Diagnostic and statistical manual of mental disorders* (4th ed.). Washington, DC: Author.

Barlow, D. H. (2002). *Anxiety and its disorders: The nature and treatment of anxiety and panic* (2nd ed.). New York: Guilford Press.

Beck, A. T. (1976). *Cognitive therapy and the emotional disorders.* New York: International Universities Press.

Beck, A. T., Freeman, A., Davis, D. D., & Associates. (2003). *Cognitive therapy of personality disorders* (2nd ed.). New York: Guilford Press.

Borkovec, T. D., & Castonguay, L. G. (1998). What is the scientific meaning of empirically supported therapy? *Journal of Consulting and Clinical Psychology, 66*, 136–142.

Borkovec, T. D., & Costello, E. (1993). Efficacy of applied relaxation and cognitive-behavioral therapy in the treatment of generalized anxiety disorder. *Journal of Consulting and Clinical Psychology, 61*, 611–619.

Borkovec, T. D., & Newman, M. G. (1998). Worry and generalized anxiety disorder. In A. S. Bellack & M. Hersen (Series Eds.) & P. Salkovskis (Vol. Ed.), *Comprehensive clinical psychology: Vol. 6. Adults: Clinical formulation and treatment* (pp. 439–459). Oxford, UK: Pergamon Press.

Borkovec, T. D., Newman, M. G., & Castonguay, L. G. (1998, November). *The potential role of interpersonal emotional processing in the treatment of generalized anxiety disorder.* Paper presented at the Association for Advancement of Behavior Therapy, Washington, DC.

Borkovec, T. D., Newman, M. G., Pincus, A. L., & Lytle, R. (2002). A component analysis of cognitive behavioral therapy for generalized anxiety disorder and the role of interpersonal problems. *Journal of Consulting and Clinical Psychology, 70*, 288–298.

Borkovec, T. D., & Ruscio, A. M. (2001). Psychotherapy for generalized anxiety disorder. *Journal of Clinical Psychiatry, 62*(Suppl. 11), 37–45.

Bowlby, J. (1982). *Attachment and loss: Vol. 1. Attachment* (2nd ed.). New York: Basic Books.

Burns, D. D. (1989). *The feeling good handbook*. New York: Morrow.

Cassidy, J. A. (1995). Attachment and generalized anxiety disorder. In D. Cicchetti & S. Toth (Eds.), *Rochester Symposium on Developmental Psychopathology: Vol. 6. Emotion, cognition, and representation* (pp. 343–370). Rochester, NY: University of Rochester Press.

Castonguay, L. G. (1996). *Integrative cognitive therapy*. Unpublished treatment manual, Pennsylvania State University, University Park.

Castonguay, L. G., & Goldfried, M. R. (1994). Psychotherapy integration: An idea whose time has come. *Applied and Preventative Psychology, 3*, 159–172.

Castonguay, L. G., Goldfried, M. R., Wiser, S., Raue, P. J., & Hayes, A. M. (1996). Predicting the effect of cognitive therapy for depression: A study of unique and common factors. *Journal of Consulting and Clinical Psychology, 64*, 497–504.

Castonguay, L. G., Hayes, A. M., Goldfried, M. R., & DeRubeis, R. J. (1995). The focus of therapist interventions in cognitive therapy for depression. *Cognitive Therapy and Research, 19*, 487–505.

Castonguay, L. G., Hayes, A. M., Goldfried, M. R., Drozd, J., Schut, A. J., & Shapiro, D. A. (1998, June). *Intrapersonal and interpersonal focus in psychodynamic-interpersonal and cognitive-behavioral therapies: A replication and extension.* Paper presented at the 29th annual meeting of the Society for Psychotherapy Research, Snowbird, UT.

Castonguay, L. G., Reid, J. J., Halperin, G. S., & Goldfried, M. R. (2003). Reconciliation and integration in psychotherapy: A strategy to address the complexity of human change. In G. Stricker, T. A. Widiger, & I. B. Weiner (Eds.), *Handbook of psychology: Vol. 8. Clinical psychology* (pp. 327–366). New York: Wiley.

Castonguay, L. G., Schut, A. J., Aikins, D., Constantino, M. J., Laurenceau, J. P., Bologh, L., et al. (in press). Integrative cognitive therapy: A preliminary investigation. *Journal of Psychotherapy Integration.*

Chorpita, B. F., & Barlow, D. H. (1998). The development of anxiety: The role of control in the early environment. *Psychological Bulletin, 124*, 3–21.

Coyne, J. C., & Gotlib, I. H. (1983). The role of cognition in depression: A critical appraisal. *Psychological Bulletin, 94*, 472–505.

Durham, R. C., Allan, T., & Hackett, C. A. (1997). On predicting improvement and relapse in generalized anxiety disorder following psychotherapy. *British Journal of Clinical Psychology, 36*, 101–119.

Elkin, I. (1991). Varieties of psychotherapy integration research. *Journal of Psychotherapy Integration, 1*, 27–33.

Foa, E. B., & Kozak, M. J. (1986). Emotional processing of fear: Exposure to corrective information. *Psychological Bulletin, 99*, 20–35.

Foa, E. B., Riggs, D. S., Massie, E. D., & Yarczower, M. (1995). The impact of fear activation and anger on the efficacy of exposure treatment for posttraumatic stress disorder. *Behavior Therapy, 26*, 487–499.

Glass, C. R., Victor, B. J., & Arnkoff, D. B. (1993). Empirical research on factors in psychotherapy change. In G. Stricker & J. R. Gold (Eds.), *Comprehensive handbook of psychotherapy integration* (pp. 9–25). New York: Plenum Press.

Goldfried, M. R. (1980). Toward the delineation of therapeutic change principles. *American Psychologist, 35*, 991–999.

Goldfried, M. R., & Castonguay, L. G. (1993). Behavior therapy: redefining clinical strengths and limitations. *Behavior Therapy, 24*, 505–526.

Goldfried, M. R., Castonguay, L. G., Hayes, A. M., Drozd, J. F., & Shapiro, D. A. (1997).

A comparative analysis of the therapeutic focus in cognitive-behavioral and psychodynamic–interpersonal sessions. *Journal of Consulting and Clinical Psychology, 65*, 740–748.

Goldfried, M. R., & Davison, G. C. (1994). *Clinical behavior therapy*. New York: Wiley.

Greenberg, L. S., Rice, L. N., & Elliott, R. K. (1996). *Facilitating emotional change: The moment-by-moment process*. New York: Guilford Press.

Greenberg, L. S., & Safran, J. D. (1987). *Emotion in psychotherapy: Affect, cognition, and the process of change*. New York: Guilford Press.

Guidano, V. F., & Liotti, G. (1983). *Cognitive processes and emotional disorders*. New York: Guilford Press.

Hayes, A. H., Castonguay, L. G., & Goldfried, M. R. (1996). The effectiveness of targeting the vulnerability factors of depression in cognitive therapy. *Journal of Consulting and Clinical Psychology, 64*, 623–627.

Hofmann, S. G., Newman, M. G., Becker, E., Taylor, C. B., & Roth, W. T. (1995). Social phobia with and without avoidant personality disorder: Preliminary behavior therapy outcome findings. *Journal of Anxiety Disorders, 9*, 427–438.

Jones, E. E., & Pulos, S. M. (1993). Comparing the process in psychodynamic and cognitive-behavioral therapies. *Journal of Consulting and Clinical Psychology, 61*, 306–316.

Kerr, S., Goldfried, M. R., Hayes, A. M., Castonguay, L. G., & Goldsamt, L. A. (1992). Interpersonal and intrapersonal focus in cognitive-behavioral and psychodynamic–interpersonal therapies: A preliminary analysis of the Sheffield project. *Psychotherapy Research, 2*, 266–276.

Linehan, M. M. (1993). *Cognitive-behavioral treatment of borderline personality disorder*. New York: Guilford Press.

Mahoney, M. J. (1980). Psychotherapy and the structure of personal revolutions. In M. J. Mahoney (Ed.), *Psychotherapy process: Current issues and future directions* (pp. 157–180). New York: Plenum Press.

Mahoney, M. J. (1991). *Human change processes*. New York: Basic Books.

Newman, M. G. (1999). The clinical use of palmtop computers in the treatment of generalized anxiety disorder. *Cognitive and Behavioral Practice, 6*, 222–234.

Newman, M. G. (2000a). Generalized anxiety disorder. In M. Hersen & M. Biaggio (Eds.), *Effective brief therapies: A clinician's guide* (pp. 157–178). San Diego, CA: Academic Press.

Newman, M. G. (2000b). Recommendations for a cost offset model of psychotherapy allocation using generalized anxiety disorder as an example. *Journal of Consulting and Clinical Psychology, 68*, 549–555.

Newman, M. G., Castonguay, L. G., & Borkovec, T. D. (1999, March). *New dimensions in the treatment of generalized anxiety disorder: Interpersonal focus and emotional deepening*. Paper presented at the annual meeting of the Society for the Exploration of Psychotherapy Integration, Miami, FL.

Newman, M. G., Castonguay, L. G., Borkovec, T. D., & Schut, A. J. (1999, November). *Integrating cognitive-behavioral, interpersonal, and humanistic interventions: Why should we and how can we?* Paper presented at the First Mid-Atlantic Chapter meeting of the Society for Psychotherapy Research, College Park, MD.

Newman, M. G., Consoli, A., & Taylor, C. B. (1997). Computers in the assessment and cognitive-behavioral treatment of clinical disorders: Anxiety as a case in point. *Behavior Therapy, 28*, 211–235.

Newman, M. G., Consoli, A., & Taylor, C. B. (1999). A palmtop computer program for the treatment of generalized anxiety disorder. *Behavior Modification, 23*, 597–619.

Newman, M. G., Kenardy, J., Herman, S., & Taylor, C. B. (1997). Comparison of cognitive-behavioral treatment of panic disorder with computer assisted brief cognitive behavioral treatment. *Journal of Consulting and Clinical Psychology, 65*, 178–183.

Norcross, J. C., & Goldfried, M. R. (Eds.). (1992). *Handbook of psychotherapy integration.* New York: Basic Books.

Pennebaker, J. W., & Traue, H. C. (1993). Inhibition and psychosomatic processes. In H. C. Traue & J. W. Pennebaker (Eds.), *Emotion, inhibition, and health* (pp. 146–163). Göttingen, Germany: Hogrefe & Huber.

Pincus, A. L., & Borkovec, T. D. (1994, June). *Interpersonal problems in generalized anxiety disorder: Preliminary clustering of patients' interpersonal dysfunction.* Paper presented at the annual meeting of the American Psychological Society, New York.

Piper, W. E., Ogrodniczuk, J. S., Joyce, A., McCallum, M., Rosie, J. S., O'Kelly, J. G., & Steinberg, P. I. (1999). Prediction of dropping out in time-limited, interpretative individual psychotherapy. *Psychotherapy, 36*, 114–122.

Rachman, S. (1980). Emotional processing. *Behaviour Research and Therapy, 18*, 51–60.

Raue, P. J., & Goldfried, M. R. (1994). The therapeutic alliance in cognitive-behavior therapy. In A. O. Horvath & L. S. Greenberg (Eds.), *The working alliance: Theory, research, and practice* (pp. 131–152). New York: Wiley.

Robins, C. J., & Hayes, A. M. (1993). An appraisal of cognitive therapy. *Journal of Consulting and Clinical Psychology, 61*, 205–214.

Roemer, L., Molina, S., & Borkovec, T. D. (1997). An investigation of worry content among generally anxious individuals. *Journal of Nervous and Mental Disease, 185*, 314–319.

Rogers, C. R. (1961). *On becoming a person.* Boston: Houghton Mifflin.

Safran, J. D., Crocker, P., McMain, S., & Murray, P. (1990). Therapeutic alliance rupture as a therapy event for empirical investigation. *Psychotherapy, 27*, 154–165.

Safran, J. D., & Greenberg, L. S. (Eds.). (1991). *Emotion, psychotherapy, and change.* New York: Guilford Press.

Safran, J. D., & Segal, Z. V. (1990). *Interpersonal process in cognitive therapy.* New York: Basic Books.

Sanderson, W. C., Wetzler, S., Beck, A. T., & Betz, F. (1994). Prevalence of personality disorders among patients with anxiety disorders. *Psychiatry Research, 51*, 167–174.

Stricker, G., & Gold, J. R. (Eds.). (1993). *Comprehensive handbook of psychotherapy integration.* New York: Plenum Press.

Sullivan, H. S. (1953). *The interpersonal theory of psychiatry.* New York: Norton.

Wiser, S., & Goldfried, M. R. (1993). Comparative study of emotional experiencing in psychodynamic-interpersonal and cognitive-behavioral therapies. *Journal of Consulting and Clinical Psychology, 61*, 892–895.

CHAPTER 14

Pharmacological Treatment

R. BRUCE LYDIARD
JEANNINE MONNIER

This chapter provides an overview of the pharmacological treatment of generalized anxiety disorder (GAD). Specific recommendations for the optimal pharmacological treatment of GAD emphasize the empirical literature, but are supplemented by our own clinical experience when appropriate. Diagnostic heterogeneity in the patient samples in many early studies of the treatment of GAD (Swinson, Cox, & Fergus, 1993) limits their relevance to the treatment of GAD as defined in the *Diagnostic and Statistical Manual of Mental Disorders*, fourth edition (DSM-IV; American Psychiatric Association [APA], 1994). The publication of the present volume is timely, since recent research has significantly advanced our knowledge about the natural history, prognosis, and pharmacological treatment of DSM-IV GAD.

The importance of optimizing treatment for GAD is underscored by evidence that GAD is associated with significant morbidity, chronicity, and poor long-term prognosis. The DSM-III-R (APA, 1987) described GAD as a "mild disorder." However, it is now clear that non-comorbid (i.e., "pure") GAD confers a level of functional impairment comparable to major depression (Kessler, DuPont, Berglund, & Wittchen, 1999), negatively affects more functional domains than either panic disorder or major depression (Stout, Dolan, Dyck, Eisen, & Keller, 2001), and confers increased risk for major depression in both women and men (Breslau, Schultz, & Peterson, 1995). If current GAD is a risk factor for or "pathway" to comorbidity, early intervention and treatment of GAD may prevent the accrual of additional disorders (depression and other anxiety disorders) and the morbidity associated with them (Kessler & Price, 1993).

Data from the National Comorbidity Survey were recently reanalyzed to look for any empirical evidence that this might be the case. The findings suggested that persons with GAD who took a psychotropic medication at least four times had a significantly reduced risk for subsequent development of major depression, compared to those persons with GAD who never took psychotropic medication (Goodwin & Gorman, 2002). Although these findings should be interpreted cautiously, they are encouraging because they provide some empirical evidence that early intervention may reduce the accrual of subsequent comorbid psychiatric disorders.

Many persons with GAD never seek treatment; the majority who do seek help from their primary care physicians (Kessler & Wittchen, 2002; Wittchen et al., 2002). Even when properly identified, GAD appears to persist over time. Yonkers, Dyck, Warshaw, and Keller (2000) recently reported a remission rate of only 38% among patients with DSM-III-R GAD over a 5-year naturalistic follow-up of treated patients; if there was a comorbid disorder, the rate of recovery was reduced by 50%. Salzman, Goldenberg, Bruce, and Keller (2001) reported on the longitudinal treatment status of the same cohort of patients examined by Yonkers and colleagues. Approximately two-thirds of the patients who entered the longitudinal study during 1989–1991 were receiving medication. By 1996, the percentage of patients receiving medication treatment had increased marginally to 73%. This is quite remarkable, since adequate pharmacological treatment of GAD can result in complete recovery (remission) from core symptoms and disability in up to 70% of those with uncomplicated GAD within about 6 months (Pollack, 2002). Although information is limited, the literature strongly suggests that there is a high probability that GAD will recur within 6–12 months after discontinuation of effective pharmacological treatment (Pollack, 2002; Rickels, Case, & Diamond, 1980).

Thus it may be possible to prevent progressive comorbidity, alleviate illness-related impairment, and improve quality of life for many persons who suffer from GAD. Clearly, educational efforts aimed at increasing the recognition and aggressive treatment (especially in primary care settings) of this common and potentially disabling disorder should be a public health priority. An important part of this effort will require effective pharmacological treatment.

MEASURING THE EFFECTS OF PHARMACOLOGICAL TREATMENT OF GAD

It should be mentioned here that most of the information on drug efficacy in GAD is derived from clinical trials supporting applications for regulatory approval. These studies necessarily exclude patients with disorders other than GAD. Accordingly, we must extrapolate from the treatment of GAD in these studies to treating GAD in the "real world."

Pharmacotherapy is targeted at the short-term control of core GAD symptoms (excessive worry, irritability, fatigue, insomnia, muscular tension) and control of symptoms of coexisting psychiatric disorders. The longer-term goals of pharmacotherapy are to eliminate functional impairment associated with GAD and associated comorbid disorders (if any), and to maximize overall quality of life (see Table 14.1).

In Chapter 9 of this volume, Turk, Heimberg, and Mennin comprehensively review assessment tools for GAD. Here we pay special attention to measurement of GAD symptoms in clinical (medication) trials. Clinical trials are intended to test the hypothesis that the experimental agent will be superior to a placebo and equal or superior to a comparison agent (if one is included) in producing improvement as measured by the primary outcome variable. Secondary outcome variables are more varied and provide useful clinical data, which are informative but not critical for regulatory purposes. The studies examining the outcome of pharmacological treatment for GAD almost invariably employ the Hamilton Anxiety Rating Scale (HAM-A; Hamilton, 1959) or a derivative measure as the primary outcome variable. Despite the limitations of this assessment tool, its continued use is based on its demonstrated validity and reliability (see Turk et al., Chapter 9, this volume), the desirability of allowing comparison across studies, and the need to expedite the approval process for new anxiolytics. The overall decrease in the group mean HAM-A total from pretreatment to posttreatment remains the most commonly used primary outcome variable. Most studies require prestudy HAM-A scores of 20 or greater. The typical group mean HAM-A score in samples with GAD falls in the 24–27 range (moderately to severely ill).

TABLE 14.1. Goals of Pharmacotherapy for GAD

Short-term goals: Control of core symptoms of GAD and comorbid disorders
- Excessive worry
- Irritability
- Fatigue
- Sleep disturbance
- Muscular tension
- Excessive autonomic symptoms
- Symptoms attributable to comorbid disorders (depression, other anxiety disorders)

Long-term goals: Improved quality of life
- Maintaining treatment gains
- Optimizing compliance with long-term treatment
- Eliminating illness-related impairment in family, social, and occupational functioning
- Improving overall emotional and physical functioning
- Improving patient's subjective sense of life satisfaction

A variety of assessment tools are commonly employed as secondary variables in studies of the pharmacotherapy of GAD. The Clinical Global Impression (CGI) rating scales for severity of illness and improvement (Guy, 1976) are intended to provide a more global clinical picture. Each is a 7-point scale ranging from 1 ("not ill") to 7 ("among the most extremely ill patients") on the CGI severity (CGI-S) rating, and from 1 ("very much improved") to 7 ("very much worse") on the CGI improvement (CGI-I) rating. Clinical studies usually require that patients are rated at least "moderately ill" on the CGI-S, which is represented by a score of 4 or more.

Another measure that is commonly used as a secondary outcome measure is the percentage of patients referred to as "responders" or "remitters." Patients who show a 50% reduction from the prestudy HAM-A score or a CGI-I rating of either 1 ("very much improved") or 2 ("much improved") are considered "responders." Both definitions allow a range of clinical improvements to be included as "response." For the HAM-A, "remission" is typically defined as a final score less than or equal to 7. This is the clinical equivalent of a CGI-S score of 1 ("not ill"). In contrast to the definitions of response, the definitions of remission are guided by rating cutoffs or clinical benchmarks arbitrarily designated as "normal," which are much less clinically ambiguous.

Since the duration of treatment in acute trials is too short to allow for identifying all of the patients who might eventually achieve remission, remission rates are typically lower than response rates. Nevertheless, assessing remission can be useful for estimating and comparing "robustness" of treatment(s) by examining the percentage of patients fully recovered in a relatively short period of time. For longer-term (i.e., 6-month or more) treatment studies in which maximum improvement may be expected, remission is a very useful measure. As might be expected, the rate of response increases more rapidly and plateaus at a higher level than remission.

There has been increasing focus on improving life satisfaction and reducing or eliminating illness-related impairment as treatment outcomes. Many instruments referred to as "quality of life" scales in reality assess illness-related functional impairment in one or more domains (Hays, Sherbourne, & Mazel, 1993; Sheehan, Harnett-Sheehan, & Raj, 1996). Other tools are available to assess patients' perceived life satisfaction (see Turk et al., Chapter 9, this volume; Endicott, Nee, Harrison, & Blumenthal, 1993).

CLINICAL APPROACH TO THE PATIENT WITH GAD

The first contact with a patient with GAD is important in establishing a therapeutic alliance. Some patients with GAD are aware that this is a problem with excessive anxiety and worry, and are ready to discuss treatment with the clinician. However, a substantial percentage of patients with anxiety disorders initially present to their primary care physician with one or more medically unexplained physical complaints. Kroenke and colleagues (1994) reported that these patients presented with a variety of physical chief complaints, including insomnia (38%), chest pain (33%), abdominal pain (31%), headache (29%), or fatigue (26%). Most have been ill for years, and many have had unsuccessful, sometimes unpleasant contacts with health care providers (Katon et al., 1990; Roy-Byrne, 1996). They may have resisted referral for consultation with a psychiatrist or psychologist, and may feel misunderstood by their referring physician and embarrassed or ashamed that their problems were deemed "mental." A significant percentage of these patients will present with concurrent GAD and major depression, which they may report as depression or stress, usually with one or more somatic complaints.

A thorough review of medical conditions that mimic or exaggerate anxiety symptoms, current prescribed or over-the-counter medications or herbal preparations, use of caffeine (including soft drinks) or other stimulants, and alcohol consumption should be completed. Physical examination, routine laboratory studies, and an electrocardiogram serve to rule out medical illnesses that may mimic anxiety and to reassure the patient. History focused on the longitudinal pattern of worry and what effect it has in the patient is important. Many patients endure being called a "worrywart" by spouses, children, or friends.

At the point of correct diagnosis, it is important to convey to the patient that both emotional and physical distress are commonly observed in individuals with GAD. Anxious patients often cannot accept that their bothersome physical symptoms reflect problems "in their brains." In this situation, it is helpful to tell patients that the same areas of the brain that mediate their stress response also play an important role in anxiety and depression and in modulating the function of the heart, respiratory system, gastrointestinal system, and other important physical functions (Coplan & Lydiard, 1998).

It may be useful to review the diagnostic criteria for GAD with the patient, explaining that physical symptoms are an important part of the diagnosis. To further illustrate the overlap of GAD with bothersome physical symptoms, a discussion of functional disorders commonly associated with GAD (e.g., irritable bowel syndrome, chronic fatigue syndrome, fibromyalgia) may be useful (Hudson & Pope, 1994; Whitehead, Palsson, & Jones, 2002).

Providing information on the familial and inherited vulnerability to GAD is also helpful (Kendler, Neale, Kessler, Heath, & Eaves, 1992). This strategy can serve to relieve the patient of his or her perceived responsibility for the illness and help him or her consider medication as a reasonable first step. We recommend that an effort be made early to provide information about GAD and its treatments. Reviewing the pros and cons of each class of anxiolytic medications (Table 14.2), and stressing that the effective dose for an individual may range from 10% to 250% of the officially "recommended" antidepressant dose, can enhance confidence and (ideally) increase compliance.

Some GAD patients can be sensitive to side effects, due in part to the same hyperreactivity to visceral sensations that originally brought them to their primary care physician. Discussion of potential side effects can prevent surprises and reduce fearful anticipation of adverse events. Patients will invariably have questions about the treatment plan and possible medication side effects. Some patients may consult other health care professionals and/or search the Internet for information. It is especially important that the clinician be especially patient and available (either by telephone or in person) early in treatment, to answer questions, provide moral support, and encourage cautious optimism. Such initial availability for questions can help build confidence in the clinician, and in our experience it may ultimately save time and increase compliance.

PHARMACOTHERAPY FOR PATIENTS WITH GAD

Antidepressants

The likelihood of current or future psychiatric comorbidity, especially comorbid depression, has led to the recommendation that "broad-spectrum" (i.e., effective for GAD and the commonly associated comorbid psychiatric disorders) antidepressants—such as the selective serotonin reuptake inhibitors (SSRIs), venlafaxine, and possibly nefazodone—be utilized as "first-line" medication treatments for GAD (Davidson, 2001; Lydiard, 2000; Pollack, 2001). Short-term benzodiazepines were the treatment of choice for many years prior to the demonstration of antidepressants' efficacy for GAD (Lydiard, Brawman-Mintzer, & Ballenger, 1996; Rickels, Downing, Schweizer, & Hassman, 1993). Benzodiazepines are now suggested as adjunctive short-term treatments; their use as primary long-term treatments should be reserved for patients who have an unfavorable response to or are intolerant of antidepressants (Davidson, 2001; Pollack, 2001; Schweizer, 1995).

Venlafaxine

Venlafaxine was the first marketed antidepressant to receive regulatory approval for the treatment of GAD, and has been the most widely studied agent tested in nondepressed patient samples with DSM-IV GAD. Venlafaxine inhibits presynatpic neuronal reuptake of both norepinephrine and serotonin (Andrews, Ninan, & Nemeroff, 1996). Because of its "dual

TABLE 14.2. Agents Used in the Pharmacological Treatment of GAD

Agent	Daily dosage range (mg)	Advantages	Disadvantages
Benzodiazepines			
Alprazolam	1–6	Rapid onset of action; favorable side effect profile	Sedation, initial impaired coordination, subjective memory difficulty; multiple doses for shorter-acting agents; dependence/ withdrawal; limited antidepressant effect; sexual side effects; abuse potential (limited)
Clonazepam	1–3		
Lorazepam	4–10		
Diazepam	15–30		
Tricyclic antidepressants			
Imipramine	150–300	Once-daily dosage; antidepressant	Limited range of efficacy; delayed onset; activation; anticholinergic effects; orthostatic hypotension; weight gain; sexual side effects
Triazolo-piperidines			
Trazodone	150–600	Once-daily dosage; low anticholinergic effectsx; fewer sexual side effects; no effect on sleep architecture	Controlled data for trazodone, not nefazodone; delayed onset; orthostatic hypotension; priapism (rare); sedation; very rare but serious hepatotoxicity (nefazodone)
Nefazodone			
Azapirones			
Buspirone	30–60	No physical dependence or withdrawal; favorable side effect profile	Multiple doses; limited range of efficacy; antidepressant efficacy not clear; long-term tolerability unclear; dizziness, nausea, headache
Selective serotonin reuptake inhibitors			
Fluoxetine	20–40	Broad spectrum of efficacy for anxiety and depression; efficacy in GAD (not proven for all); favorable side effect profile	Gastrointestinal side effects; activation; delayed onset; sexual side effects
Sertraline	50–200		
Paroxetine	10–50		
Fluvoxamine	100–300		
Citalopram	20–40		
Escitalopram	10–20		

(continued)

TABLE 14.2. *(continued)*

Agent	Daily dosage range (mg)	Advantages	Disadvantages
Serotonin–norepinephrine reuptake inhibitors			
Venlafaxine (XR)	15–45	Clear efficacy in GAD, depression; some data for other anxiety disorders	Sexual dysfunction; nausea common but transient
Mirtazapine	75–225		Efficacy data lacking; no controlled studies; sedation; weight gain
Other agents			
Hydroxyzine	37.5–50	Tolerable; no dependence	Sedation; anticholinergic effects
Pregabalin	200–600	Well tolerated; efficacy and comparative efficacy shown; limited drug–drug interactions	Not yet available; limited experience; antidepressant efficacy unclear

Note. These data are based on controlled studies and our own clinical experience.

reuptake" effect, it has been classified as a serotonin–norepinephrine reuptake inhibitor.

Regulatory approval of venlafaxine for treatment of GAD was based on evidence from multicenter, placebo-controlled studies conducted in the United States, Canada, and Europe (Allgulander, Hackett, & Salinas, 2001; Davidson, DuPont, Hedges, & Haskins, 1999; Gelenberg et al., 2000; Rickels, Pollack, Sheehan, & Haskins, 2000; Sheehan, 1999). Table 14.3 summarizes these (and other) studies of the pharmacotherapy of GAD. These data collectively represent the largest data set obtained to date from patients with DSM-IV GAD without any important psychiatric comorbidity. The patient samples and design of all these studies were quite similar. Included were nondepressed, medically stable men and women aged 18 years or more, with DSM-IV GAD of at least moderate severity, who gave both written and oral consent for participation in the study. Patients with major depression, or other psychiatric or medical conditions that would interfere with interpretation of outcome, were excluded.

The fixed-dose studies each included slightly different dose ranges of venlafaxine, revealing a pattern of increasing improvement with higher

TABLE 14.3. Studies of the Pharmacotherapy of GAD

Study	Type, weeks	Agent, mg/day	n	% Female	Age	Years ill	HAM-A pre	HAM-A post	HAM-A resp, %	CGI-I Resp, %	Comments
Gelenberg et al. (2000)	Flexible, 26	Venlafaxine 75–225 Pbo	113 123	68 72	41 38	7.5 6.2	25.0 25.0	11.6 16.3	69* 40	67* 33	52% venlafaxine, 36% Pbo completed; venlafaxine > Pbo on all primary outcome measures; mean dose venlafaxine = 176 mg/day.
Davidson et al. (1999)	Fixed, 8	Venlafaxine 75 Venlafaxine 150 Buspirone 30 Pbo	87 87 93 91	52 60 51 61	38 37 37 39	8.3 5.7 7.8 6.8	23.7 23.0 23.8 23.7	13.0 13.8 14.1 15.6	49 49 55 39	62* 49 55* 39	Venlafaxine 75 and buspirone > Pbo on CGI-I; no between-group differences on HAM-A.
Allgulander et al. (2001)	Fixed, 24	Venlafaxine 37.5 Venlafaxine 75 Venlfaxine 150 Pbo	138 130 137 130	57 62 65 58	45 44 45 46	10.9 9.1 8.2 9.4	26.6 26.3 26.3 26.7	12.8 11.8 10.1 15.5	60* 70* 79* 42	69* 77* 80* 46	All doses > Pbo on HAM-A by Week 2, CGI-I by Week 3; 75 and 150 mg > Pbo on all outcome measures.
Rickels, Pollack, et al. (2000)	Fixed, 8	Venlafaxine 75 Venlafaxine 150 Venlafaxine 225 Pbo	86 81 86 96	58 56 52 57	40 40 42 41	6.7 6.7 8.9 9.3	24.7 24.5 23.6 24.1	13.8 12.1* 12.0* 14.6	NA	NA	75 mg = Pbo on most measures; 150 and 225 mg doses Pbo on all measures.
Pollack et al. (2001)	Flexible, 8	Paroxetine 20–50 Pbo	161 163	61 66	39 41	11.0 11.0	24.2 24.1	12.6 NA	64* 44	62* 47	Mean dose paroxetine 26.8 mg; final dose–20 mg, 26%; 0 mg, 26%; 40 mg, 20%; 50 mg, 26%; ejaculatory disturbance in 34.9% of males.

(continued)

359

TABLE 14.3. (continued)

Study	Type, weeks	Agent, mg/day	n	% Female	Age	Years ill	HAM-A pre	HAM-A post	HAM-A resp, %	CGI-I Resp, %	Comments
Bellew et al. (2000)	Fixed, 8	Paroxetine 20 Paroxetine 40 Pbo	188 197 180	NA	NA	NA	24.0 23.8 24.0	12.1 11.0 13.3	81* 68* 52	NA	Sheehan Disability ratings improved at both doses; suggested initial dose 20 mg for most patients.
Pohl et al. (2002)	Fixed, 6	Pregabalin 100 bid Pregabalin 200 bid Pregabalin 150 tid Pbo	344 total	NA	NA	NA	NA	NA	NA	56* 55* 59* 34	Showed twice-daily and three-times-daily dosing to be effective.
Rickels et al. (2002)	Fixed, 4	Pregabalin 100 tid Pregabalin150 tid Pregabalin 200 tid Alprazolam 0.5 tid Pbo	455 total		38 39 39 40 41	12 12 14 12 13	25 25 25 25 24			61* 44* 51* 45* 31	Only 4 weeks duration; all doses of pregabalin and alprazolam > Pbo: pregabalin 300 mg/day (−12.2), pregabalin 450 mg/day (−11.0), pregabalin 600 mg/day (−11.8), alprazolam 1.5 mg/day (−10.9), and placebo (−8.4).
Davidson et al. (2002)	Flexible, 8	Escitalopram 10–20 Pbo	124 128	60 63	40 41	11.4 13.1	22.8 22.1	12.8 15.9	NA	NA	Single-blind Pbo run-in; initial dose 10 mg, could increase to 20 mg at Week 4; main three adverse events: nausea, headache, insomnia.
Allgulander et al. (2002)	Flexible, 12	Sertraline 50–150 Pbo	182 188	59 51	40 42	25 25	25 25	13.3 17.0	NA	63* 37	Single-blind Pbo run-in; dropout due to adverse events— 7.6% sertraline, 9.6% Pbo;

360

sertraline > Pbo on QLES-Q patient-rated life satisfaction.

Study	Design	Drug/dose	N			Pre	Post	Resp %	Comments
Rickels et al. (1993)	Flexible, 8	Diazepam 27	56	NA	NA	NA	NA	66*	Patients had DSM-III-R GAD; results are for completers; intent-to-treat outcome was similar; imipramine superior to diazepam; diazepam had more rapid onset.
		Imipramine 143	58					73*	
		Trazodone 245	61					69*	
		Pbo	55					47	
Moller et al. (2001)	Fixed, 4	Alprazolam 2	102	67 (three-group mean)	48 (three-group mean)	27.9	12.6	64*	HAM-A minimum = 17; ICD-10 F41.1 used for GAD diagnosis, semistructured interview; primary care MDs supervised by psychiatrists; excluded major depression and panic disorder; only 4 weeks; dropouts comparable across all groups (about 30%).
		Opipramol 200[a]	100			27.7	13.1	63*	
		Pbo	105			29.3	16.2	47	
Lader & Scotto (1998)	Fixed, 4	Hydroxyzine 37.5	81	69	42	26.6	14.8	50*	Pbo lead-in and washout, single-blind. Conducted in six primary care practices, supervised by psychiatrists. Buspirone not greater than Pbo on reduction in mean HAM-A, but statistically significant on secondary measures.
		Buspirone 30	82	78	41	26.7	17.9	NA	
		Pbo	81	63	40	26.2	19.0	30	

Note. NA, information not available; HAM-A, Hamilton Anxiety Rating Scale; CGI, Clinical Global Impression improvement scale; Pre, pretreatment; Post, posttreatment; Resp, responders; Pbo, placebo; bid, twice a day; tid, three times a day.
[a]Not available in the United States.
*Statistically superior to placebo.

doses. Satisfactory completion rates for all the short-term studies were noted.

LONG-TERM TREATMENT. The results of the Gelenberg and colleagues (2000) study are shown in Figure 14.1. This study showed that benefits of venlafaxine can be maintained over a long period in patients with GAD, with HAM-A response rates of 69% for venlafaxine extended release (XR) at Weeks 6 through 28, versus 42–46% for the placebo group. Remission rates were lower than response rates and achieved the highest level later in the study period. A 6-month randomized, fixed-dose study by Allgulander and colleagues (2001) further supported the long-term efficacy of venlafaxine XR in the treatment of GAD at doses as low as 75 mg/day. In the Gelenberg and colleagues study, 52% of the group receiving venlafaxine versus 36% of placebo recipients completed this 6-month study. In contrast, in the Allgulander and colleagues study, conducted in Europe,

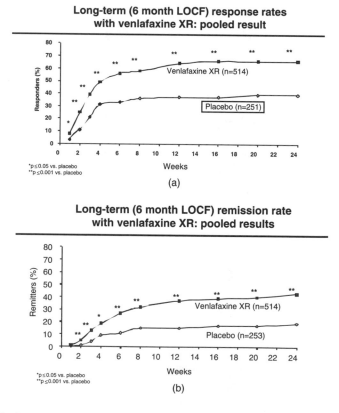

FIGURE 14.1. Rates of response (a) and remission (b) in patients receiving either venlafaxine or placebo over 24 weeks. LOCF, last observation carried forward. Data from Gelenberg et al. (2000).

higher completion rates of 73–78% across groups receiving venlafaxine and 66% of placebo recipients were reported. It is interesting to speculate that cultural differences may have played a role in these different completion rates.

The fixed-dose studies suggest that both short-term and long-term efficacy is greater at higher doses; because dosages could not be adjusted, this may reflect lower response rates than a similarly designed study with flexible dosing might have obtained. The maximum dose allowed in the flexible-design Gelenberg and colleagues (2000) study was 225 mg daily, and the mean dose at endpoint was 176 mg daily. This suggests that there is a fairly large range of "optimal" dosages, and that titration for each individual patient is important.

Paroxetine

The efficacy of paroxetine as a treatment for GAD has been reported in both flexible-dose (Pollack et al., 2001) and fixed-dose (Bellew, McCafferty, Iyengar, & Zaninelli, 2000) multicenter placebo-controlled studies (see Table 14.3). Both studies showed a significant difference favoring paroxetine over placebo in the percentage of patients achieving at least a 50% reduction in HAM-A ratings by the end of the study. Pollack and colleagues (2001) reported the results of an 8-week, flexible-dose study of 20–50 mg daily paroxetine versus placebo, using 10 mg as the initial dose. As with the venlafaxine studies, the primary outcome measure was the mean change in the HAM-A total score from baseline. For the primary and all secondary outcome measures, paroxetine was significantly more effective than placebo. In this study, the Sheehan Disability Scale (Sheehan et al., 1996) was administered, and significant reductions in impairment in functioning were noted as early as the first week. The percentages of responders and remitters in this study were also significantly greater among paroxetine-treated patients than among placebo recipients. Bellew and colleagues (2000) compared 20 and 40 mg paroxetine with placebo in a fixed-dose design. In this study, both groups receiving paroxetine showed significantly greater reduction in total HAM-A scores than the placebo recipients.

LONG-TERM TREATMENT. In a long-term study, 559 patients who were rated as remitters after 8 weeks of single-blind treatment with 20–50 mg paroxetine daily were randomly assigned to continue paroxetine or placebo (Stocchi et al., 2003). Those who received placebo relapsed at a significantly higher rate than did those who continued paroxetine. As can be seen in Figure 14.2, patients who continued to receive paroxetine were more likely to achieve remission over time than were those who were randomly assigned to placebo.

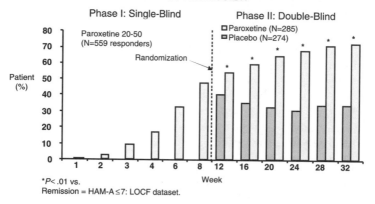

FIGURE 14.2. Full relapse of remitted paroxetine-treated patients with GAD following double-blind placebo substitution versus continuing paroxetine. From F. Stocchi, G. Nordera, R. H. Jokinen, U. M. Lepola, K. Hewitt, H. Bryson, M. K. Iyengar, and the Paroxetine Generalized Anxiety Workgroup, "Efficacy and Tolerability of Paroxetine for the Long-Term Treatment of Generalized Anxiety Disorder," *Journal of Clinical Psychiatry, 64,* 250–258, 2003. Copyright 2003 by Physicians Postgraduate Press. Reprinted by permission.

Sertraline

The SSRI sertraline has also been studied in large samples of patients with DSM-IV GAD. The first large, controlled, multicenter study has recently been completed (Allgulander et al., 2002; see Table 14.3). This flexible-dose study was quite similar in design to those reviewed above. These investigators employed 50–150 mg sertraline daily versus placebo. Sertraline was superior to placebo on primary and secondary outcome measures, including measures of quality of life and patient satisfaction.

In a 9-week double-blind study, 22 children aged 5–17 with DSM-IV GAD received either 50 mg sertraline or placebo (Rynn, Siqueland, & Rickels, 2001). In this small study, the clinical response as assessed by HAM-A scores did not differ between children with low ($n = 9$) and high ($n = 13$) depression scores. The findings showed statistically significant superiority for the sertraline-treated group versus those receiving placebo.

Escitalopram

Escitalopram, which is the active isomer of the SSRI citalopram, is the SSRI most recently marketed for the treatment of depression. A preliminary report of a recent multicenter study of patients with DSM-IV GAD showed that 10–20 mg escitalopram was superior to placebo in reducing HAM-A scores (Davidson, Bose, & Su, 2002; Table 14.3). Patients were given 10 mg escitalopram for the first 4 weeks; the dose could be increased thereafter to 20 mg if there was inadequate response. There were significant drug–placebo differences after 4 weeks of treatment with 10 mg escitalopram, providing some preliminary evidence that this lower dosage may be sufficient for a significant percentage of patients with GAD. Determination of the optimal dosage will require dose-finding (i.e., fixed-dose) studies to test this hypothesis.

Other SSRIs

There are no controlled data regarding the efficacy of other SSRIs in the treatment of GAD. It is likely that these agents would also be effective.

Tricyclic Antidepressants (Imipramine)

Since the introduction of the newer antidepressants, investigations of the efficacy of the tricyclic antidepressants (TCAs) in the treatment of GAD have been almost completely abandoned. To date, there has been only one study in which patients with DSM-IV GAD were treated with a TCA (Rocca, Fonzo, Scotta, Zanalda, & Ravizza, 1997). In this 8-week, uncontrolled comparative study, imipramine was compared with desmethyl-diazepam (similar to diazepam) and paroxetine in a total of 81 patients with DSM-IV GAD. The three groups were comparably ill (mean HAM-A values about 25 at baseline). All three groups fared comparably well, with approximately two-thirds of each group being classified as responders by the study's end. There was a differential effect favoring both antidepressants over the benzodiazepine in treating psychic symptoms, while the benzodiazepine was more effective in alleviating somatic symptoms in this study. This finding is consistent with earlier reports of studies in patients with DSM-III-R GAD, although reduction in HAM-A scores was similar, both in a non-placebo-controlled comparison (Hoehn-Saric, McLeod, & Zimmerli, 1988) and in a placebo-controlled study (Rickels et al., 1993). Also consistently reported was a greater side effect burden associated with the TCA than with the benzodiazepine (Andrews et al., 1996; Feighner, 1999). This is a major disadvantage of the TCAs, especially since many patients with GAD need long-term treatment.

Other Antidepressants

The data supporting the effectiveness of other antidepressants are limited to case reports and small open studies (Goodnick, Puig, DeVane, & Freund, 1999; Hedges, Reimherr, Strong, Halls, & Rust, 1996). Table 14.2

summarizes the available evidence for efficacy of antidepressants in GAD and other anxiety disorders. This is based on the existing literature and our own clinical experience.

Benzodiazepines

The benzodiazepines have been extensively studied in the treatment of DSM-III-R GAD (Enkelmann, 1991; Feighner, 1999; Lydiard et al., 1996; Rickels et al., 1993; Wilcox et al., 1994). One of the main advantages of benzodiazepines over other anxiolytic agents is the rapid onset of action—often statistically superior to that of antidepressants after 1 week—while the overall efficacy is comparable by the end of a study (see Figure 14.3).

Both of the studies in which patients with DSM-IV GAD were treated with benzodiazepines employed alprazolam (Moller, Volz, Reimann, & Stoll, 2001; Rickels et al., 2002; see Table 14.3). In both fixed-dose, double-blind studies, alprazolam at daily doses of either 1.5 mg (Rickels et al., 2002) or 2 mg (Moller et al., 2001) was superior to placebo. These results are quite comparable with the older literature on benzodiazepine treatment of DSM-III-R GAD: Benzodiazepine treatment is effective for short-term treatment of GAD.

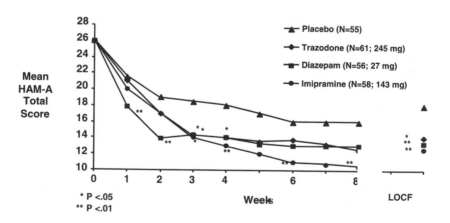

FIGURE 14.3. Comparative efficacy of trazodone, imipramine, and diazepam in the treatment of patients with DSM-III-R GAD over 8 weeks. From "Antidepressants for the Treatment of Generalized Anxiety Disorder: A Placebo-Controlled Comparison of Imipramine, Trazodone, and Diazepam" by K. Rickels, R. Downing, E. Schweizer, and H. Hassman, 1993, *Archives of General Psychiatry, 50,* 884–895. Copyright 1993 by the American Medical Association. All rights reserved. Reprinted by permission.

LONG-TERM TREATMENT. Because of the chronic nature of GAD, clinicians increasingly need to consider long-term pharmacotherapy as part of the overall treatment plan. Despite objective evidence to the contrary, persistent concerns among both clinicians and patients about long-term treatment with benzodiazepines are common. These include the development of tolerance, potential abuse, and inability to discontinue benzodiazepines after long-term treatment. Unfortunately, the literature relating to long-term treatment with benzodiazepines is almost exclusively focused on panic disorder. The empirical evidence provides no indication that tolerance to the anxiolytic effect of the benzodiazepines occurs, that abuse is an significant clinical problem in anxious patients, or that patients cannot discontinue benzodiazepines over time (Nagy, Krystal, Charney, Merikangas, & Woods, 1993; Uhlenhuth, Balter, Ban, & Yang, 1999; Uhlenhuth, DeWit, Balter, Johanson, & Mellinger, 1988). Although comparable data for patients with GAD are unfortunately lacking, our clinical experience is consistent with the above observations. Despite decades of research and controversy, long-term benzodiazepine treatment of patients with GAD has yet to be adequately investigated (Mahe & Balogh, 2000).

Current recommendations that antidepressants are superior to the benzodiazepines as a first-line treatment for GAD usually refer to the need for long-term treatments that will prevent or treat emergent depression (Ballenger et al., 2001; Culpepper, 2002; Davidson, 2001; Gorman, 2002; Lydiard, 2000; Pollack, 2001). It was somewhat surprising that a recent report from the Harvard/Brown Anxiety Research Program's study of anxiety disorders indicated that significantly more patients with GAD received benzodiazepines alone than SSRIs alone or in combination with benzodiazepines both in 1990 and in 1996 (Salzman et al., 2001). Also important was the trend the authors observed: a slightly greater percentage of combined benzodiazepines and SSRIs, and slightly less monotherapy, as a pattern emerging over the two time points examined. Unfortunately, the report did not include patient response information for the different groups, making it impossible to determine whether monotherapy or a combination of treatments was more effective.

Although emergent depression in patients taking benzodiazepines alone is a clinical concern, there is significant evidence that benzodiazepines can be coadministered with SSRIs in the treatment of major depression, with no apparent adverse consequences. In fact, the combination appears to enhance the rate of improvement of depressive symptoms and to increase compliance over both the short and the longer term (Buysse et al., 1997; Londborg, Smith, Glaudin, & Painter, 2000; Smith, Londborg, Glaudin, & Painter, 2002). Thus it appears that the benzodiazepines enhance both the response to and tolerability of SSRI treatment in patients with major depression. We found no information on the use of combined benzodiazepines and antidepressants in GAD. This is clearly an area in which research could inform us further about optimal long-term treatment of GAD.

DISCONTINUATION AFTER LONG-TERM USE. It is the responsibility of the clinician to present the facts clearly and fairly to the patient for whom long-term prescription of a benzodiazepine is being considered. With proper supervision, any patient can stop a benzodiazepine, even if an alternative treatment is required (DuPont, 1990). During the course of long-term treatment, the clinician is responsible for periodic assessment of the continued requirement for medication. Planning a very gradual taper schedule (e.g., over 3–6 months or more), and slowing the taper rate after reaching about 50% of the original dose, will enhance the likelihood of a positive outcome (Rickels, Schweizer, Case, & Greenblatt, 1990). We also recommend continuing to use divided doses of short- to intermediate-half-life benzodiazepines (e.g., alprazolam, lorazepam) during the taper, to avoid fluctuations in plasma benzodiazepine concentrations over a 24-hour period. If bothersome anxiety symptoms emerge during the taper, it is important to learn whether they represent rebound anxiety due to dose reduction or a reemergence of GAD symptoms. In such a situation, we recommend stopping the taper and raising the benzodiazepine dose as needed to minimize discomfort. Symptoms due to rebound anxiety related to the taper should abate within 2–3 weeks of stopping the taper, while those that persist or worsen are more likely related to reemergence of the anxiety symptoms initially treated. This "differential diagnostic" point is critical in determining the next step in treatment (i.e., continuing to taper, or stopping the taper and reinstituting benzodiazepine treatment).

Patients who are motivated to discontinue benzodiazepines can usually accomplish their goal if they are allowed the necessary time for a gradual taper and have the cooperation of the clinician during this sometimes difficult process. In our experience, patients who are stabilized on an antidepressant known to treat GAD are more likely to complete a benzodiazepine taper successfully (Rickels, De Martinis, et al., 2000).

It is important that the clinician and patient begin this process during a time when predictable stress will be minimal. Furthermore, it should be made explicit that demonstration of the continued need for benzodiazepine treatment should also be considered a satisfactory end result. Adjunctive cognitive-behavioral treatments during benzodiazepine discontinuation have been helpful for patients with panic disorder (Otto et al., 1993); this may be useful for patients with GAD as well.

Azapirones

Buspirone is the only marketed azapirone; it is a nonbenzodiazepine anxiolytic that is currently approved for the treatment of GAD. Buspirone's antianxiety effects are mediated at least in part via partial agonist effects at the serotonin 1a receptor on serotonergic neurons. The studies in which buspirone was demonstrated to be useful for GAD were largely conducted in patients with DSM-III (Enkelmann, 1991; Laakmann et al., 1998; Olajide & Lader, 1987; Pecknold et al., 1989) or DSM-III-R (Pollack, Worthington, Manfro, Otto, & Zucker, 1997) GAD. In the initial studies, doses as low as 15 mg buspirone were as effective as diazepam and superior to placebo. In clinical practice, 15 mg buspirone daily was often ineffective, and clinical experience indicated that 30 mg or more buspirone daily was more likely to be efficacious. Two studies in patients with DSM-IV GAD were identified. Buspirone was compared with venlafaxine and placebo by Davidson and colleagues (1999). In that study, there were no differences between any treatment and placebo on the main outcome variable. In the second (Lader & Scotto, 1998), the efficacy of buspirone was compared with hydroxyzine and placebo in six primary care settings, each of which was supervised by a psychiatrist. Buspirone (30 mg daily) was not statistically significantly different from placebo, while hydroxyzine (37.5 mg) was shown to be superior on the primary outcome variable. The time period for treatment was short (4 weeks), and the relatively small sample size (approximately 80 patients per group) may have contributed to a Type II error.

A main disadvantage, relative to the other available anxiolytics, is that buspirone is ineffective in the treatment of panic disorder (Schweizer & Rickels, 1988; Sheehan, Raj, Sheehan, & Soto, 1988, 1990) and social anxiety disorder (van Vliet, den Boer, Westenberg, & Pian, 1997), which are the two most commonly coexisting anxiety disorders in patients with GAD. In studies reporting efficacy of buspirone in major depression, the effects appear to be less robust than with the TCAs (Fabre 1990; Rickels, Amsterdam, Clary, Puzzuoli, & Schweizer, 1991; Schweizer, Rickels, Hassman, & Garcia-Espana, 1998), and doses may be as high as 90 mg daily, with up to 60% of patients dropping out due to adverse effects prior to the end of a study.

The narrow range of anxiolytic efficacy of buspirone and its questionable usefulness in depression limit clinicians' enthusiasm for its use as a first-line treatment for GAD. Therefore, the role of buspirone in the treatment of GAD is probably limited to patients with uncomplicated GAD who are intolerant of or unresponsive to other agents. For patients with a history of substance abuse, buspirone might provide some benefits. However, the efficacy of buspirone in patients who have received benzodiazepines within a month appears to be less than in patients without recent prior benzodiazepine use (DeMartinis, Rynn, Rickels, & Mandos, 2000). The most prominent adverse effects of buspirone include headache, nonvertigo dizziness, and nausea/other gastrointestinal distress.

Novel Agents

After the discovery that gabapentin, an antiepileptic with novel anxiolytic properties, was clinically effective in anxiety disorders (Pande et al., 1999; Pande, Davidson, et al., 2000), the effectiveness of a related agent, pregabalin as a treatment for GAD was studied in large numbers of patients with DSM-IV GAD. Preliminary findings of two completed studies (Pohl et al., 2002; Rickels et al., 2002) are shown in Table 14.3. As can be seen, Rickels and colleagues (2002) showed that pregabalin (200–600 mg daily) was equally effective and possibly superior to alprazolam over 4 weeks of treatment; both active agents were statistically significantly superior to placebo. In the study by Pohl and colleagues (2002), the effectiveness of twice-daily dosing was confirmed over a 6-week treatment period, with good efficacy of pregabalin compared with placebo. Preliminary data from a third completed study, which compared pregabalin (200 and 300 mg twice daily), venlafaxine (37.5 mg twice daily), and placebo, showed that both doses of pregabalin and venlafaxine were superior to placebo (Lydiard, Zimbroff, Tobias, & Zornberg, 2003). Although the effectiveness of pregabalin in major depression is not yet clear, it reduces mild symptoms of depression in patients with GAD to a greater extent than placebo (Kavoussi, Crockatt, Werth, Liu-Dumaw, & Pande, 2000) and is superior to placebo in the treatment of social anxiety disorder (Pande, Feltner, Jefferson, Davidson, & Lydiard, 1999). Pregabalin is currently undergoing evaluation for approval for the treatment of GAD. The large database that already exists for this agent provides substantial evidence for its efficacy in GAD. Information on its effectiveness as an antidepressant and as a treatment for other anxiety disorders (especially panic disorder) will be useful in filling the remaining gaps in our knowledge regarding this interesting compound.

Other Agents

Hydroxyzine is an antihistamine with sedating properties which is prescribed by primary care clinicians as an anxiolytic. Lader and Scotto (1998) reported that hydroxyzine (37.5 mg daily) was superior to placebo over a 4-week period in the treatment of patients with GAD (Table 14.3).

Herbal Agents

Anxious patients frequently seek alternative medicine treatments in addition to "standard" treatment (Eisenberg et al., 1998). Despite the number of individuals in the United States who take herbal medicine on one or more occasions, training in alternative medicine is not offered as a standard part of medical training, though it is occasionally available as an elective (Wetzel, Eisenberg, & Kaptchuk, 1998). Individuals with anxiety disorders are among those most likely to seek alternative treatments in addition to conventional treatment (Kessler et al., 2001).

Many claims for the therapeutic benefits of herbal products for a variety of conditions are made, and some clinical reports support their usefulness (Yager, Siegfreid, & DiMatteo, 1999). There is now controlled evidence that kava is effective in the treatment of human anxiety (Volz & Kieser, 1997). The physiological effects of kava in patients with GAD has recently been reported by Watkins, Connor, and Davidson (2001), who demonstrated that baroreceptor cardiac rate control, a measure of vagal activity shown to be abnormal in GAD, was normalized significantly more in patients receiving kava than those who received placebo. The authors noted that degree of change in this measure correlated with clinical benefit. Although these recent data are encouraging, the scientific database demonstrating the effectiveness of other herbal products for anxiety disorders is lacking. Moreover, unexpected adverse effects from adding herbal preparations to ongoing pharmacotherapy have been reported (Yager et al., 1999).

It seems prudent for clinicians treating patients with GAD to become acquainted with the basic uses of herbal products for emotional symptoms. If the clinician can offer information and asks to be included in a patient's decisions about using herbal products during ongoing pharmacotherapy for GAD, it will increase the likelihood of the clinician's staying informed, and thus the likelihood of serious adverse events.

SUMMARY OF RECOMMENDATIONS

Table 14.2 lists the dosage range and the advantages and disadvantages of the various pharmacological agents for the treatment of GAD. The bulk of the empirical data on the pharmacological treatment of GAD is derived from published literature and abstracts from the extensive research on venlafaxine and paroxetine. Other studies will be appearing in the literature in the near future. Based on the available literature, there is no evidence to indicate either benzodiazepines or antidepressants as superior over the short or long term. At this point, largely on the basis of our clinical experience, broad-spectrum antidepressants are recommended as first-line pharmacological treatments for GAD. We recommend benzodiazepines as useful adjunctive treatments in combination with antidepressants for many patients with GAD. In addition, for those patients who are intolerant of or unresponsive to antidepressants, the benzodiazepines represent a useful treatment alternative. For patients with current or prior substance abuse, nonbenzodiazepine anxiolytics should be used. The current recommendations for the use of benzodiazepines versus antidepressants versus the combination for the treatment of GAD are based more on clinical judgment than empirical data. Further research on the efficacy of these agents would have important implications for clinical practice.

COMORBID PSYCHIATRIC DISORDERS

As has been reviewed by Kessler, Walters, and Wittchen in Chapter 2 of this volume, GAD very frequently precedes and coexists with major depression (Kessler & Wittchen, 2002) and/or other anxiety disorders (Judd et al., 1998). Patients with comorbid anxiety and depression are more depressed and anxious, are more impaired, and have a poorer prognosis than patients with either anxiety or depression (Lydiard, 1991; Yonkers, Warshaw, Massion, & Keller, 1996); they also tend to terminate treatment prematurely more often than patients with depression alone do (Brown, Schulberg, Madonia, Shear, & Houck, 1996). In one of the few studies to address treatment of patients with comorbidity, Brown and colleagues (1996) compared patients with depression alone to those who had depression with GAD or with panic disorder. When treated in a systematic fashion with either nortriptyline or manualized psychotherapy for depression, patients with depression and GAD exhibited slower recovery rates than patients with depression only, but they eventually responded. In contrast, patients with depression and lifetime panic disorder responded poorly to both treatments. Silverstone and Salinas (2001) reanalyzed data from a multicenter, placebo-controlled comparison of venlafaxine and fluoxetine in 368 patients with major depression. The subgroup of 98 patients who had comorbid DSM-IV GAD were compared with the 276 patients in that study with depression without comorbidity. Consistent with the Brown and colleagues study, venlafaxine was superior to placebo in patients with comorbid GAD; the comorbid patients had a slower rate of response than did those without comorbid anxiety. In this study, the response to fluoxetine was less robust, but a pattern of slower onset in the comorbid patients (similar to such patients' response to venlafaxine) was observed. These studies both suggest that practitioners should be prepared to encourage patients with comorbid GAD and depression to wait longer for improvement prior to changing treatment.

With respect to GAD that coexists with other anxiety disorders or to multiple comorbidity (i.e., depression plus one or more additional disorders), there are no empirical data. In our experience, the use of agents that are effective in the treatment of each disorder present produces the most positive outcome. Clinicians should keep in mind that the time required for improvement is likely to be longer than for patients with only one disorder. In addition, we have found that it is often necessary to use dosages two to three times higher than the usual antidepressant dose in such patients, and that the use of more than one agent (e.g., a broad-spectrum antidepressant plus a benzodiazepine) is more frequently necessary to provide optimal benefit.

CONCLUSIONS

The empirical database on the treatment of DSM-IV GAD has expanded significantly in the past several years. Most significant is the evolution of GAD, through skepticism about the validity of the diagnosis to the finding that it is a serious and chronic disorder that is prevalent in the U.S. population. This chapter has provided an overview of the rationale and empirical basis for pharmacological treatment of GAD. Large gaps in the literature include the lack of any empirical evidence to demonstrate that benzodiazepines are less efficacious than antidepressants over the long term. This controversy can be resolved with hypothesis-testing studies in patients with DSM-IV GAD. Comorbidity, which is the rule rather than the exception, has been largely ignored in the experimental literature, and the clinician is still left with much more "art" than "science" in determining the optimal treatment approach in those patients with the greatest burden of illness. Continued efforts based on community survey data, treatment studies (medications alone and in combination with psychotherapy), and long-term follow-up studies are sorely needed to fill in the remaining gaps in our knowledge of optimal treatment of GAD with medication.

REFERENCES

Allgulander, C., Dahl, A. A., Morris, P., Kutcher, S., Sogaard, J., Clary, C., & Austin, C. (2002, December). *Sertraline for the treatment of generalized anxiety disorder: Results of a multicenter double-blind, placebo-controlled trial.* Paper presented at the annual meeting of the American College of Neuropsychopharmacology, San Juan, PR.

Allgulander, C., Hackett, D., & Salinas, E. (2001). Venlafaxine extended release (ER) in the treatment of generalized anxiety disorder: Twenty-four-week placebo-controlled dose-ranging study. *British Journal of Psychiatry, 179,* 15–22.

Andrews, J. M., Ninan, P. T., & Nemeroff, C. B. (1996). Venlafaxine: A novel antidepressant that has a dual mechanism of action. *Depression, 4,* 48–56.

American Psychiatric Association (APA). (1987). *Diagnostic and statistical manual of mental disorders* (3rd ed., rev.). Washington, DC: Author.

American Psychiatric Association (APA). (1994). *Diagnostic and statistical manual for mental disorders* (4th ed.). Washington, DC: Author.

Ballenger, J. C., Davidson, J. R., Lecrubier, Y., Nutt, D. J., Borkovec, T. D., Rickels, K., Stein, D. J., & Wittchen, H. U. (2001). Consensus statement on generalized anxiety disorder from the International Consensus Group on Depression and Anxiety. *Journal of Clinical Psychiatry, 62*(Suppl. 11), 53–58.

Bellew, K. M., McCafferty, J. P., Iyengar, M., & Zaninelli, R. M. (2000, June). *Paroxetine treatment of GAD: A double-blind, placebo-controlled trial.* Paper presented at the annual meeting of the American Psychiatric Association, Chicago.

Breslau, N., Schultz, L., & Peterson, E. (1995). Sex differences in depression: A role for preexisting anxiety. *Psychiatry Research, 58,* 1–12.

Brown, C., Schulberg, H. C., Madonia, M. J., Shear, M. K., & Houck, P. R. (1996). Treatment outcomes for primary care patients with major depression and lifetime anxiety disorders. *American Journal of Psychiatry, 153,* 1293–1300.

Buysse, D. J., Reynolds, C. F., III, Houck, P. R., Perel, J. M., Frank, E., Begley, A. E., Mazumdar, S., & Kupfer, D. J. (1997). Does lorazepam impair the antidepressant response to nortriptyline and psychotherapy? *Journal of Clinical Psychiatry, 58,* 426–432.

Coplan, J. D., & Lydiard, R. B. (1998). Brain circuits in panic disorder. *Biological Psychiatry, 44,* 1264–1276.

Culpepper, L. (2002). Generalized anxiety disorder in primary care: Emerging issues in management and treatment. *Journal of Clinical Psychiatry, 63*(Suppl. 8), 35–42.

Davidson, J. R. (2001). Pharmacotherapy of generalized anxiety disorder. *Journal of Clinical Psychiatry, 62*(Suppl. 11), 46–50.

Davidson, J. R., DuPont, R. L., Hedges, D., & Haskins, J. T. (1999). Efficacy, safety, and tolerability of venlafaxine extended release and buspirone in outpatients with generalized anxiety disorder. *Journal of Clinical Psychiatry, 60,* 528–535.

Davidson, J. R. T., Bose, A., & Su, G. (2002, March). *Escitalopram in the treatment of generalized anxiety disorder.* Paper presented at the annual meeting of the Anxiety Disorders Association of America, Austin, TX.

DeMartinis, N., Rynn, M., Rickels, K., & Mandos, L. (2000). Prior benzodiazepine use and buspirone response in the treatment of generalized anxiety disorder. *Journal of Clinical Psychiatry, 61,* 91–94.

DuPont, R. L. (1990). A physician's guide to discontinuing benzodiazepine therapy. *Western Journal of Medicine, 152,* 600–603.

Eisenberg, D. M., Davis, R. B., Ettner, S. L., Appel, S., Wilkey, S., Van Rompay, M., & Kessler, R. C. (1998). Trends in alternative medicine use in the United States, 1990–1997: Results of a follow-up national survey. *Journal of the American Medical Association, 280,* 1569–1575.

Endicott, J., Nee, J., Harrison, W., & Blumenthal, R. (1993). Quality of Life Enjoyment and Satisfaction Questionnaire: A new measure. *Psychopharmacology Bulletin, 29,* 321–326.

Enkelmann, R. (1991). Alprazolam versus buspirone in the treatment of outpatients with generalized anxiety disorder. *Psychopharmacology, 105,* 428–432.

Fabre, L. F. (1990). Buspirone in the management of major depression: A placebo-controlled comparison. *Journal of Clinical Psychiatry, 51*(Suppl.), 55–61.

Feighner, J. P. (1999). Overview of antidepressants currently used to treat anxiety disorders. *Journal of Clinical Psychiatry, 60*(Suppl. 22), 18–22.

Gelenberg, A. J., Lydiard, R. B., Rudolph, R. L., Aguiar, L., Haskins, J. T., & Salinas, E. (2000). Efficacy of venlafaxine extended-release capsules in nondepressed outpatients with generalized anxiety disorder: A 6-month randomized controlled trial. *Journal of the American Medical Association, 283,* 3082–3088.

Goodnick, P. J., Puig, A., DeVane, C. L., & Freund, B. V. (1999). Mirtazapine in major depression with comorbid generalized anxiety disorder. *Journal of Clinical Psychiatry, 60,* 446–448.

Goodwin, R. D., & Gorman, J. M. (2002). Psychopharmacologic treatment of generalized anxiety disorder and the risk of major depression. *American Journal of Psychiatry, 159,* 1935–1937.

Gorman, J. M. (2002). Treatment of generalized anxiety disorder. *Journal of Clinical Psychiatry, 63*(Suppl. 8), 17–23.

Guy, W. (1976). *ECDEU assessment manual for psychopharmacology.* Washington, DC: U.S. Department of Health, Education and Welfare.

Hamilton, M. (1959). The assessment of anxiety states by rating. *British Journal of Psychiatry, 32,* 50–55.

Hays, R. D., Sherbourne, C. D., & Mazel, R. M. (1993). The RAND 36-Item Health Survey 1.0. *Health Economics, 2,* 217–227.

Hedges, D. W., Reimherr, F. W., Strong, R. E., Halls, C. H., & Rust, C. (1996). An open trial of nefazodone in adult patients with generalized anxiety disorder. *Psychopharmacology Bulletin, 32,* 671–676.

Hoehn-Saric, R., McLeod, D. R., & Zimmerli, W. D. (1988). Differential effects of alprazolam and imipramine in generalized anxiety disorder: Somatic versus psychic symptoms. *Journal of Clinical Psychiatry, 49,* 293–301.

Hudson, J. I., & Pope, H. G. (1994). The concept of affective spectrum disorder: Relationship to fibromyalgia and other syndromes of chronic fatigue and chronic muscle pain. *Baillière's Clinical Rheumatology, 8,* 839–856.

Judd, L. L., Kessler, R. C., Paulus, M. P., Zeller, P. V., Wittchen, H. U., & Kunovac, J. L. (1998). Comorbidity as a fundamental feature of generalized anxiety disorders: Results from the National Comorbidity Study (NCS). *Acta Psychiatrica Scandinavica, 393*(Suppl.), 6–11.

Katon, W., Von Korff, M., Lin, E., Lipscomb, P., Russo, J., Wagner, E., & Polk, E. (1990). Distressed high utilizers of medical care: DSM-III-R diagnoses and treatment needs. *General Hospital Psychiatry, 12,* 355–362.

Kavoussi, R. J., Crockatt, J. G., Werth, J. L., Liu-Dumaw, M., & Pande, A. C. (2000, December). *Pregabalin reduces depressive symptomatology in patients with generalized anxiety disorder.* Paper presented at the annual meeting of the American College of Neuropsychopharmacology, San Juan, PR.

Kendler, K. S., Neale, M. C., Kessler, R. C., Heath, A. C., & Eaves, L. J. (1992). Generalized anxiety disorder in women: A population-based twin study. *Archives of General Psychiatry, 49,* 267–272.

Kessler, R. C., DuPont, R. L., Berglund, P., & Wittchen, H.-U. (1999). Impairment in pure and comorbid generalized anxiety disorder and major depression at 12 months in two national surveys. *American Journal of Psychiatry, 156,* 1915–1923.

Kessler, R. C., & Price, R. H. (1993). Primary prevention of secondary disorders: A proposal and agenda. *American Journal of Community Psychology, 21,* 607–633.

Kessler, R. C., Soukup, J., Davis, R. B., Foster, D. F., Wilkey, S. A., Van Rompay, M. M., & Eisenberg, D. M. (2001). The use of complementary and alternative therapies to treat anxiety and depression in the United States. *American Journal of Psychiatry, 158,* 289–294.

Kessler, R. C., & Wittchen, H.-U. (2002). Patterns and correlates of generalized anxiety disorder in community samples. *Journal of Clinical Psychiatry, 63*(Suppl. 8), 4–10.

Kroenke, K., Spitzer, R. L., Williams, J. B. W., Linzer, M., Hahn, S. R., de Gruy, F. V., III, & Brody, D. (1994). Physical symptoms in primary care: Predictors of psychiatric disorders and functional impairment. *Archives of Family Medicine, 3,* 774–779.

Laakmann, G., Schule, C., Lorkowski, G., Baghai, T., Kuhn, K., & Ehrentraut, S. (1998). Buspirone and lorazepam in the treatment of generalized anxiety disorder in outpatients. *Psychopharmacology, 136,* 357–366.

Lader, M., & Scotto, J. C. (1998). A multicentre double-blind comparison of hydroxy-zine, buspirone and placebo in patients with generalized anxiety disorder. *Psycho-pharmacology, 139,* 402–406.

Londborg, P. D., Smith, W. T., Glaudin, V., & Painter, R. (2000). Short-term cotherapy with clonazepam and fluoxetine: Anxiety, sleep disturbance and core symptoms of depression. *Journal of Affective Disorders, 61,* 73–79

Lydiard, R. B. (1991). Coexisting depression and anxiety: Special diagnostic and treat-ment issues. *Journal of Clinical Psychiatry, 52*(Suppl.), 48–54.

Lydiard, R. B. (2000). An overview of generalized anxiety disorder: Disease state-appropriate therapy. *Clinical Therapeutics, 22*(Suppl. A), A3–A19.

Lydiard, R. B., Brawman-Mintzer, O., & Ballenger, J. C. (1996). Recent developments in the psychopharmacology of anxiety disorders. *Journal of Consulting and Clinical Psychology, 64,* 660–668.

Lydiard, R. B., Zimbroff, D., Tobias, T., & Zornberg, G. L. (2003, May). *Efficacy of pregabalin in treating psychic and somatic symptoms in generalized anxiety disorder.* Pa-per presented at the annual meeting of the American Psychiatric Association, San Francisco.

Mahe, V., & Balogh, A. (2000). Long-term pharmacological treatment of generalized anxiety disorder. *International Clinical Psychopharmacology, 15,* 99–105.

Moller, H. J., Volz, H. P., Reimann, I. W., & Stoll, K. D. (2001). Opipramol for the treat-ment of generalized anxiety disorder: A placebo-controlled trial including an alprazolam-treated group. *Journal of Clinical Psychopharmacology, 21,* 59–65.

Nagy, L. M., Krystal, J. H., Charney, D. S., Merikangas, K. R., & Woods, S. W. (1993). Long-term outcome of panic disorder after short-term imipramine and behavior-al group treatment: 2.9-year naturalistic follow-up study. *Journal of Clinical Psycho-pharmacology, 13,* 16–24.

Olajide, D., & Lader, M. (1987). A comparison of buspirone, diazepam, and placebo in patients with chronic anxiety states. *Journal of Clinical Psychopharmacology, 7,* 148–152.

Otto, M. W., Pollack, M. H., Sachs, G. S., Reiter, S. R., Meltzer-Brody, S., & Rosenbaum, J. F. (1993). Discontinuation of benzodiazepine treatment: Efficacy of cognitive-behavioral therapy for patients with panic disorder. *American Journal of Psychiatry, 150,* 1485–1490.

Pande, A. C., Davidson, J. R., Jefferson, J. W., Janney, C. A., Katzelnick, D. J., Weisler, R. H., Greist, J. H., & Sutherland, S. M. (1999). Treatment of social phobia with gabapentin: A placebo-controlled study. *Journal of Clinical Psychopharmacology, 19,* 341–348.

Pande, A. C., Feltner, D., Jefferson, J., Davidson, J. R. T., & Lydiard, R. B. (1999). Pregabalin, a novel anxiolytic, in the treatment of generalized social anxiety disor-der: A placebo-controlled, multicenter study. *Journal of Clinical Psychopharmacol-ogy, 19,* 341–348.

Pande, A. C., Pollack, M. H., Crockatt, J., Greiner, M., Chouinard, G., Lydiard, R. B., Taylor, C. B., Dager, S. R., & Shiovitz, T. (2000). Placebo-controlled study of gabapentin treatment of panic disorder. *Journal of Clinical Psychopharmacology, 20,* 467–471.

Pecknold, J. C., Matas, M., Howarth, B. G., Ross, C., Swinson, R., Vezeau, C., & Ungar, W. (1989). Evaluation of buspirone as an antianxiety agent: Buspirone and diaze-pam versus placebo. *Canadian Journal of Psychiatry, 34,* 766–771.

Pohl, R. B., Zimbroff, D., Hartford, J. T., Fieve, R., Feltner, D., Pande, A. C., & Kavoussi, R. (2002, June). *Pregabalin: Efficacy in generalized anxiety disorder using a*

BID regimen. Paper presented at the annual meeting of the American Psychiatric Association, Philadelphia.

Pollack, M. H. (2001). Optimizing pharmacotherapy of generalized anxiety disorder to achieve remission. *Journal of Clinical Psychiatry, 62*(Suppl. 19), 20–25.

Pollack, M. H. (2002, June). *Generalized anxiety disorder: Long-term treatment to improve outcome.* Paper presented at the annual meeting of the American Psychiatric Association, Philadelphia.

Pollack, M. H., Worthington, J. J., Manfro, G. G., Otto, M. W., & Zucker, B. G. (1997). Abecarnil for the treatment of generalized anxiety disorder: A placebo-controlled comparison of two dosage ranges of abecarnil and buspirone. *Journal of Clinical Psychiatry, 58*(Suppl. 11), 19–23.

Pollack, M. H., Zaninelli, R., Goddard, A., McCafferty, J. P., Bellew, K. M., Burnham, D. B., & Iyengar, M. K. (2001). Paroxetine in the treatment of generalized anxiety disorder: Results of a placebo-controlled, flexible-dosage trial. *Journal of Clinical Psychiatry, 62,* 350–357.

Rickels, K., Amsterdam, J. D., Clary, C., Puzzuoli, G., & Schweizer, E. (1991). Buspirone in major depression: A controlled study. *Journal of Clinical Psychiatry, 52,* 34–38.

Rickels, K., Case, W. G., & Diamond, L. (1980). Relapse after short-term drug therapy in neurotic outpatients. *International Pharmacopsychiatry, 15,* 186–192.

Rickels, K., DeMartinis, N., Garcia-Espana, F., Greenblatt, D. J., Mandos, L. A., & Rynn, M. (2000). Imipramine and buspirone in treatment of patients with generalized anxiety disorder who are discontinuing long-term benzodiazepine therapy. *American Journal of Psychiatry, 157,* 1973–1979.

Rickels, K., Downing, R., Schweizer, E., & Hassman, H. (1993). Antidepressants for the treatment of generalized anxiety disorder: A placebo-controlled comparison of imipramine, trazodone, and diazepam. *Archives of General Psychiatry, 50,* 884–895.

Rickels, K., Pollack, M. H., Lydiard, R. B., Bielski, R. J., Feltner, D. E., Pande, A. C., & Kavoussi, R. J. (2002, June). *Efficacy and safety of pregabalin and alprazolam in generalized anxiety disorder.* Paper presented at the annual meeting of the American Psychiatric Association, Philadelphia.

Rickels, K., Pollack, M. H., Sheehan, D. V., & Haskins, J. T. (2000). Efficacy of extended-release venlafaxine in nondepressed outpatients with generalized anxiety disorder. *American Journal of Psychiatry, 157,* 968–974.

Rickels, K., Schweizer, E., Case, W. G., & Greenblatt, D. J. (1990). Long-term therapeutic use of benzodiazepines: I. Effects of abrupt discontinuation. *Archives of General Psychiatry, 47,* 899–907.

Rocca, P., Fonzo, V., Scotta, M., Zanalda, E., & Ravizza, L. (1997). Paroxetine efficacy in the treatment of generalized anxiety disorder. *Acta Psychiatrica Scandinavica, 95,* 444–450.

Roy-Byrne, P. P. (1996). Generalized anxiety and mixed anxiety–depression: Association with disability and health care utilization. *Journal of Clinical Psychiatry, 57*(Suppl. 7), 86–91.

Rynn, M. A., Siqueland, L., & Rickels, K. (2001). Placebo-controlled trial of sertraline in the treatment of children with generalized anxiety disorder. *American Journal of Psychiatry, 158,* 2008–2014.

Salzman, C., Goldenberg, I., Bruce, S. E., & Keller, M. B. (2001). Pharmacologic treatment of anxiety disorders in 1989 versus 1996: Results from the Harvard/Brown Anxiety Disorders Research Program. *Journal of Clinical Psychiatry, 62,* 149–152.

Schweizer, E. (1995). Generalized anxiety disorder: Longitudinal course and pharmacologic treatment. *Psychiatric Clinics of North America, 18,* 843–857.

Schweizer, E., & Rickels, K. (1988). Buspirone in the treatment of panic disorder: A controlled pilot comparison with clorazepate. *Journal of Clinical Psychopharmacology, 8,* 303.

Schweizer, E., Rickels, K., Hassman, H., & Garcia-Espana, F. (1998). Buspirone and imipramine for the treatment of major depression in the elderly. *Journal of Clinical Psychiatry, 59,* 175–183.

Sheehan, D. V. (1999). Venlafaxine extended release (XR) in the treatment of generalized anxiety disorder. *Journal of Clinical Psychiatry, 60*(Suppl. 22), 23–28.

Sheehan, D. V., Harnett-Sheehan, K., & Raj, B. A. (1996). The measurement of disability. *International Clinical Psychopharmacology, 11*(Suppl. 3), 89–95.

Sheehan, D. V., Raj, A. B., Sheehan, K. H., & Soto, S. (1988). The relative efficacy of buspirone, imipramine and placebo in panic disorder: A preliminary report. *Pharmacology, Biochemistry, and Behavior, 29,* 815–817.

Sheehan, D. V., Raj, A. B., Sheehan, K. H., & Soto, S. (1990). Is buspirone effective for panic disorder? *Journal of Clinical Psychopharmacology, 10,* 3–11.

Silverstone, P. H., & Salinas, E. (2001). Efficacy of venlafaxine extended release in patients with major depressive disorder and comorbid generalized anxiety disorder. *Journal of Clinical Psychiatry, 62,* 523–529.

Smith, W. T., Londborg, P. D., Glaudin, V., & Painter, J. R. (2002). Is extended clonazepam cotherapy of fluoxetine effective for outpatients with major depression? *Journal of Affective Disorders, 70,* 251–259.

Stocchi, F., Nordera, G., Jokinen, R. H., Lepola, U. M., Hewett, K., Brysoin, H., Iyengar, M. K., & the Paroxetine Generalized Anxiety Workgroup. (2003). Efficacy and tolerability of paroxetine for the long-term treatment of generalized anxiety disorder. *Journal of Clinical Psychiatry, 64,* 250–258.

Stout, R. L., Dolan, R., Dyck, I., Eisen, J., & Keller, M. B. (2001). Course of social functioning after remission from panic disorder. *Comprehensive Psychiatry, 42,* 441–447.

Swinson, R. P., Cox, B. J., & Fergus, K. D. (1993). Diagnostic criteria in generalized anxiety disorder treatment studies. *Journal of Clinical Psychopharmacology, 13,* 455.

Uhlenhuth, E. H., Balter, M. B., Ban, T. A., & Yang, K. (1999). International study of expert judgment on therapeutic use of benzodiazepines and other psychotherapeutic medications: IV. Therapeutic dose dependence and abuse liability of benzodiazepines in the long-term treatment of anxiety disorders. *Journal of Clinical Psychopharmacology, 19*(Suppl. 2), 23S–29S.

Uhlenhuth, E. H., DeWit, H., Balter, M. B., Johanson, C. E., & Mellinger, G. D. (1988). Risks and benefits of long-term benzodiazepine use. *Journal of Clinical Psychopharmacology, 8,* 161–167.

van Vliet, I. M., den Boer, J. A., Westenberg, H. G., & Pian, K. L. (1997). Clinical effects of buspirone in social phobia: A double-blind placebo- controlled study. *Journal of Clinical Psychiatry, 58,* 164–168.

Volz, H. P., & Kieser, M. (1997). Kava-kava extract WS 1490 versus placebo in anxiety disorders: A randomized placebo-controlled 25–week outpatient trial. *Pharmacopsychiatry, 30,* 1–5.

Watkins, L. L., Connor, K. M., & Davidson, J. R. (2001). Effect of kava extract on vagal cardiac control in generalized anxiety disorder: Preliminary findings. *Journal of Psychopharmacology, 15,* 283–286.

Wetzel, M. S., Eisenberg, D. M., & Kaptchuk, T. J. (1998). Courses involving complementary and alternative medicine at US medical schools. *Journal of the American Medical Association, 280,* 784–787.

Whitehead, W. E., Palsson, O., & Jones, K. R. (2002). Systematic review of the comorbidity of irritable bowel syndrome with other disorders: What are the causes and implications? *Gastroenterology, 122,* 1140–1156.

Wilcox, C. S., Ryan, P. J., Morrissey, J. L., Cohn, J. B., DeFrancisco, D. F., Linden, R. D., & Heiser, J. F. (1994). A fixed-dose study of adinazolam-SR tablets in generalized anxiety disorder. *Progress in Neuropsychopharmacology and Biological Psychiatry, 18,* 979–993.

Wittchen, H.-U., Kessler, R. C., Beesdo, K., Krause, P., Hofler, M., & Hoyer, J. (2002). Generalized anxiety and depression in primary care: Prevalence, recognition, and management. *Journal of Clinical Psychiatry, 63*(Suppl. 8), 24–34.

Yager, J., Siegfreid, S. L., & DiMatteo, T. L. (1999). Use of alternative remedies by psychiatric patients: Illustrative vignettes and a discussion of the issues. *American Journal of Psychiatry, 156,* 1432–1438.

Yonkers, K. A., Dyck, I. R., Warshaw, M., & Keller, M. B. (2000). Factors predicting the clinical course of generalized anxiety disorder. *British Journal of Psychiatry, 176,* 544–549.

Yonkers, K. A., Warshaw, M. G., Massion, A. O., & Keller, M. B. (1996). Phenomenology and course of generalized anxiety disorder. *British Journal of Psychiatry, 168,* 308–313.

PART IV
Special Populations

CHAPTER 15

Children and Adolescents

ANNE MARIE ALBANO
SABINE HACK

One of the most vexing issues in psychopathology research is the quest to establish the reliability and validity of diagnostic categories when these are applied to children and adolescents, and generalized anxiety disorder (GAD) has been the "leader of the pack" when it comes to stumping clinical scientists. In this chapter, we present a brief overview of the evolution of the diagnosis of GAD in youth, and describe the essential features and associated conditions of the diagnosis as they are currently understood. We review disorder-specific information on prevalence, age, gender, and sociodemographic factors, as well as the long-term course and sequelae of GAD. The current status of treatment research and clinical applications of cognitive-behavioral therapy and pharmacotherapy are then reviewed. We conclude with a summary and discussion of future directions.

HISTORY AND DESCRIPTION OF THE DISORDER IN YOUTH

The study of anxiety in children has a long history dating back to the late 19th century (see Albano, Chorpita, & Barlow, 2003). It was not until the publication of the *Diagnostic and Statistical Manual of Mental Disorders*, second edition (DSM-II; American Psychiatric Association [APA], 1968), however, that "overanxious reaction of childhood" was introduced as a distinct diagnostic category under the umbrella of "phobic neuroses." As noted in many texts outlining the history of psychiatric classification, the early DSM systems presented diagnostic categories that were heavily tied to psychoanalytic theory. Thus childhood overanxious reaction was assumed to arise from an unconscious process or conflict (Barlow, 2002). Although the combination of theory and diagnosis muddied the waters for clinicians who did not ascribe to analytic theory, the inclusion of overanxious reaction in the DSM-II ushered in a new appreciation for, and attention to, the study of clinical manifestations of anxiety in children and adolescents.

DSM-III (APA, 1980), with its attempt at an atheoretical and empirically derived diagnostic system, introduced a separate category of childhood anxiety disorders, including "overanxious disorder of childhood or adolescence" (OAD). OAD was meant to capture in children and adolescents the early form of the adult anxiety category of GAD, although youth could also be diagnosed with GAD if they fit the diagnostic criteria. The essential features of OAD involved worry more days than not for at least 6 months, about a number of issues, events, or activities. Although OAD proved to be a diagnosis of high prevalence and high comorbidity in clinical and epidemiological samples, it proved to be highly unreliable and unstable (Silverman & Eisen, 1992; Silverman & Nelles, 1988). This was partially attributed to an overlap with symptoms of other diagnoses (e.g., social phobia), resulting in difficulty making a differential diagnosis between GAD and other disorders (Kendall, Krain, & Treadwell, 1999). Consequently, OAD was dropped from the psychiatric nomenclature in DSM-IV (APA, 1994) and subsumed under GAD.

Diagnostic Criteria

As noted throughout this volume, the essential feature of GAD in DSM-IV is excessive and uncontrollable anxiety and worry about a number of events and activities, occurring more days than not for at least 6 months. Research on the DSM-IV GAD criteria as applied to children found that whereas nonreferred youth report as many worries as children with GAD, the groups differ in their self-reported perception of the intensity of the worry (Muris, Meesters, Merckelbach, Sermon, & Zwakhalen, 1998; Perrin & Last, 1997; Weems, Silverman, & La Greca, 2000). Hence feelings of being unable to control or stop the worry process are probably related to the degree of distress and excessive anxiety generated by the worry, as opposed to the number of worries that a child may experience. These studies thus support the application of the "uncontrollable worry" criterion to youth.

As with other anxiety disorders, the symptoms of GAD must cause significant impairment in one or more areas of functioning in order to meet diagnostic criteria. One change from OAD to GAD is the requirement of the presence of at least one physiological symptom. Although the presence of any physiological symptom was included as a criterion for OAD, a child could meet the minimum number of criteria (four of seven) to receive the diagnosis without endorsing a physiological complaint. Notably, complaints such as headaches and stomachaches are missing from this list, despite being among the most commonly reported physical complaints of children with OAD (Eisen & Engler, 1995). The DSM-IV physiological symptom list for GAD was derived from studies of adults, and further evaluation of these criteria in youth is warranted (Kendall et al., 1999). In an evaluation of the changed the diagnostic criteria in children, Tracey, Chorpita, Douban, and Barlow (1997) found evidence supporting the convergent and divergent validity of the GAD diagnosis in children aged 7–17. However, the children had difficulty deciding whether their worry was uncontrollable, and hence parental report was especially important in evaluating this symptom. Moreover, in contrast to the report of adults with GAD, both children and parents infrequently endorsed muscle tension as a symptom of the diagnosis in youth. Kendall and Warman (1996) found nonsignificant differences between DSM-III-R (APA, 1987) and DSM-IV anxiety diagnoses in children, suggesting that past research on OAD can be applied to understanding GAD in youth. However, future studies must more fully examine the validity of these criteria as applied to the broad age range of children and adolescents.

Clinical Features

The thoughts of children with GAD are characterized by recurrent worries typically expressed in the form of a "what if" question. These worries revolve around classic cognitive distortions, such as all-or-nothing thinking, catastrophizing, disqualifying the positive, and probability overestimation. In clinical samples of anxious children, including those with GAD, negative self-talk predominates (e.g., Howard & Kendall, 1996; Ronan & Kendall, 1997), and parents of children with GAD often refer to them as "worry warts." Youth with GAD worry excessively about a range of general issues, including the future, family issues (e.g., finances, the parental relationship), and competence in areas such as school achievement and performance-based activities (e.g., sports, music). As opposed to the child with social phobia, who is concerned with looking foolish and fears the negative evaluation of others, the child with GAD sets an excessively high standard of achievement that is usually unrealistic or unnecessary. The straight-A student, for example, will worry about failing a class, despite all evidence to the contrary. Children with GAD will, however, worry about social competence and social relationships, making the distinction between GAD and social phobia difficult at times. Also common to children with GAD are worries about safety ("Will a robber get into our house?"), world events ("What if a war happens in the United States?"), and health ("What if Mom gets cancer?"). Studies of children with OAD found them to worry excessively about events having a low probability of occurrence, while simultaneously not recognizing the distorted probability overestimation (Silverman, La Greca, & Wasserstein, 1995).

Children with GAD have been described as pseudomature, appearing to be "little adults" because of their anxieties about keeping appointments, worry about little things, and concerns with following rules (Kendall et al., 1999). In addition, children with GAD are markedly self-conscious and require frequent reassurance from others (Eisen & Kearney, 1995; Silverman & Ginsburg, 1995), although parents often report that no amount of reassurance is ever enough (Kearney & Albano, 2000; Kendall et al., 1999). This need for constant reassurance can be particularly impairing in academic contexts, where the child with GAD may be found at the teacher's desk repeatedly throughout the school day, disrupting the class routine and potentially garnering a negative reaction from the teacher. Moreover, children and adolescents with GAD may struggle for hours on end with homework assignments, due to perfectionism, self-doubt, self-imposed high standards, and fear of failure. One striking example was an eighth-grade student with GAD seen in our clinic who had straight A's, worked continually each day from 4:00 P.M. until after midnight on homework, and was constantly fearful of failing a test. Her school counselor referred her for treatment after she collapsed in tears because her teachers would not write letters of recommendation for her *college* applications.

Physical complaints are common in youth with GAD (Eisen & Engler, 1995). In contrast to the symptoms of a panic attack or the sudden onset of fear associated with confronting a feared stimulus for children with specific phobias, youth with GAD often report diffuse physical complaints such as headaches, stomachaches, enuresis, and restlessness (Eisen & Engler, 1995; Kendall et al., 1991). Moreover, these symptoms appear despite the absence of documentable physical cause (Kendall et al., 1999), and physicians often refer children with GAD to mental health practitioners (Bell-Dolan & Brazeal, 1993).

Associated Features and Comorbidity

Children with GAD may have difficulty with attention and concentration, due to the intrusion of uncontrollable worry and/or physical symptoms; thus their school performance can be disrupted. Perfectionism and other worries about academic competence can likewise interfere with effective study habits, completion of homework, participation in group learning activities, and test-taking behavior. Youth with GAD may also present with disruption in sleep patterns, nervous habits such as nail biting or skin picking, affective lability, and increased irritability (Albano et al., 2003; Kendall et al., 1999). These youth may make frequent visits to the school nurse, express distress and a desire to miss school, and often develop school refusal behavior (Kearney, 2001).

A pattern of escalating avoidance may occur for social and athletic activities, as worry concerning competence in these areas may also lead to withdrawal from participation in these events. Children with GAD report lower levels of self-confidence in social and performance situations, along with correspondingly higher levels of social anxiety and expectations for social failure (Chansky & Kendall, 1997; Strauss, Lahey, Frick, Frame, & Hynd, 1988). A vicious cycle can then result whereby withdrawal from peer activities can result in a child being less well known and liked by peers (Strauss, Lahey, et al., 1988); this in turn can result in the exclusion of the child with GAD from future events, thus compounding the child's sense of being ostracized by peers.

Early studies of youth with OAD found younger children (aged 5–11) to present with comorbid separation anxiety disorder (SAD) and attention-deficit/hyperactivity disorder (ADHD), whereas older children (aged 12–19) presented more often with comorbid phobic disorders and major depressive disorder (Strauss, Last, Hersen, & Kazdin, 1988; Strauss, Lease, Last, & Francis, 1988). One study found adolescents with GAD, especially girls, to report disturbing dreams (Nielsen et al., 2000). Depression is a common associated feature of GAD and one that complicates the clinical picture by intensifying a child's distress and impairment. In a study of 108 children and adolescents with GAD, Masi, Favilla, Mucci, and Millipiedi (2000) found those with comorbid depression to report significantly more anxiety symptoms and to be more severely impaired across a range of functional domains than youth without depression

EPIDEMIOLOGY

Two cross-sectional epidemiological studies (Kashani & Orvaschel, 1988; Kashani, Orvaschel, Rosenberg, & Reid, 1989) sampled children aged 8, 12, or 17 years for DSM-III anxiety disorders. Results indicated that 21% of children reported enough symptoms for a diagnosis of an anxiety disorder. In examining individual diagnostic categories, prevalence rates reported for these samples were 12.9% and 12.4% for SAD and OAD, respectively, with lower rates for the phobic disorders (3.3% for simple phobia, 1.1% for social phobia). An ongoing longitudinal study conducted in New Zealand (Anderson, Williams, McGee, & Silva, 1987; McGee et al., 1990) sampled 792 children at age 11 years and again at age 15 years. At age 11, prevalence rates for DSM-III anxiety disorders were 3.5% for SAD, 2.9% for OAD, 2.4% for simple phobia, and 1.0% for social phobia; at age 15 years (McGee et al., 1990), the overall prevalence rates were 5.9% for OAD/GAD, 2.0% for SAD, 3.6% for simple phobia, and 1.1% for social phobia. Other investigators report rates of OAD/GAD in children and adolescents to range from 2.4% to 10.8% (Bell-Dolan & Brazeal, 1993; Bowen, Offord, & Boyle, 1990; Costello, Stouthamer-Loeber, & DeRosier, 1993), with prevalence increasing with age. In addition to these population studies, clinic-referred samples of children and adolescents have found prevalence rates ranging from 2.8% to 15% (Cantwell & Baker, 1989; Last, Strauss, & Francis, 1987; Silverman & Nelles, 1988). Again, GAD is more prevalent in older referred youth (Albano, Chorpita, DiBartolo, & Barlow, 1995).

DEVELOPMENTAL COURSE AND LONG-TERM OUTCOMES

There is still limited information on the developmental course of GAD and its associated long-term outcomes. An exploratory factor-analytic study of parental report of anxiety symptoms in preschool children (age range 2½ to 6½ years) in Australia suggested that separation anxiety symptoms and generalized anxiety symptoms were not readily differentiated into distinct factors (Spence, Rapee, McDonald, & Ingram, 2001). Using a confirmatory factor-analytic strategy, the authors generated a five-factor solution, reflecting the DSM-IV anxiety disorders (including GAD). However, they found superior fit for a higher-order model, explained by a single anxiety factor. There were no differences found between boys and girls for the total symptom ratings or factor scores, contrary to the frequent finding that girls present with higher levels of anxiety than boys (see Albano et al., 2003). Moreover, Spence (1997) found minimal support for a distinct generalized anxiety factor in a study of primary school children. The results of these studies suggest that anxiety in early childhood may best reflect a nonspecific factor related to high trait anxiety, with differentiation into specific diagnostic categories occurring later in development (Spence et al., 2001).

In two studies by Ialongo and colleagues (Ialongo, Edelsohn, Werthamer-Larsson, Crockett, & Kellam, 1994, 1995), 2.5% of a sample of 5-year-old children manifested severe anxiety symptoms that remained relatively stable over a 4-month period. In addition, anxiety symptoms at 5 years of age predicted adaptive functioning at a 4-year follow-up. After controlling for level of adaptive functioning, children in the high-anxiety group (the top third of anxious symptoms in first grade) were 10 times more likely to be in the bottom third for achievement in fifth grade. Earlier studies of OAD/GAD suggested a variable and unstable course. Although some studies suggested a minority of youth followed over time retained the diagnosis, most children received an alternative diagnosis of an anxiety or mood disorder at follow-up, suggesting that OAD/GAD may be a precursor to other disorders of negative affect (Cantwell & Baker, 1989; Last, Hersen, Kazdin, Finkelstein, & Strauss, 1987; Last, Perrin, Hersen, & Kazdin, 1992). These studies must be interpreted with caution, however, due to issues of sample size and/or methodological limitations.

An association between anxiety and alcohol use has been demonstrated in recent studies. For example, Lewinsohn, Zinbarg, Seeley, Lewinsohn, & Sack (1997) found significant associations between the DSM-IV anxiety disorders (except panic disorder and specific phobia) and alcohol abuse/dependence in their longitudinal cohort of adolescents. The specific relationship of GAD to the initiation of alcohol use was examined in a prospective, longitudinal study of 936 children evaluated at age 9, 11, or 13, and again 4 years later (Kaplow, Curran, Angold, & Costello, 2001). When depressive symptomatology was controlled for, youth with early symptoms of GAD were found to be at an increased risk for the initiation of alcohol use, in contrast to youth with early symptoms of SAD, who were found to be at a decreased risk. There were no moderating effects due to gender. The authors suggest that youth with GAD may use alcohol at an earlier age to be accepted by peers, due to worry surrounding issues of social competence and peer acceptance (see also Clark, Parker, & Lynch, 1999). However, once the youth are involved in the peer group, alcohol use may then continue as a self-medication strategy to attenuate worries and physical symptoms (Kaplow et al., 2001). This study did not address the degree of (frequency, quantity) use or the impairment associated with the youth's alcohol use. The authors caution that additional research is indicated to examine the associations between the early onset of GAD and alcohol use.

An association of GAD with suicidal ideation has been demonstrated in several studies. A clinical sample of 1,979 outpatients (aged 5–19 years) presenting to a clinic for mood and anxiety disorders revealed that older children (age > 15 years) with suicidal ideation were more likely to be diagnosed with GAD than nonsuicidal patients were (Strauss et al., 2000). Interestingly, youth with suicide attempts had a lower prevalence of SAD than those with ideation. A separate study examined the relationship among anxiety disorders, comorbidity, and suicide attempts in a sample of 80 adolescent female outpatients (Pawlak, Pascual-Sanchez, Rae, Fischer, & Ladame, 1999). GAD was the most frequent specific anxiety disorder in this sample. Of youth with anxiety disorders who attempted suicide, the large majority (95%) had comorbid major depression. Similar findings were reported by Lewinsohn, Rohde, and Seeley (1995), demonstrating that youth with a lifetime history of anxiety disorder (including

GAD) comorbid with major depression were more likely to have made a suicide attempt than youth without this comorbidity. These studies suggest that clinicians treating youth with anxiety disorders should closely monitor their patients for suicidal ideation, especially when GAD and depression are present.

DIAGNOSIS AND ASSESSMENT OF GAD IN CHILDREN AND ADOLESCENTS

Prior to our review of treatments for GAD, we first outline certain differential diagnostic issues, followed by a discussion of current diagnostic and assessment methodologies for GAD in youth.

Differential Diagnosis

As noted above, youth with GAD present with a variety of comorbid conditions and associated impairments (Brady & Kendall, 1992). Younger children may report more diffuse symptoms and complaints (e.g., "I don't feel well," "I need you [Mommy or Daddy] to stay with me," "I don't want to go to school"), which may be easily confused with SAD. A careful diagnostic evaluation should probe for whether the child's fears are focused on separation situations, such as getting lost and not being able to find loved ones, or the possibility that something untoward will happen to result in a permanent separation from the family. In such cases, SAD is the more appropriate diagnosis. Youth with GAD may report fears of burglars, wars, accidents, or other tragedies that could result in a separation, but the focus is not specifically on separation per se.

In older children and adolescents, concerns about social standing, social competence, academic progress, and physical appearance may suggest the presence of social phobia rather than GAD. Indeed, the criteria for GAD specify worry that is excessive and uncontrollable about a number of areas, including social and performance situations. Although there are no hard-and-fast decision rules for differentiating social phobia from GAD, certain questions should be considered when one is making the diagnostic distinction. First, are the worries limited to social and/or evaluative situations? If they are, then the diagnosis should be social phobia. Second, are the worries focused on what other people may think or how the child believes others will evaluate him or her, or is the child fearful of failing some self-imposed, unrealistic standard? If the worries are focused mostly on what others think, then a diagnosis of social phobia may be warranted. However, if the worries are fears of not meeting some inappropriate standard or goal, GAD is the appropriate diagnosis. Third, are there social or competence worries, but also evidence for other worries that are not specific to social-evaluative situations? If so, one should consider GAD and the possible additional diagnosis of social phobia.

In addition to symptoms in common with social phobia, youth with GAD may present with any number of physiological and vegetative symptoms that are shared by ADHD and depression. A child who has difficulty sustaining attention, staying still, relaxing and settling down, and completing assigned tasks may appear to have ADHD. However, ADHD symptoms must begin before age 7, be stable over time, and occur in more than one context (e.g., home and school). These symptoms may appear in the child with GAD in response to specific stressors, such as exams, starting school or other changes in routine, or psychosocial stressors. Thus their onset may be more acute and their course more variable in youth with GAD. Depression and GAD also share symptoms, such as changes in sleep habits, lack of energy, and increased irritability. Depression is more likely to occur in older children and adolescents; to be accompanied by sad or irritable mood, as opposed to anxious apprehension and worry; and to result in more withdrawal, as opposed to the excessive help-seeking behavior and need for reassurance found in GAD. Obviously, when sufficient symptom clusters and intensity are found, both diagnoses should be assigned.

Assessment Overview

From the cognitive-behavioral perspective, assessment is the cornerstone of effective treatment (Barrios & O'Dell, 1998). Assessment is necessary to guide the development of a comprehensive treatment plan, to pinpoint symptoms and behaviors for selected interventions, and to outline goals for the course of treatment. Assessment continues throughout treatment in many forms, which are discussed below, and provides the clinician with data by which to evaluate treatment response and outcome. Assessment must involve multiple informants and multiple methods; must be conducted with the aim of understanding the individual child in an idiographic manner; and must take demographic variables, developmental level, family factors, cultural contexts, environmental variables, and appropriate normative comparisons into account (Albano et al., 2003; Barrios & Hartmann, 1997; Kendall et al., 1999). A multimethod, multi-informant approach to assessment is imperative in order to gain a clear understanding of the child's clinical picture (e.g., Barrios & Hartmann, 1997; March & Albano, 2002). In general, a comprehensive evaluation involves a diagnostic interview, self-report and parent report measures, teacher report, and (when feasible) behavioral observation methods (see Mash & Terdal, 1997). Table 15.1 presents an overview of the most common assessment methods utilized in the diagnosis and assessment of GAD in youth.

TABLE 15.1. Selected Diagnostic and Assessment Instruments for GAD in Youth

Measure	Targets	Informant(s)	Comments
Diagnostic interview			
Anxiety Disorders Interview Schedule for DSM-IV, Child Version (ADIS-IV-C; Silverman & Albano, 1996)	DSM-IV disorders: anxiety disorders, mood disorders, ADHD, oppositional defiant disorder, conduct disorder; screening questions for learning and developmental disorders, substance abuse, eating disorders, psychotic symptoms, and somatoform disorders. Also assesses school refusal behavior, social relationships, and relevant demographic and historical information.	Separate interviews for child and parent, with decision rules and guidelines for combining data into a composite diagnosis.	Provides a clinician's severity rating on a 0–8 scale (indicating increasing distress and impairment) for each identified diagnosis. Allows clinician to identify principal (most disabling) and additional disorders to track course of disorder and treatment response.
Self-report measures			
Revised Children's Manifest Anxiety Scale (RCMAS; Reynolds & Richmond, 1979)	General levels of anxiety, with three subscales (fear, worry/ concentration, physiological arousal) and a validity scale (lie scale).	Child only	Considered a measure of negative affect more broadly, as opposed to specific to anxiety, due to poor discriminative validity; little utility for clinical practice.
State–Trait Anxiety Inventory for Children (STAIC; Spielberger, 1973)	State and trait levels of general anxiety.	Child only	Useful for general research purposes, but does not have high utility in clinical settings.
Multidimensional Anxiety Scale for Children (MASC; March et al., 1997)	Four broad factors: physiological symptoms (tense/restless and somatic/ autonomic), harm avoidance (perfectionism and anxious coping behaviors), social anxiety (humiliation fears and performance anxiety), and separation anxiety.	Child only	Good psychometric properties and mapping to DSM-IV diagnoses in research trials. Potential for high utility as a clinical screening tool.
Screen for Child Anxiety Related Emotional Disorders (SCARED; Birmaher et al., 1997)	Assesses DSM-IV symptoms of panic disorder, generalized anxiety disorder, separation anxiety disorder, social phobia, and school refusal behavior.	Child and parent report	Good psychometric properties, with potential for high utility in clinical settings.
Penn State Worry Questionnaire for Children (PSWQ-C; Chorpita et al., 1997)	Severity of child's worry.	Child only	Still under development, but potential for high utility as a screening measure of children's worry.

Diagnostic Interview

The use of a diagnostic interview schedule, whether structured or semistructured, provides a format for establishing the presence or absence of symptoms, level of impairment, and time course for the disorder, as well as for excluding alternative diagnoses. Diagnostic interviews may be particularly important in the case of GAD, as earlier studies examining the psychometric properties of instruments assessing OAD demonstrated poor interrater reliability, test–retest reliability, and parent–child concordance (see, e.g., Silverman & Eisen, 1992; Silverman & Nelles, 1988). These studies suggested that the category of OAD was poorly defined, as opposed to the interview method being flawed, as other anxiety disorder categories demonstrated good to excellent psychometric properties. However, recent studies utilizing DSM-IV criteria within the updated Anxiety Disorders Interview Schedule for DSM-IV, Child Version (ADIS-IV-C; Silverman & Albano, 1996) indicate good psychometric properties for the GAD category (Silverman, Saavadra, & Pina, 2001). Although the ADIS-IV-C and its predecessor, the ADIS-C, have been the most widely used clinical interviews for assessing anxiety disorders in both clinical and research settings (Dadds, Heard, & Rapee, 1992; Kendall et al., 1997; Stallings & March, 1995), various interview schedules are available for deriving diagnoses in youth (see Barrios & Hartmann, 1997, for a review).

Questionnaire Methods

Interviews are clinician-administered and driven by the evaluation of diagnostic criteria, whereas self-report measures provide a relatively cost- and time-efficient means for gathering dimensional information related to fear, worry, anxiety, and related constructs in youth. Although self-report measures cannot provide the data necessary to establish a clinical diagnosis, they have high utility in establishing baseline ratings and tracking changes across time. Among the oldest and most widely disseminated self-report measures of anxiety in youth are the Revised Children's Manifest Anxiety Scale (RCMAS; Reynolds & Richmond, 1979) and the State–Trait Anxiety Inventory for Children (STAIC; Spielberger, 1973). Primarily utilized in research settings, both the RCMAS and the STAIC assess the broad construct of negative affectivity in youth. The RCMAS contains subscales that cover fear, physiological arousal, and worry/oversensitivity, whereas the STAIC consists of forms for state anxiety and trait (generalized) anxiety. The major criticisms of these two instruments are that they correlate highly with measures of depression and negative affectivity (e.g., anger) and perform poorly with regards to specificity and sensitivity for identifying anxiety disordered youth (March & Albano, 2002; Perrin & Last, 1992).

More recently, two self-report scales for assessing anxiety in youth were introduced to address the shortcomings of existing measures. The Multidimensional Anxiety Scale for Children (MASC; March, Parker, Sullivan, Stallings, & Conners, 1997) and the Screen for Child Anxiety and Related Emotional Disorders (SCARED; Birmaher et al., 1997, 1999) were designed to assess DSM-IV symptoms of anxiety in youth. The MASC is a 39-item, 4-point Likert self-report rating scale for use in children and adolescents aged 8 through 17, and includes four factors: physical symptoms (tense/restless and somatic/autonomic subfactors), social anxiety (humiliation/rejection and public performance subfactors), harm avoidance (anxious coping and perfectionism subfactors) and separation/panic anxiety. Three-week test–retest reliability for the MASC is .79 in clinical samples (March et al., 1997) and .88 in school-based samples (March & Sullivan, 1999). The MASC is widely used in clinical and epidemiological studies of anxious youth (e.g., Research Units in Pediatric Psychopharmacology [RUPP] Anxiety Work Group, 2001). Moreover, the MASC was found to identify nonreferred youth with anxiety disorders (primarily GAD and social phobia) and to discriminate youth with anxiety disorders from those with depression or no disorder (Dierker et al., 2001).

The SCARED (Birmaher et al., 1997, 1999) is a 41-item scale for youth aged 7–17, assessing DSM-IV symptoms of panic disorder, SAD, social phobia, and GAD, as well as symptoms of school refusal behavior. The SCARED has corresponding child and parent self-report forms, both of which have shown robust psychometric properties in large clinical samples (Birmaher et al., 1997, 1999) and in a community sample (Muris, Merckelbach, et al., 1998). Both the MASC and SCARED are appropriate for assessing symptoms of DSM-IV GAD in youth and for tracking changes in this symptom cluster over time. In contrast to these scales, the Penn State Worry Questionnaire for Children (PSWQ-C; Chorpita, Tracey, Brown, Collica, & Barlow, 1997) is a new scale, still under development, designed specifically to assess the severity of worry—the hallmark symptom of GAD.

Various other self-report scales assess constructs related to generalized anxiety in youth, including specific fears (Fear Survey Schedule for Children—Revised; Ollendick, 1983), depression (Children's Depression Inventory; Kovacs, 1981), and problems related to school attendance (School Refusal Assessment Scale; Kearney & Silverman, 1993).

Various cognitive-developmental factors, such as age, intellectual level, and language abilities, may have an impact on children's or adolescents' reporting of their private internal states. Because of these issues and the private and subjective nature of anxiety, parent and teacher information are important and useful in providing a complete understanding of a young person's functioning. With the exception of the parent versions of the SCARED, there are no GAD-specific measures for assessing youth by parent or teacher report. However, well-developed parent and teacher rating scales assess anxiety within a broader range of childhood problems, such as the Child Behavior Checklist (Achenbach & Edelbrock, 1983) and the Teacher Report Form (Achenbach, 1991). These broad measures of psychopathology provide an overall assessment of youth's anxiety concerns in relation to other aspects of their behavior and potential comorbidities.

Behavioral Observation Methods

In addition to diagnostic interviews and standardized questionnaire methods, a variety of observational methods for gathering information concerning specific triggers to the child's worry, along with patterns of response, reinforcement, and consequences of the worry, can be utilized. These methods are not standardized, however, due in part to the complexity and variety of anxiety symptoms that occur across individuals and the innumerable triggers that can prompt an anxiety response. Thus, although no behavioral observation system exists for identifying and quantifying anxiety in youth, idiographic diary forms are useful for assessing the intensity of anxiety, antecedents to and consequences of anxious behaviors, and specific thoughts characteristic of the child and anxiety in question (e.g., Beidel, Neal, & Lederer, 1991). Further development of behavioral rating systems is necessary, as observational systems may uncover classes of stimuli (triggers/antecedents), child (symptom) response, and subsequent consequences of the anxiety, enabling clinical scientists to modify and refine existing treatment paradigms and perhaps to develop preventive intervention programs.

TREATMENTS FOR GAD IN CHILDREN AND ADOLESCENTS

In keeping with the *Zeitgeist* surrounding the treatment of emotional disorders in general, the trend in the treatment of anxiety disorders in youth is to move away from nonspecific, open-ended psychotherapies and toward the application of empirically based, flexibly applied treatment approaches (Albano & Kendall, 2002). The fields of clinical child psychology and child psychiatry stand poised at a critical and exciting juncture with regard to the development and dissemination of effective treatments for GAD and related anxiety disorders in youth. The last 20 years of the 20th century witnessed two parallel scientific endeavors: Cognitive-behavioral therapy (CBT) emerged as the most promising psychosocial approach for youth, and the selective serotonin reuptake inhibitors (SSRIs) gained wide acceptance from the medical community. In this section we review the literature on the CBT and pharmacological approaches to the treatment of GAD in youth.

Cognitive-Behavioral Therapy

Behavior therapy and CBT have a long tradition of effective treatments for fears, phobias, and anxieties in children and adolescents (see Barrios & O'Dell, 1998, for a review). With the introduction of the childhood anxiety section of the DSM-III in 1980, attention turned toward the testing of CBT for these disorders in children. CBT for childhood anxiety disorders involves several essential components: psychoeducation, somatic management skills training, cognitive restructuring, exposure methods, and relapse prevention methods (see Table 15.2). Psychoeducation introduces youth to an understanding of the range of human emotions and provides corrective information about anxiety and feared stimuli. Somatic management techniques address autonomic arousal and related physiological responses through such methods such as progressive muscle relaxation training and deep breathing. Cognitive restructuring skills, geared to the child's or adolescent's age and developmental level, are focused on identifying maladaptive thoughts and teaching realistic, coping-focused thinking. Exposure techniques involve graduated, systematic, and controlled exposure to the stimuli that evoke the worry response. These skills, when put together into a "coping template" or plan, provide the child or teen with tools for recognizing the onset of worry, examining and challenging unhelpful thoughts with realistic responses, and changing avoidance reactions to proactive coping. Finally, relapse prevention plans are geared toward consolidating and generalizing treatment gains over time. Of note, procedures used in the treatment of adults with GAD, such as worry exposure (Craske, Barlow, & O'Leary, 1992), experiential and interpersonal techniques (see Newman, Castonguay, Borkovec, & Molnar, Chapter 13, this volume), and mindfulness techniques (Roemer & Orsillo, 2002), have not as yet been subjected to systematic testing in children and adolescents with this disorder.

Although a CBT program focused solely on youth with GAD does not exist at this time, several investigators have evaluated the effectiveness of CBT for youth with GAD and related anxiety disorders. The first systematic study of CBT for youth with anxiety disorders utilized a manualized treatment program, the Coping Cat, developed by Kendall and colleagues for youth aged 8–13 years (Kendall, Kane, Howard, & Siqueland, 1990). Forty-seven children aged 8–13 years meeting criteria for SAD, OAD/GAD, and social phobia (including the DSM-III diagnosis of avoidant disorder of childhood) on the ADIS-C (Silverman & Nelles, 1988) were randomly assigned to either CBT or a wait-list condition

TABLE 15.2. Psychosocial Treatment Components for GAD in Children and Adolescents

Component	Aims of intervention	Key techniques
Psycho-education	Presenting information about helpful and unhelpful anxiety; presenting a three-component model of anxiety; normalizing anxiety response; identifying anxiety triggers and patterns of response.	Didactic instruction facilitated by use of drawings, workbooks, and/or relevant readings; use of self-monitoring through diary forms or notebooks; Socratic questioning to assess child's comprehension.
Somatic management	Targeting autonomic arousal and related physiological symptoms; providing means for calming self and relieving tension and anxious arousal.	Progressive muscle relaxation training, assigned daily; deep diaphragmatic breathing, for "portable" use throughout the day.
Cognitive restructuring	Teaching child to identify unhelpful (anxiety-provoking) thoughts, beliefs, and images, and to evaluate their validity and generate helpful, coping thoughts.	Use of diaries for monitoring the relationship between anxiety triggers and anxious thoughts; Socratic questioning, role play, and behavioral exposure to generate alternative, realistic, coping thoughts.
Exposure	Identifying situations or stimuli that trigger anxiety (worry hierarchy); using graduated, well-defined, and controlled exposure to anxiety-provoking situation(s), to provide experience with using anxiety management skills.	Collaboration with the child in defining the anxiety-provoking task to "enter" or confront while using somatic management and cognitive restructuring skills. Beginning with least anxiety-provoking situation, and gradually moving "up" to more challenging tasks. Use of imaginal exposure, role plays, and *in vivo* exposure as child is able to manage these situations.
Family involvement	Addressing parental anxiety, overcontrol, reinforcement of escape or avoidance, reassurance, and rescue behavior; breaking cycle of anxiety in family system.	Education directed specifically to parents; assigned readings; encouragement for accessing therapy when needed for parents' anxiety and/or marital issues; role-playing (with therapist) handling GAD-related situations; use of behavioral contracts; teaching parenting skills such as reinforcement techniques.
Relapse prevention	Promoting maintenance of gains and continued improvement after the conclusion of therapy; providing means for adapting learned skills in new situations as they arise; anticipating upcoming challenges or developmental changes to give child a "heads up" or sense of predictability and control over these events.	Throughout treatment, having child keep a log or diary of techniques and progress; developing a "storybook" wherein child writes about overcoming various anxiety issues through therapy; conducting role reversal exercise, where child "treats" therapist for GAD concerns; using a "coping plan" system for anticipating upcoming events (e.g., exams, change to new school) and writing out skills to use to manage these events; scheduling booster sessions at times of transition or high stress.

(Kendall, 1994). Children in the CBT condition demonstrated significant improvement from pre- to posttreatment on both self-report and parent report of emotional distress and coping abilities. In addition, 66% of treated children no longer met criteria for their primary anxiety diagnosis at posttreatment, based on diagnostic severity ratings from the ADIS-C. Results were robust and were maintained at a 1-year follow-up. Moreover, an additional follow-up of the treated youth (2- to 5-year follow-up, $m = 3.5$ yrs; $n = 36$) revealed maintenance of treatment gains on self-report, parent report, and diagnostic interview measures (Kendall & Southam-Gerow, 1996). In a second controlled test of the Coping Cat program, 94 children with the three diagnoses, aged 9–13 years, were randomly assigned to the CBT protocol or a wait-list condition. At posttreatment, over 50% of the treated group no longer met criteria for their entry diagnosis, with significant reductions in clinical severity for youth who continued to report anxiety symptoms. Gains were again maintained at a 1-year follow-up, with the majority of youth evidencing greater improvement over time (Kendall et al., 1997).

The Kendall treatment package has proven to be both transportable and adaptable to other countries/cultures, such as Australia (e.g., Barrett, Dadds, & Rapee, 1996) and Canada (Mendlowitz et al., 1999). CBT protocols for youth with GAD, SAD, and social phobia, including the Coping Cat, have also demonstrated efficacy when delivered in groups of anxious youth aged 7–14 (Barrett, 1998; Cobham, Dadds, & Spence, 1998; Flannery-Schroeder & Kendall, 2000; Silverman, Kurtines, Ginsburg, Weems, Lumpkin, et al., 1999).

Although the CBT studies described above are considered exemplary because of their methodological rigor (inclusion of rigorous and standardized assessment procedures, comparison of the active treatment with a control condition, clinically meaningful outcome criteria, and long-term follow-up; see Kazdin & Weisz, 1998), results must be interpreted carefully, as each study can be criticized for one or more methodological flaws. For example, outcomes are sometimes cited only for youth who completed a study, not for the intent-to-treat sample; the latter outcomes are typically more modest. For example, Flannery-Schroeder and Kendall (2000) reported response rates of 50% and 73% for those who completed group and individual CBT, respectively, yet in the intent-to-treat analyses, the response rates were 46% and 50%, respectively. The greatest challenge to studies examining the efficacy of CBT involves choosing a credible control condition, as both wait-list control and educational support conditions have been criticized as inadequate (Klein, 1997). For example, relatively equivocal effects for CBT as compared to control conditions were found in two randomized trials—not because of the lack of efficacy of the active treatment, but because of a high response rate to the educational support control (e.g., Last, Hansen, & Franco, 1998; Silverman, Kurtines,

Ginsburg, Weems, Rabian, et al., 1999). These results may indicate that educational support contains enough "active ingredients" of CBT to prompt positive effects.

Pharmacotherapy

There are limited data on the psychopharmacological treatment of anxiety disorders in youth, with the exception of obsessive–compulsive disorder (RUPP Anxiety Work Group, 2001). Overall, there are few well-controlled medication studies involving youth with OAD/GAD, separation anxiety disorder, or social phobia, and for those that are published, the results have been equivocal (March, 1999). There is mixed evidence of efficacy for the tricyclic antidepressants (Bernstein et al., 2000; Klein, Koplewicz, & Kanner, 1992); however, risks of cardiotoxicity limit their use in children (Wilens et al., 1996). Benzodiazepines are often prescribed for adult anxiety disorders, especially GAD and panic disorder. However, three small trials of these medications in children did not demonstrate efficacy (Bernstein, Garfinkel, & Borchardt, 1990; Graae, Milner, Rizzotto, & Klein, 1994; Simeon et al., 1992). In addition, the benzodiazepines are also infrequently prescribed for youth due to their potential side effects, such as cognitive blunting and memory problems, along with a high potential for addiction and discontinuation difficulties (Graae et al., 1994).

Studies of adults with anxiety disorders and children with OCD indicated good efficacy, tolerable side effects, and a good safety profile for the SSRIs (Rynn, Siqueland, & Rickels, 2001). Several studies enrolling youth with GAD, SAD, and/or social phobia yielded positive results for fluoxetine (Birmaher et al., 1994; Fairbanks et al., 1997) and fluvoxamine (RUPP Anxiety Work Group, 2001). Only one recent study focused solely on youth with GAD. Rynn and colleagues (2001) reported on 22 children aged 5–17 years who met criteria for GAD, based on the ADIS-IV-C interview and an adult Hamilton Anxiety Rating Scale (Hamilton, 1959) score ≥16. Following a 2- to 3-week prestudy lead-in period, youth were randomly assigned to either sertraline or a pill placebo for a 9-week double-blind treatment phase. By the fourth week of treatment, positive effects for the active medication were evident. Overall, by the end of treatment, 90% of the group receiving sertraline improved as compared to only 10% of the youth receiving placebo. Moreover, the authors reported no differences between groups in side effects, and sertraline caused a significant reduction in both the psychic and somatic symptoms of GAD. Although this study was limited by small sample size and the use of the adult Hamilton Anxiety Rating Scale (which is not standardized for children), results are promising, and further study with larger samples are indicated.

Table 15.3 presents a summary of medications often prescribed for the treatment of GAD in youth. However, it should be noted that none of

TABLE 15.3. Medications for GAD in Children and Adolescents

Medication	Initial dosing (mg)	Dosing range (mg/day) [Target (mg/kg/day)]	Dosing schedule	Indications	Side effects
Selective serotonin reuptake inhibitors (SSRIs)				First-line treatment for GAD; nonaddictive and generally well tolerated; does not provide immediate relief.	Nausea, diarrhea, insomnia or somnolence, headaches, activation, sexual dysfunction, sweating, tremor.
Citalopram	10–20 QD	10–60	QD–BID		
Fluoxetine	10–20 Qam	10–80	QD–BID		
Fluvoxamine	25–50 QHS	25–300	BID		
Paroxetine	5–10 Qam	5–50	QD–BID		
Sertraline	25–50 Qam	25–200	QD–BID		
Tricyclic antidepressants (TCAs)				Second-line treatment for GAD; nonaddictive but often difficult to tolerate; requires blood level and electrocardiographic monitoring; does not provide immediate relief.	Sedation, headaches, dry mouth, constipation, nausea, orthostatic hypotension, blurred vision, urinary retention, cardiac conduction delays.
Amitriptyline	10–25 QHS	10–300 [2–5]	QHS–BID		
Clomipramine	25 QHS	25–250 [2–5]	QHS–BID		
Desipramine	10–25 QHS	10–300 [2–5]	QHS–BID		
Imipramine	10–25 QHS	10–300 [2–5]	QHS–BID		
Nortriptyline	10 QHS	10–150 [1–3]	QHS–BID		
Protriptyline	5–10 QHS	5–60 [0.5–2]	BID–QID		
Other antidepressants				Second-line treatment for GAD; nonaddictive with midrange tolerability; does not provide immediate relief.	Sedation, constipation, dry mouth, nausea, orthostatic hypotension, blurred vision, hypertension (venlafaxine only).
Mirtazapine	15 QHS	15–45	QHS		
Nefazodone	25–50 BID	25–600	BID		
Venlafaxine	25–37.5 BID	25–375	BID–TID		
Benzodiazepines				Third-line treatment for GAD; addictive potential and cognitive blunting limit use in children. Provides immediate relief; best used in time-limited circumstances.	Sedation, cognitive blunting, dizziness, ataxia, memory disturbance, constipation, diplopia, hypotension.
Alprazolam	0.25 TID	0.25–4	TID		
Diazepam	1–2 TID	0.12–0.8	TID–QID		
Clonazepam	0.25–0.5 BID	0.1–0.2	BID–TID		
Lorazepam	0.25–0.5 TID	0.25–8	TID–QID		
Other anxiolytics				First-line treatment for GAD; nonaddictive and generally well tolerated; does not provide immediate relief.	Headache, nausea, dizziness, light-headedness, somnolence.
Buspirone	5 BID	5–60	BID		

Note. QD, once daily; BID, twice per day; QHS, at bedtime; TID, three times per day; Qam, in the morning. Data from Birmaher and Waterman (1994) and Fairbanks et al. (1997).

these formulations have as yet gained the U.S. Food and Drug Administration's indication for GAD in children, and all medications are prescribed "off-label" at this time.

SUMMARY AND FUTURE DIRECTIONS

GAD in children and adolescents is characterized by intrusive and uncontrollable worry that causes significant distress and impairment in daily functioning. Both prospective and retrospective studies suggest that GAD runs a chronic course from childhood through adulthood and may place an individual at risk for additional anxiety disorders, mood disorders, and a variety of psychosocial and emotional liabilities. Youth with GAD, when onset occurs early, are prone to impairments in academic functioning in the elementary school years, while associations between GAD, alcohol abuse, and suicidality have been found in adolescent samples. Further research into the natural history and course of GAD in youth is warranted, especially as refinements occur in our ability to identify youth at risk for, or in the early stages of, this anxiety disorder. Thus research must continue along the lines of developing effective and sensitive screening instruments for identifying cases of this disorder.

Exciting developments are emerging on the treatment front with regard to GAD and related anxiety disorders in youth. CBT has demonstrated efficacy in the treatment of GAD through a number of controlled randomized trials. Long-term follow-up of treated youth suggest maintenance of treatment gains, in addition to further improvement over time. There must be a further evaluation of CBT programs for GAD, and a developmental psychopathology perspective must be taken when future treatment studies are considered. In this sense, the efficacy of CBT should be examined in youth with a variety of risk factors, adversities, protective factors, variations in cognitive and developmental functioning, severity levels, and contexts; this will help clinicians to refine or revise the existing protocols to meet the needs of patients presenting to community-based clinics and mental health professionals. In other words, effectiveness research is needed.

Concurrently, clinical child psychologists and child psychiatrists are now engaged in a collaborative effort, supported by the National Institute of Mental Health, to conduct the first large-scale, randomized controlled clinical trial evaluating the relative efficacy of CBT, medication, combination treatment, and pill placebo in youth aged 7–16 with GAD, SAD, or social phobia (J. Walkup, personal communication, October 2002). This study should propel clinical scientists into the next generation of treatment studies—those evaluating treatment algorithms, discontinuation procedures, and the "staying power" of treatments over the long term. This is not a stakeholder issue, where psychologists will line up to cheer for CBT or psychiatrists for medication to "win the race." Rather, clinical scientists are engaged in a collaborative effort that will (let us hope) prove fruitful in informing front-line clinicians on strategies to effectively treat and relieve the suffering and long-term consequences experienced by youth with GAD.

REFERENCES

Achenbach, T. M. (1991). *Manual for the Child Behavior Checklist 4–18 and 1991 Profile.* Burlington: Department of Psychiatry, University of Vermont.

Achenbach, T. M., & Edelbrock, C. (1983). *Manual for the Child Behavior Checklist and Revised Child Behavior Profile.* Burlington: Department of Psychiatry, University of Vermont.

Albano, A. M., Chorpita, B. F., & Barlow, D. H. (2003). Childhood anxiety disorders. In E. J. Mash & R. A. Barkley (Eds.), *Child psychopathology* (2nd ed., pp. 279–329). New York: Guilford Press.

Albano, A. M., Chorpita, B. F., DiBartolo, P. M., & Barlow, D. H. (1995). *Comorbidity among anxiety disorders in youth.* Unpublished manuscript.

Albano, A. M., & Kendall, P. C. (2002). Cognitive behavioural therapy for children and adolescents with anxiety disorders: Clinical research advances. *International Review of Psychiatry, 14,* 128–133.

American Psychiatric Association (APA). (1968). *Diagnostic and statistical manual of mental disorders* (2nd ed.). Washington, DC: Author.

American Psychiatric Association (APA). (1980). *Diagnostic and statistical manual of mental disorders* (3rd ed.). Washington, DC: Author.

American Psychiatric Association (APA). (1987). *Diagnostic and statistical manual of mental disorders* (3rd ed., rev.). Washington, DC: Author.

American Psychiatric Association (APA). (1994). *Diagnostic and statistical manual of mental disorders* (4th ed.). Washington, DC: Author.

Anderson, D. J., Williams, S., McGee, R., & Silva, P. A. (1987). DSM-III disorders in preadolescent children: Prevalence in a large sample from the general population. *Archives of General Psychiatry, 44,* 69–76.

Barlow, D. H. (2002). *Anxiety and its disorders* (2nd ed.). New York: Guilford Press.

Barrett, P. M. (1998). Evaluation of cognitive-behavioral group treatments for childhood anxiety disorders. *Journal of Clinical Child Psychology, 27,* 459–468.

Barrett, P. M., Dadds, M. M., & Rapee, R. M. (1996). Family treatment of childhood anxiety: A controlled trial. *Journal of Consulting and Clinical Psychology, 64,* 333–342.

Barrios, B. A., & Hartmann, D. P. (1997). Fears and anxieties. In E. J. Mash & L. G. Terdal (Eds.), *Assessment of childhood disorders* (3rd ed., pp. 230–327). New York: Guilford Press.

Barrios, B. A., & O'Dell, S. L. (1998). Fears and anxieties. In E. J. Mash & R. A. Barkley (Eds.), *Treatment of childhood disorders* (2nd ed., pp. 249–337). New York: Guilford Press.

Beidel, D., Neal, A. M., & Lederer, A. S. (1991). The feasibility and validity of a daily diary for the assessment of anxiety in children. *Behavior Therapy, 22,* 505–517.

Bell-Dolan, D., & Brazeal, T. J. (1993). Separation anxiety disorder, overanxious disorder, and school refusal. *Child and Adolescent Psychiatric Clinics of North America, 2,* 563–580.

Bernstein, G. A. Borchardt, C. M., Perwien, A. R., Crosby, R. D., Kushner, M. G., Thuras, P. D., & Last, C. G. (2000). Imipramines plus cognitive-behavioral therapy in the treatment of school refusal. *Journal of the American Academy of Child and Adolescent Psychiatry, 39,* 276–283.

Bernstein, G. A., Garfinkel, B. D., & Borchardt, C. M. (1990). Comparative studies of pharmacotherapy for school refusal. *Journal of the American Academy of Child and Adolescent Psychiatry, 29,* 773–781.

Birmaher, B., Brent, D. A., Chiappetta, L., Bridge, J., Monga, S., & Baugher, M. (1999). Psychometric properties of the Screen for Child Anxiety Related Emotional Disorders (SCARED): A replication study. *Journal of the American Academy of Child and Adolescent Psychiatry, 38,* 1230–1236.

Birmaher, B., Khetarpal, S., Brent, D. A., Cully, M., Balach, L., Kaufman, J., & McKenzie-Neer, S. (1997). The Screen for Child Anxiety Related Emotional Disorders (SCARED): Scale construction and psychometric characteristics. *Journal of the American Academy of Child and Adolescent Psychiatry, 36,* 545–553.

Birmaher, B., & Waterman, S. (1994). Fluoxetine in childhood anxiety disorders. *Journal of the American Academy of Child and Adolescent Psychiatry, 33,* 993–999.

Birmaher, B., Waterman, G. S., Ryan, N., Cully, M., Balach, L., Ingram, J., & Brodsky, M. (1994). Fluoxetine for childhood anxiety disorders. *Journal of the American Academy of Child and Adolescent Psychiatry, 33,* 993–999.

Bowen, R. C., Offord, D. R., & Boyle, M. H. (1990). The prevalence of overanxious disorder and separation anxiety disorder: Results from the Ontario Child Health Study. *Journal of the American Academy of Child and Adolescent Psychiatry, 29,* 753–758.

Brady, E. U., & Kendall, P. C. (1992). Comorbidity of anxiety and depression in children and adolescents. *Psychological Bulletin, 111,* 244–255.

Cantwell, D. P., & Baker, L. (1989). Stability and natural history of DSM-III childhood diagnoses. *Journal of the American Academy of Child and Adolescent Psychiatry, 29,* 691–700.

Chansky, T. E., & Kendall, P. C. (1997). Social expectancies and self-perceptions in anxiety disordered children. *Journal of Anxiety Disorders, 11,* 347–364.

Chorpita, B. F., Tracey, S. A., Brown, T. A., Collica, T. J., & Barlow, D. H. (1997). Assessment of worry in children and adolescents: An adaptation of the Penn State Worry Questionnaire. *Behaviour Research and Therapy, 35,* 569–581.

Clark, D. B., Parker, A. M., & Lynch, K. G. (1999). Psychopathology and substance-related problems during early adolescence: A survival analysis. *Journal of Clinical Child Psychology, 28,* 333–341.

Cobham, V. E., Dadds, M. R., & Spence, S. H. (1998). The role of parental anxiety in the treatment of childhood anxiety. *Journal of Consulting and Clinical Psychology, 66,* 893–905.

Costello, E. J., Stouthamer-Loeber, M., & DeRosier, M. (1993). *Continuity and change in psychopathology from childhood to adolescence.* Paper presented at the annual meeting of the Society for Research in Child and Adolescent Psychopathology, Santa Fe, NM.

Craske, M. G., Barlow, D. H., & O'Leary, T. (1992). *Master of your anxiety and worry.* San Antonio, TX: Psychological Corporation.

Dadds, M. R., Heard, P. M., & Rapee, R. M. (1992). The role of family intervention in the treatment of child anxiety disorders: Some preliminary findings. *Behaviour Change, 20,* 171–177.

Dierker, L., Albano, A. M., Clarke, G. N., Heimberg, R. G., Kendall, P. C., Merikangas, K. R., Lewinsohn, P. M., Offord, D. R., Kessler, R., & Kupfer, D. J. (2001). Screening for anxiety and depression in early adolescence. *Journal of the American Academy of Child and Adolescent Psychiatry, 40,* 929–936.

Eisen, A. R., & Engler, L. B. (1995). Chronic anxiety. In A. R. Eisen, C. A. Kearney, & C. A. Schaefer (Eds.), *Clinical handbook of anxiety disorders in children and adolescents* (pp. 223–250). Northvale, NJ: Aronson.

Eisen, A. R., & Kearney, C. A. (1995). *Practitioner's guide to treating fear and anxiety in children and adolescents: A cognitive-behavioral approach.* Northvale, NJ: Aronson.

Fairbanks, J. M., Pine, D. S., Tancer, N. K., Dummit, E. S., III, Kentgen, L. M., Martin, J., Asche, B. K., & Klein, R. G. (1997). Open fluoxetine treatment of mixed anxiety disorders in children and adolescents. *Journal of Child and Adolescent Psychopharmacology, 7,* 17–29.

Flannery-Schroeder, E., & Kendall, P. C. (2000). Group and individual cognitive-behavioral treatments for youth with anxiety disorders: A randomized clinical trial. *Cognitive Therapy and Research, 24,* 251–278.

Graae, F., Milner, J., Rizzotto, L., & Klein, R. G. (1994). Clonazepam in childhood anxiety disorders. *Journal of the American Academy of Child and Adolescent Psychiatry, 33,* 372–376.

Hamilton, M. (1959). The assessment of anxiety states by rating. *British Journal of Medical Psychology, 32,* 50–55.

Howard, B. L., & Kendall, P. C. (1996). Cognitive-behavioral family therapy for anxiety-disordered children: A multiple-baseline evaluation. *Cognitive Therapy and Research, 20,* 423–443.

Ialongo, N., Edelsohn, G., Werthamer-Larsson, L., Crockett, L., & Kellam, S. (1994). The significance of self-reported anxious symptoms in first-grade children. *Journal of Abnormal Child Psychology, 22,* 441–455.

Ialongo, N., Edelsohn, G., Werthamer-Larsson, L., Crockett, L., & Kellam, S. (1995). The significance of self-reported anxious symptoms in first grade children: Prediction to anxious symptoms and adaptive functioning in fifth grade. *Journal of Child Psychology and Psychiatry, 36,* 427–437.

Kaplow, J. B., Curran, P. J., Angold, A., & Costello, E. J. (2001). The prospective relation between dimensions of anxiety and the initiation of adolescent alcohol abuse. *Journal of Clinical Child Psychology, 30,* 316–326.

Kashani, J. H., & Orvaschel, H. (1988). Anxiety disorders in midadolescence: A community sample. *American Journal of Psychiatry, 145,* 960–964.

Kashani, J. H., Orvaschel, H., Rosenberg, T. K., & Reid, J. C. (1989). Psychopathology in a community sample of children and adolescents: A developmental perspective. *Journal of the American Academy of Child and Adolescent Psychiatry, 28,* 701–706.

Kazdin, A. E., & Weisz, J. R. (1998). Identifying and developing empirically supported child and adolescent treatments. *Journal of Consulting and Clinical Psychology, 66,* 19–36.

Kearney, C. A. (2001). *School refusal behavior in youth: A functional approach to assessment and treatment.* Washington, DC: American Psychological Association.

Kearney, C. A., & Albano, A. M. (2000). *When children refuse school: A cognitive behavioral therapy approach. Therapist's manual.* San Antonio, TX: Psychological Corporation.

Kearney, C. A., & Silverman, W. K. (1993). Measuring the function of school refusal behavior: The School Refusal Assessment Scale. *Journal of Clinical Child Psychology, 22* 85–96.

Kendall, P. C. (1994). Treating anxiety disorders in children: Results of a randomized clinical trial. *Journal of Consulting and Clinical Psychology, 62,* 100–110.

Kendall, P. C., Chansky, T. E., Freidman, M., Kim, R., Kortlander, E., Sessa, F. M., & Siqueland, L. (1991). Treating anxiety disorders in children and adolescents. In P. C. Kendall (Ed.), *Child and adolescent therapy: Cognitive-behavioral procedures* (pp. 131–164). New York: Guilford Press.

Kendall, P. C., Flannery-Schroeder, E., Panicelli-Mindel, S. M., Southam-Gerow, M. A., Henin, A., & Warman, M. (1997). Therapy for youths with anxiety disorders: A second randomized clinical trial. *Journal of Consulting and Clinical Psychology, 65,* 366–380.

Kendall, P. C., Kane, M. T., Howard, B. L., & Siqueland, L. (1990). *Cognitive-behavioral therapy for anxious children: Treatment manual.* (Available from P. C. Kendall, Department of Psychology, Temple University, Philadelphia, PA)

Kendall, P. C., Krain, A., & Treadwell, K. R. (1999). Generalized anxiety disorders. In R. T. Ammerman, M. Hersen, & C. G. Last (Eds.), *Handbook of prescriptive treatments for children and adolescents* (2nd ed., pp. 155–171). Needham Heights, MA: Allyn & Bacon.

Kendall, P. C., & Southam-Gerow, M. A. (1996). Long-term follow-up of a cognitive behavioral therapy for anxiety disordered youth. *Journal of Consulting and Clinical Psychology, 64,* 724–730.

Kendall, P. C., & Warman, M. J. (1996). Anxiety disorders in youth: Diagnostic consistency across DSM-III-R and DSM-IV. *Journal of Anxiety Disorders, 10,* 453–463.

Klein, D. (1997). Control groups in pharmacotherapy and psychotherapy evaluations. *Treatment* [Online], *1.* Available: http://journals.apa.org/treatment/vol1/97_a91.html

Klein, R. G., Koplewicz, H. S., & Kanner, A. (1992). Imipramine treatment of children with separation anxiety disorder. *Journal of the American Academy of Child and Adolescent Psychiatry, 31,* 21–28.

Kovacs, M. (1981). Rating scales to assess depression in school-aged children. *Acta Paedopsychiatrica: International Journal of Child and Adolescent Psychiatry, 46,* 305–315.

Last, C. G., Hansen, C., & Franco, N. (1998). Cognitive-behavioral treatment of school phobia. *Journal of the American Academy of Child and Adolescent Psychiatry, 37,* 404–411.

Last, C. G., Hersen, M., Kazdin, A. E., Finkelstein, R., & Strauss, C. C. (1987). Comparison of DSM-III separation anxiety and overanxious disorders: Demographic characteristics and patterns of comorbidity. *Journal of the American Academy of Child and Adolescent Psychiatry, 26,* 527–531.

Last, C. G., Perrin, S., Hersen, M., & Kazdin, A. E. (1992). DSM-III-R anxiety disorders in children: Sociodemographic and clinical characteristics. *Journal of the American Academy of Child and Adolescent Psychiatry, 31,* 1070–1076.

Last, C. G., Strauss, C. C., & Francis, G. (1987). Comorbidity among childhood anxiety disorders. *Journal of Nervous and Mental Disease, 175,* 726–730.

Lewinsohn, P. M., Rohde, P., & Seeley, J. R. (1995). Adolescent psychopathology: III. The clinical consequences of comorbidity. *Journal of the American Academy of Child and Adolescent Psychiatry, 34,* 510–519.

Lewinsohn, P. M., Zinbarg, R., Seeley, J. R., Lewinsohn, M., & Sack, W. H. (1997). Lifetime comorbidity among anxiety disorders and between anxiety disorders and other mental disorders in adolescents. *Journal of Anxiety Disorders, 11,* 377–394.

March, J. S. (1999). Pharmacotherapy of pediatric anxiety disorders: A critical review. In D. Beidel (Ed.), *Treating anxiety disorders in youth: Current problems and future solutions* (pp. 42–62). Washington, DC: Anxiety Disorders Association of America.

March, J. S., & Albano, A. M. (2002). Anxiety disorders in children and adolescents. In D. J. Stein & E. Hollander (Eds.), *Textbook of anxiety disorders* (pp. 415–427). Washington, DC: American Psychiatric Press.

March, J. S., Parker, J. D. A., Sullivan, K., Stallings, P., & Connors, C. K. (1997). The Multidimensional Anxiety Scale for Children (MASC): Factor structure, reliability, and validity. *Journal of the American Academy of Child and Adolescent Psychiatry, 36,* 554–565.

March, J. S., & Sullivan, K. (1999). Test–retest reliability of the Multidimensional Anxiety Scale for Children. *Journal of Anxiety Disorders, 13,* 349–358.

Mash, E. J., & Terdal, L. G. (Eds.). (1997). *Assessment of childhood disorders* (3rd ed.). New York: Guilford Press.

Masi, G., Favilla, L., Mucci, M., & Millepiedi, S. (2000). Depressive comorbidity in children and adolescents with generalized anxiety disorder. *Child Psychiatry and Human Development, 30,* 205–215.

Mendlowitz, S. L., Manassis, K., Bradley, S., Scapillato, D., Miezitis, S., & Shaw, B. F. (1999). Cognitive-behavioral group treatments in childhood anxiety disorders: The role of parental involvement. *Journal of the American Academy of Child and Adolescent Psychiatry, 38,* 1223–1229.

McGee, R., Fehan, M., Williams, S., Partridge, F., Silva, P. A., & Kelly, J. (1990). DSM-III disorders in a large sample of adolescents. *Journal of the American Academy of Child and Adolescent Psychiatry, 29,* 611–619.

Muris, P., Meesters, C., Merckelbach, H., Sermon, A., & Zwakhalen, S. (1998). Worry in normal children. *Journal of the American Academy of Child and Adolescent Psychiatry, 37,* 703–710.

Muris, P., Merckelbach, H., Mayer, B., van Brakel, A., Thissen, S., Moulaert, V., & Gadet, B. (1998). The Screen for Child Anxiety and Related Emotional Disorders (SCARED) and traditional childhood anxiety measures. *Journal of Behavior Therapy and Experimental Psychiatry, 29,* 327–339.

Nielsen, T. A., Laberge, L., Paquet, J., Tremblay, R. E., Vitaro, F., & Montplaisir, J. (2000). Development of disturbing dreams during adolescence and their relation to anxiety symptoms. *Sleep, 23,* 727–736.

Ollendick, T. H. (1983). Fear in children and adolescents: Normative data. *Behaviour Research and Therapy, 23,* 465–467.

Pawlak, C., Pascual-Sanchez, T., Rae, P., Fischer, W., & Ladame, F. (1999). Anxiety disorders, comorbidity, and suicide attempts in adolescence: A preliminary investigation. *European Psychiatry, 14,* 132–136.

Perrin, S., & Last, C. G. (1992). Do childhood anxiety measures measure anxiety? *Journal of Abnormal Child Psychology, 20,* 567–578.

Perrin, S., & Last, C. G. (1997). Worrisome thoughts in children referred for anxiety disorder. *Journal of Clinical Child Psychology, 26,* 181–189.

Reynolds, C. R., & Richmond, B. O. (1979). Factor structure and construct validity of "What I think and feel": The Revised Children's Manifest Anxiety Scale. *Journal of Personality Assessment, 43,* 281–283.

Roemer, L., & Orsillo, S. M. (2002). Expanding our conceptualization of and treatment for generalized anxiety disorder: Integrating mindfulness/acceptance-based approaches with existing cognitive-behavioral models. *Clinical Psychology: Science and Practice, 8,* 54–68.

Ronan, K. R., & Kendall, P. C. (1997). Self-talk in distressed youth: States-of-mind and content specificity. *Journal of Clinical Child Psychology, 26,* 330–337.

RUPP Anxiety Work Group. (2001). Fluvoxamine for the treatment of anxiety disorders in children and adolescents. *New England Journal of Medicine, 344,* 1279–1285.

Rynn, M. A., Siqueland, L., & Rickels, K. (2001). Placebo-controlled trial of sertraline in the treatment of children with generalized anxiety disorder. *American Journal of Psychiatry, 158,* 2008–2014.

Silverman, W. K., & Albano, A. M. (1996). *The Anxiety Disorders Interview Schedule for DSM-IV, Child Version.* San Antonio, TX: Psychological Corporation.

Silverman, W. K., & Eisen, A. R. (1992). Age differences in the reliability of parent and child reports of child anxious symptomatology using a structured interview. *Journal of the American Academy of Child and Adolescent Psychiatry, 31,* 117–124.

Silverman, W. K., & Ginsberg, G. (1995). Specific phobia and generalized anxiety disorder. In J. S. March (Ed.), *Anxiety disorders in children and adolescents* (pp. 151–180). New York: Guilford Press.

Silverman, W. K., & Kurtines, W. M. (1996). *Anxiety and phobic disorders: A pragmatic approach.* New York: Plenum Press.

Silverman, W. K., Kurtines, W. M., Ginsburg, G. S., Weems, C. F., Lumpkin, P., White, C., & Hicks, D. (1999). Treating anxiety disorders in children with group cognitive-behavioral therapy: A randomized clinical trial. *Journal of Consulting and Clinical Psychology 67,* 995–1003.

Silverman, W. K., Kurtines, W. M., Ginsburg, G. S., Weems, C. F., Rabian, B., & Serafini, L. T. (1999). Contingency management, self-control, and education support in the treatment of childhood phobic disorders: A randomized clinical trial. *Journal of Consulting and Clinical Psychology, 67,* 675–687.

Silverman, W. K., La Greca, A., & Wasserstein, S. (1995). What do children worry about?: Worries and their relation to anxiety. *Child Development, 66,* 671–686.

Silverman, W. K., & Nelles, W. B. (1988). The Anxiety Disorders Interview Schedule for Children. *Journal of the American Academy of Child and Adolescent Psychiatry, 27,* 772–778.

Silverman, W. K., Saavedra, L. M., & Pina, A. A. (2001). Test–retest reliability of anxiety symptoms and diagnoses with the Anxiety Disorders Interview Schedule for DSM-IV: Child and Parent Versions. *Journal of the American Academy of Child and Adolescent Psychiatry, 40,* 937–944.

Simeon, J. G., Ferguson, H. B., Knott, V., Roberts, N., Gauthier, B., Dubois, C., & Wiggins, D. (1992). Clinical, cognitive, and neurophysiological effects of alprazolam in children and adolescents with overanxious and avoidant disorders. *Journal of the American Academy of Child and Adolescent Psychiatry, 31,* 29–33.

Spence, S. H. (1997). The structure of anxiety symptoms among children: A confirmatory factor analytic study. *Journal of Abnormal Psychology, 106,* 280–297.

Spence, S. H., Rapee, R., McDonald, C., & Ingram, M. (2001). The structure of anxiety symptoms among preschoolers. *Behaviour Research and Therapy, 39,* 1293–1316.

Spielberger, C. D. (1973). *Manual for the State–Trait Anxiety Inventory for Children.* Palo Alto, CA: Consulting Psychologists Press.

Stallings, P., & March, J. (1995). Assessment. In J. S. March (Ed.), *Anxiety disorders in children and adolescents* (pp. 125–147). New York: Guilford Press.

Strauss, C. C., Lahey, B. B., Frick, P., Frame, C. L., & Hynd, G. W. (1988). Peer social status of children with anxiety disorders. *Journal of Consulting and Clinical Psychology, 56,* 137–141.

Strauss, C. C., Last, C. G., Hersen, M., & Kazdin, A. F. (1988). Association between anxiety and depression in children and adolescents with anxiety disorders. *Journal of Abnormal Child Psychology, 16,* 57–68.

Strauss, C. C., Lease, C. A., Last, C. G., & Francis, G. (1988). Overanxious disorder: An examination of developmental differences. *Journal of Abnormal Child Psychology, 16,* 433–443.

Tracey, S. A., Chorpita, B. F., Douban, J., & Barlow, D. H. (1997). Empirical evaluation of DSM-IV generalized anxiety disorder criteria for children and adolescents. *Journal of Clinical Child Psychology, 26,* 404–414.

Weems, C. F., Silverman, W. K., & La Greca, A. M. (2000). What do youth referred for anxiety problems worry about?: Worry and its relation to anxiety and anxiety disorders in children and adolescents. *Journal of Abnormal Child Psychology, 28,* 63–72.

Wilens, T. E., Biederman, J., Baldessarini, R. J., Geller, B., Schleifer, D., Spencer, T. J., Birmaher, B., & Goldblatt, A. (1996). Cardiovascular effects of therapeutic doses of tricyclic antidepressants in children and adolescents. *Journal of the American Academy of Child and Adolescent Psychiatry, 35,* 1491–1501.

CHAPTER 16

Older Adults

J. GAYLE BECK
PATRICIA M. AVERILL

For many years, research on the anxiety disorders focused exclusively on the study of young and middle-aged adults. Although this concentrated effort has resulted in a large database enumerating many aspects of the psychopathology, assessment, and treatment of each of the anxiety disorders, it has created a somewhat myopic perspective on these conditions. In the past several years, there has been increasing recognition of this myopia, with ensuing efforts to expand the field to include children, culturally diverse groups, and older adults. In this chapter, we focus on issues pertaining to the conceptualization, diagnosis, assessment, and treatment of generalized anxiety disorder (GAD) in older adults (individuals aged 60 and older). In most respects, we are in the early stages of research on GAD in elderly persons. In an effort to extend the current boundaries of research on GAD in the elderly population, we interface available knowledge on GAD in older adults with the larger literature on the disorder in younger adults, as well as related gerontological literature. Certainly, a focus on geriatric populations has the potential to expand our conceptual understanding of GAD, in light of current theoretical approaches to this disorder. In particular, there appear to be multiple avenues to the development and maintenance of GAD, as we discuss. Older adults with GAD exemplify these many pathways, and as such constitute a unique study population. Moreover, several unique characteristics of older adults may have an impact on their assessment and treatment, including concurrent medical problems, decrements in cognitive and perceptual functioning, and age cohort effects. Each of these issues is discussed here, particularly with respect to available assessment and treatment strategies.

PREVALENCE, COMORBID CONDITIONS, AND ASSOCIATED FEATURES OF GAD IN ELDERLY PERSONS

Prevalence

Epidemiological studies suggest that the prevalence of anxiety disorders is lower among older than among younger adults (e.g., Blazer, George, & Hughes, 1991; Flint, 1994; Regier, et al., 1988). In Wave 2 of the Epidemiological Catchment Area (ECA) study (the only wave of this study to evaluate GAD), the 6-month and lifetime prevalence rates for GAD in older adults (age 65 and older) were reported at 1.9% and 4.6%, respectively. In contrast, for adults aged 45–64, the 6-month and lifetime prevalence rates were 3.1% and 6.7%, respectively. Despite the somewhat lower prevalence of GAD among older adults documented in the ECA and related surveys, it is conceivable that a number of factors impede recognition of anxiety-based problems among elderly persons (e.g., Palmer, Jeste, & Sheikh, 1997). For example, many authors have questioned whether the GAD criteria outlined in the various editions of the *Diagnostic and Statistical Manual of Mental Disorders* (DSM) apply to older adults (e.g., Sheikh, 1992). As argued by Flint (1994) and others (e.g., Parmelee, Katz, & Lawton, 1993), older adults are likely to report a mixture of anxiety and depressive symptoms, rather than more "pure" versions of these disorders. However, this does not imply that anxiety symptoms are a rare occurrence among older adults. As noted by Gurian and Miner, (1991, p. 31), anxiety tends to be a common symptom among elderly individuals, but an "uncommon syndrome." This would suggest that fewer older adults meet the symptom criteria for GAD, despite the presence of notable anxiety symptoms. However, Scogin (1998) and others have suggested that there is ample cause to believe that GAD is alive and well represented among the older population, and that the ECA prevalence figures are underestimates of the disorder in older adults, given data documenting atypical symptom patterns in related disorders (e.g., Katz, 1996). At present, this issue remains unresolved and awaits greater understanding of the psychopathology of GAD in older adults for its resolution.

Moreover, considerable symptom overlap exists between GAD and the mood disorders, complicating this issue further. Contrasting the symptom criteria for GAD with the criteria for a major depressive episode (MDE) illustrates this point. Of the six specific symptoms listed for GAD, three (sleep disturbance, fatigue, and difficulty concentrating) overlap with the symptom criteria for an MDE, with an additional symptom (restlessness) that is similarly described for the two. Thus there is a natural "confound" in the diagnostic criteria for GAD and depressive disorders—a confound that may be more salient in the evaluation of older adults, given their tendency to focus on somatic symptomatology (e.g., Spar & LaRue, 1990). For this reason, considerable clinical skill appears to be necessary when one is evaluating an older adult with mood-related complaints. In particular, one should be vigilant in differentiating somatic symptoms from cognitive and affective problems. The latter may be more distinctive indicators of GAD (or depressive disorders) in older adults.

Thus older patients are more likely to express anxiety symptoms in terms of somatic features (e.g., muscle tension) or behavioral changes (e.g., fidgety conduct; Spar & LaRue, 1990) than in terms of cognitive or emotional symptoms. Because the current age cohort of older adults may be less likely to discuss emotional states (Lipton & Schaffer, 1988), it will be interesting to observe whether this finding persists in the future. It is entirely possible that later cohorts will be more comfortable reporting cognitive and emotional events as they age, which would eliminate current concerns about differentiating anxiety and depression primarily on the basis of bodily symptoms. On the other hand, it is equally possible that later cohorts also may report a preponderance of somatic symptoms, which would suggest that there are some clear age-related changes in symptom profiles in GAD (and the depressive disorders). Clearly, this question awaits the "maturing" of adults who are presently young and middle-aged. At present, however, one must attempt to differentiate actual symptoms from an older patient's style of reporting, prior to drawing any conclusions about the nature of anxiety versus depressive disorders in old age.

In considering the occurrence of GAD, it is striking that there are so few published studies on the prevalence of the disorder within nursing home settings. Given that many of the "old-old" (i.e., individuals aged 75–80 and older) reside in a structured setting of some form, this is a critical shortcoming in the literature. This segment of the population has been increasing proportionally much faster than the rest of the population (U.S. Bureau of the Census, 1992). To date, several studies have reported prevalence rates ranging between 3.5% and 6% for GAD in nursing home residents (e.g., Junginger, Phelan, Cherr, & Levy, 1993; Parmelee et al., 1993). These figures, however, do not take into account important features of this population, such as comorbid dementia or related medical conditions (Howell, 1996; Pearson, 1998). It will be important for future investigations to evaluate (rather than to exclude) elderly patients with the full spectrum of aging-related disorders, in order to examine the impact of cognitive and physical decline on the course of GAD.

Comorbid Conditions

As discussed by many authors, anxiety and depressive disorders co-occur frequently, and this is certainly true in aging samples (e.g., Beekman et al., 1998). Although similar patterns of syndrome comorbidity may occur, differences may appear in symptom patterns, exposure to risk factors, and specific vulnerabilities in older adults. Beekman and colleagues (1998, 2000) report interesting data from a 10-year longitudinal study focusing on adults aged 55 and older. These authors note that 30.3% of older individuals who were identified in an initial screening with major depressive disorder also received a diagnosis of GAD during a second phase of screening. On the other hand, among those individuals initially identified with GAD during the initial screening, a very low rate of depressive disorders was noted during the second phase of screening. In addition, a risk factor analysis was conducted for both anxiety and depressive disorders (Beekman et al., 2000), indicating that an external locus of control was relevant in setting the stage for the comorbidity of these diagnoses. Given increased sophistication in our knowledge about GAD, it will be interesting to watch this line of research expand our understanding of risk factors for the development of multiple disorders in the context of GAD.

To date, the relationship between anxiety and cognitive disorders (e.g., vascular dementia, Alzheimer's disease) has not been addressed adequately. Some investigators note that the co-occurrence of these two types of disorders is common (e.g., Wands et al., 1990), although others have failed to find an association between anxiety and cognitive impairment (e.g., van Balkom et al., 2000). Consideration of the overlap between GAD and cognitive impairment reveals that this issue is complex. To begin with, there are no measures currently available to evaluate anxiety and worry in individuals with dementia. The majority of measures used to evaluate GAD rely on self-report (e.g., questionnaire, structured interview), and thus cannot be used with individuals with more advanced dementia who have lost verbal skills. This suggests a need for observational measures. However, as discussed cogently by Fisher and Noll (1996), anxious behaviors may take a different form in individuals with advanced dementia. These authors speculate that aggressive or assaultive behaviors may fall under the umbrella of "anxiety," depending on their function. If, for example, assaultive behavior represents an effort to escape from a situation that an individual finds threatening, would this not be categorized as a behavioral manifestation of anxiety? Clearly, considerably more work needs to be done on the development of observational assessment techniques. It appears that this can best be accomplished via functional analysis, given the possibility that anxiety may manifest itself in a very different fashion in demented individuals (see Fisher & Noll, 1996, for further discussion).

A variety of medical conditions may also be present in the older adult with GAD. Because of the overlap between anxiety and some medical illnesses, careful evaluation is necessary when one is considering GAD in an older adult. It is important to remain mindful that anxiety symptoms can be an emotional response to a serious medical illness, a facet of certain medical conditions (such as cardiac diseases, hypertension, or chronic obstructive pulmonary disease; Zarit & Zarit, 1998), or a reflection of older adults' tendency to focus on somatic symptoms. As highlighted by many authors (e.g., Gurian & Miner, 1991; Katz, 1996), a substantial amount of work has examined the interplay between depression and medical problems in elderly persons. Unfortunately, this work is not paralleled in the anxiety arena. Clinically, a thorough medical evaluation is important in the differential diagnosis of GAD. For example, if excessive anxiety and worry represent an emotional response to a major medical problem, the treatment formulation may be quite different from the approach utilized to address GAD. The development of clinical guidelines to differentiate anxiety and medical conditions would be a tremendously useful addition.

An interesting question is whether the presence of GAD affects medical resource utilization (e.g., length of hospital stay, frequency of hospitalization). The literature is quite mixed on this point, with some studies reporting that anxiety is associated with a longer duration of hospital stay (e.g., Levenson, Hamer, & Rossiter, 1990), and other studies failing to support this interrelationship (e.g., Fulop, Strain, Fahs, Schmeidler, & Snyder, 1998). The public health implications of this topic are clear, and thus we can expect more empirical data on this issue to emerge.

Associated Features

A number of features appear to be associated with GAD in older adults. As in younger samples, women with the disorder appear to outnumber men, with an approximate ratio of 2:1 (Regier et al., 1988). Although this gender ratio appears to be continuous across the lifespan, it may not be. Women live longer on average than men (National Center for Health Statistics, 1993), and this gap in life expectancy is found cross-culturally (Kinsella & Taeuber, 1993). As a result, women outnumber men by a ratio of 3:2 among people over age 65 (Zarit & Zarit, 1998). In light of this information on life expectancy, it may be that a lower proportion of older women than of younger women report GAD, relative to the population base rate. At present, consideration of base rates (life expectancy) has not accompanied work on associated features and risk factors for GAD. Additional features that appear to be associated with GAD in older adults include being unmarried, having a low income, and having less education (see Stanley & Beck, 1998, for further discussion of demographic features).

A related feature of GAD in elderly persons involves age of onset. As noted in the ECA study, GAD appears to have a bimodal distribution in older adults, with 39% reporting that uncontrollable worry has been a problem for 21 years or longer (Blazer, Hughes, & George, 1987). Although some have argued that these figures may suggest that GAD should be conceptualized as an Axis II personality disorder rather than an

Axis I condition within the DSM (e.g., Sanderson & Wetzler, 1991), this chronicity may simply be an associated feature of the disorder. Another 52% of participants in the ECA study reported the onset of GAD within 5 years of their research involvement. It is possible that GAD began as a response to stressful life events for this latter subsample, as related research has documented that exposure to a catastrophic financial loss can serve as a key stressor for the development of anxiety problems in older adults (Ganzini, McFarland, & Culter, 1990). This bimodal age-of-onset pattern has been replicated in related samples of older adults with GAD (J. G. Beck, Stanley, & Zebb, 1996). In this report, few differences were noted in clinical features (e.g., anxiety, depression, phobias) when patients with onset of GAD before age 15 were contrasted with those reporting onset after age 39. This would suggest that although there may be at least two pathways for the development of GAD, we remain uncertain as to whether early versus late onset distinguishes symptom profiles, clinical presentation, and related facets of GAD in older patients. Further work on this issue would be well advised to integrate available theoretical ideas, which are discussed in the next section.

THEORETICAL CONSIDERATIONS

Although there have been notable advances in our conceptualization and theoretical formulations of GAD, there have been few efforts to extend these concepts to older patients with this disorder. In some respects, current theories have interesting implications for shaping the study of GAD in elderly individuals. Below, several of these implications are discussed.

The Nature of Worry and Anxiety in Elderly Persons

A central issue in emerging work on GAD in elderly persons is whether the nature of worry and anxiety remains invariant across the life cycle. Although one could assume that worry and anxiety should remain essentially the same as people age, the opposite could also appear true—namely, that the nature of anxiety changes as people mature. To date, interesting preliminary studies have been conducted in this regard. Lawton, Kleban, and Dean (1993) examined potential differences in the factor structure of affect in three groups of community-dwelling adults: younger (aged 18–30), middle-aged (aged 31–59), and older (aged 60 and over) adults. When the investigators examined the relative rates of endorsement of these affective states, older adults were found to report less of almost every negative emotional state (including anxiety) relative to the other two age groups, although few between-group differences were noted for positive affect terms. However, examination of the structure of these affect terms (via confirmatory factor analyses) indicated differences in factor correlations and item loading across the three groups. The primary differences occurred between the younger and older adults with respect to factors measuring positive affect, depression, and anxiety–guilt. In particular, affect terms describing guilt (e.g., "ashamed," "guilty") were more salient and clustered with anxiety terms for younger adults, and did not load as highly with the anxiety items for older adults.

These findings are amplified by a related report (Shapiro, Roberts, & Beck, 1999), which examined the factor structure of the Cognitive Checklist (CCL; A. T. Beck, Brown, Steer, Eidelson, & Riskind, 1987) in 283 community-dwelling older participants. Results indicated a three-factor solution (Anxiety, Social Loss, and Negative Self-Evaluation/Worthlessness), and these cognitive factors were not uniquely related to anxiety and depression. More recently, we (J. G. Beck et al., 2003) addressed this question in a sample of 83 older patients with GAD. These results suggested a factor structure for the CCL similar to that noted in younger adults. The CCL Depression subscale showed strong correlations with measures of depression, although the CCL Anxiety subscale did not show unique correlations with measures of anxiety. Clearly, additional work needs to be conducted to resolve this discrepancy in findings. In a related vein, Lowe and Reynolds (2000) observed three factors when examining the factor structure of the Adult Manifest Anxiety Scale—Elderly version, a self-report questionnaire modeled after the Revised Children's Manifest Anxiety Scale (RCMAS; Reynolds & Richmond, 1978). These authors' three-factor solution reflected worry, fear of aging, and physiological manifestations of anxiety. They noted overlap with the observed factor structure of the RCMAS, which reflects worry, physiological anxiety symptoms, and fear/concentration items. Although one might question whether it is appropriate to compare data from older adults with those obtained from children, these findings indicate areas of both overlap and separation in the structure of anxiety across age groups. Taken together, these studies suggest that distinctions between the cognitive and affective facets of depression and anxiety may have a different organization in younger versus older adults, at least in the current age cohort. It thus appears safe to suggest that the nature of anxiety cannot be assumed to remain invariant across the lifespan. Continued efforts in this domain could benefit our available conceptual models of anxiety, worry, and GAD in older adults.

The most recent study to amplify this conclusion was reported by Wetherell, Gatz, and Pederson (2001). These authors conducted a longitudinal modeling analysis of anxiety and depression among 1,391 community-dwelling adults. Participants ranged in age from 29 to 95 (average age = 60.9) and participated as part of the Swedish Adoption/Twin Study of Aging investigation. Over two 3-year intervals, anxiety symptoms led to depressive symptoms, but the converse was not true. Anxiety symptoms were more stable than depressive symptoms, suggesting that anxiety may be more indicative of a personality dimension. Ideally, this type of analysis can be extended to samples of older patients with GAD, since it will be helpful to understand the interplay between chronic anxiety and depression as these two mood states are expressed over time.

Examination of the content of elderly persons' worries suggest that *what* one worries about is reflective of developmentally appropriate themes. For example, community-dwelling older adults appear to worry about physical health, whereas younger adults appear more preoccupied with worries about finances and social events (Person & Borkovec, 1995; Powers, Wisocki, & Whitbourne, 1992). Consideration of this issue in patients with GAD suggests that older patients spend more time worrying about health issues and less about work issues, relative to younger patients (Diefenbach, Stanley, & Beck, 2001). As the conceptualization of GAD has evolved, we have come to recognize that *what* people worry about is not perhaps the most central aspect of worry; rather, the perceived uncontrollability of the worry, the degree to which worry disrupts ongoing activities, and related dimensions are more central to GAD (American Psychiatric Association, 1994). It will be interesting for future work to examine these features of excessive worry in older patients with GAD.

It is also important to examine factors that have been identified by current theories of GAD, with respect to their potential applicability for older adults with the disorder. Although there have been no direct studies of these theories using samples of elderly patients with GAD, related experimental data suggests that this avenue of investigation would be useful.

Information-Processing Models

As discussed by MacLeod and Rutherford (Chapter 5, this volume), information-processing models have provided a rich context for research on the anxiety disorders and on GAD. Considerable evidence suggests that anxiety-based deficits in cognitive performance may be limited to tasks involving working memory (e.g., MacLeod, 1999), and that these deficits include selective encoding, interpretative biases, and possible biases in implicit memory (see MacLeod & Rutherford, Chapter 5). In brief, information-processing models focus on specific facets of cognitive processing biases as these contribute to the development and maintenance of excessive worry and anxiety. At the heart of these models is the presumption that a cognitive vulnerability exists in the form of a "schema" (e.g., A. T. Beck & Emery with Greenberg, 1985), or cognitive blueprint, which guides information processing. This schema is stated to have existed since childhood and is activated during exposure to stressful or threatening events. These models were not developed with aging adults in mind, and one may ask how well they apply to older adults with GAD. Although ultimately this is an empirical question, this issue is complicated from both a methodological and a conceptual standpoint. For example, the bimodal age of onset of GAD in older adults would need to be incorporated within any information-processing account of GAD in elderly persons, as would consideration of normative patterns of aging. As well, the fact that greater heterogeneity in cognitive functioning exists among older individuals than among younger ones would need to be integrated into empirical methods. In many respects, this represents an exciting new avenue for theoretical developments within the literature on aging and anxiety disorders.

Although use of these specific laboratory paradigms (e.g., the modified Stroop paradigm, dot probe methodology) to test information-processing models of GAD has not yet expanded to include older adults, work within cognitive psychology on memory processes in aging may inform clinical research in this arena. For example, Christensen and colleagues (1999) followed 426 elderly community dwellers over a 3½-year interval, in order to examine individual-difference factors that would be associated with changes in four domains of cognitive ability. This report noted that higher levels of depression were associated with greater variability in cognitive performance, although anxiety was not predictive of cognitive performance. Given the noted comorbidity between GAD and the depressive disorders, some form of control for depression is necessary in research on this issue, in order to reduce the impact of this potential confound. Relatedly, a small collection of findings has accrued concerning the impact of lowered self-efficacy on memory in elderly persons, with mixed findings (see Light, 1996). It is conceivable that greater collaboration between clinical and cognitive researchers will facilitate an increased understanding of how anxiety influences information processing across the lifespan—a topic that has particular theoretical importance and many potential clinical applications.

Problem Solving

The role of impairments in problem solving has been emphasized in theories on the etiology and maintenance of GAD (e.g., Davey, 1994). As discussed by Dugas, Gagnon, Ladouceur, and Freeston (1998), GAD appears to be associated with poor "problem orientation"—a set of processes reflecting awareness and appraisal of everyday problems and one's ability to solve them. As initially discussed by Davey (1994), worry appears to be associated with low confidence in one's problem-solving abilities, as well as low perceived control over the problem-solving process. Dugas and colleagues (1998) have integrated this factor within a larger conceptual model of GAD, emphasizing how poor problem orientation interacts with intolerance for uncertainty, dysfunctional beliefs about worry, and cognitive avoidance. Early empirical examinations of this model have been supportive (e.g., Dugas et al., 1998; Dugas, Freeston, & Ladouceur, 1997), although these studies have not involved older adults.

In some respects, the concept of poor problem orientation has intuitive appeal when one is considering elevated anxiety and worry in older adults. Given the numerous changes that have occurred in technology, business, and finance in the past decade, one could assume that today's older adults require good problem-solving skills (and confidence in their abilities) to negotiate these cultural advances. Is it possible that this factor is salient in the development of GAD during middle to later adulthood? One empirical study suggests that the answer to this question might be "yes." Kant, D'Zurilla, and Maydeu-Olivares (1997) compared the social problem-solving skills of middle-aged (aged 40–55) and elderly (aged 60–80) community residents. Problem-solving deficits were related significantly to both anxiety and depression in the two subsamples. In addition, support was found for the idea that problem solving serves a mediational role in the relationship between everyday problems and ensuing depression and anxiety. A natural next step would be to extend this paradigm to older patients with GAD, in order to examine whether these interrelationships continue to be noted. This type of finding has clear implications for the refinement of treatments for GAD in elderly persons.

Avoidance Theory

According to the avoidance theory of worry and GAD (e.g., Borkovec, Shadick, & Hopkins, 1991), worry is a verbal/linguistic process that appears to inhibit strong negative feelings, emotional imagery, and physiological arousal. Worry represents an abstract, conceptual form of thought that appears to serve an avoidance function. When an individual "thinks" (worries) about an issue in a remote, theoretical way, little or no negative emotion, disturbing imagery, or physiological arousal will occur (e.g., Vrana, Cuthbert, & Lang, 1986). This is immediately reinforcing, particularly when the content of the worry has the potential to create negative emotions (e.g., the poor health of a loved one). Unfortunately, avoidance of the emotional nature of the worry carries with it a price—namely, a lack of resolution of the original emotional disturbance (Borkovec, Roemer, & Kinyon, 1995). Data from this research group extend this conceptualization. As reported by Borkovec and colleagues (1995), when asked about possible reasons for worry, patients with GAD noted that they worried in order to distract themselves from even more emotional topics—issues that they did not want to face. This finding suggests that worry serves an avoidance function on multiple levels. Borkovec and colleagues have extended this formulation further, in an effort to understand what such patients are trying to avoid. Their current speculations hypothesize that because some patients with GAD report disturbing childhood experiences, chronic worry may have developed as a strategy that allows the patients to stay away emotionally from painful memories. Although empirical evidence is not yet available on this issue, this speculation might help to explain the subset of older patients with GAD who report that worry began during their early childhood years. This would suggest that there could be at least two possible pathways in the development of GAD: learned avoidance stemming back to a dysfunctional childhood, and onset following a stressful life event in adulthood. If this speculation is accurate, it has the potential to refine our understanding of the psychopathology (and possibly the treatment) of GAD in older adults.

Summary

Although the field is rich with theoretical ideas concerning the etiology and maintenance of GAD, these ideas have not played a central role in guiding research on the disorder in older adults. This is particularly unfortunate, given the fact that much of the available research on GAD in elderly individuals has been descriptive in nature. Ideally, greater integration of the theoretical constructs and paradigms that have proved useful in the study of GAD among younger adults will occur in the study of older adults. In many respects, the development and refinement of assessment tools for older adults with GAD will assist in these efforts. Next, we review the status of assessment of worry and anxiety in elderly persons.

ASSESSMENT OF WORRY AND GAD IN OLDER ADULTS

Given the array of unique considerations involved in the evaluation of GAD in elderly persons, the need for psychometrically sound assessment instruments becomes clear. To date, two strategies have evolved in the evaluation of assessment instruments for older adults: (1) developing measures specifically for use with older adults, in an effort to capture those aspects of anxiety that are specific to older adults; and (2) evaluating existing measures with an eye toward determining their psychometric properties in older adults. To date, only clinician-rated measures and self-report questionnaires have been considered in these pursuits, as we note below. As discussed in a previous section, the need for observational measures is clear, particularly if the field is going to consider aging-related conditions (such as dementia) in conjunction with elevated anxiety and worry. Although preliminary steps have been taken in this regard (Novy et al., 1997), considerably more effort needs to be devoted to this undertaking. In reviewing the available data on measures for the assessment of worry and GAD in older adults, it is important to recognize that this arena is ripe for future development.

Clinician-Rated Measures

Among the clinician-rated measures that have been examined for elderly individuals are previously established structured diagnostic interviews and rating scales. Both the Anxiety Disorders Interview Schedule—Revised (ADIS-R; DiNardo, Moras, Barlow, Rapee, & Brown, 1993) and the Structured Clinical Interview for DSM-III-R (SCID; Spitzer, Williams, Gibbon, & First, 1988) have been shown to be potentially useful in diagnosing older adults according to DSM-III-R criteria (e.g., J. G. Beck et al., 1996; Segal, Hersen, VanHasselt, Kabacoff, & Roth, 1993). In particular, Segal et al. included 73 older adults from both inpatient and outpatient settings who were not preselected on the basis of presenting symptomatology. Results indicated adequate to strong interdiagnostician agreement on the SCID for the anxiety and somatoform disorders, as well as major depressive disorder. In addition, the Diagnostic Interview Schedule (DIS; Robins, Helzer, Croughan, & Ratcliff, 1981) has been used with community-dwelling elders (Regier et al, 1988). Because numerous general drawbacks of the DIS have been discussed (e.g., Beidel & Turner, 1991; Knauper & Wittchen, 1994), this instrument should not be the first choice of a structured interview for use with older adults. Given the changes in the diagnostic criteria for GAD that occurred between DSM-III-R and DSM-IV, it will be important to ascertain whether the current versions of all these structured interviews continue to allow reliable diagnoses.

One topic that has received little attention in this domain is whether family informants can provide data that will allow accurate diagnoses. Given the fact that some older adults may not be able to complete structured diagnostic interviews (owing to stroke-related speech problems, dementia, etc.), this issue bears considerable relevance for evaluation of worry and GAD in elderly individuals. Heun and Muller (1998) examined this issue with 283 participants, grouped according to whether they could be diagnosed with Alzheimer's dementia, a depressive disorder, or no psychiatric diagnoses. These individuals and their available first-degree relatives were interviewed with the Composite International Diagnostic Interview (World Health Organization, 1990). Results indicated low reliability for the anxiety disorders (kappa = .19) between family informants, although interinformant reliability was higher for dementia (kappa = .58). These data should be replicated with an eye toward identifying sources of unreliability. For example, do family informants report worry and associated symptomatology consistently, or could inconsistency across individuals account for these findings? Ideally, future work can begin to develop accurate and reliable methods for interviewing family informants about anxiety in their older relatives.

In addition to structured interviews, investigators have examined clinician-administered rating scales, such as the Hamilton Anxiety Rating Scale (HARS; Hamilton, 1959) and the Hamilton Rating Scale for Depression (HRSD; Hamilton, 1960). In one study, J. G. Beck, Stanley, and Zebb (1999) administered the HARS to 50 elderly patients with GAD and 93 control participants without psychiatric diagnoses. The HARS was scored according to both the original and revised (Riskind, Beck, Brown, & Steer, 1987) criteria, the latter of which were designed to differentiate symptoms of depression and anxiety more clearly. Internal consistency was good for both samples, and the HARS was able to classify 90% of participants correctly into diagnostic groups. Unfortunately, overlap with the HRSD was high for both the original and revised HARS scoring methods (r's = .78 and .64, respectively), suggesting that the Hamilton scales are not optimal for differentiating anxiety and depression in older adults. We (Diefenbach, Stanley, Beck, Novy, et al., 2001) subsequently replicated these findings. A related report by Clayton, Holroyd, and Sheldon-Keller (1997) suggests that the HRSD may not be sensitive to those symptoms of depression that elderly respondents most frequently report, such as diminished social activities, malaise, and boredom. In this report, the HRSD correlated poorly (r = .33) with the Geriatric Depression Scale (GDS), a well-validated self-report measure of gerontological depression (Yesavage et al., 1983). Data were derived from a sample of well-diagnosed older patients with GAD, further suggesting that clinician-rated affect scales deserve a closer look in older adults. Although various explanations exist for these findings, it appears that considerably more work is needed to develop clinician-administered rating scales to evaluate anxiety and depression separately in older adults. Clearly, this work will need to accompany related psychopathology research, in order to determine the degree to which mood and anxiety disorders overlap in later life.

Preliminary efforts have also been made to develop brief clinician-administered screening instruments for the detection of anxiety in the elderly. Sinoff, Ore, Zlotogorsky, and Tamir (1999) report initial validation of the Short Anxiety Screening Test (SAST), a 10-item instrument designed to detect anxiety symptoms, especially in the presence of depression. The SAST was compared with clinician-derived diagnoses (derived via the ADIS-IV; Brown, DiNardo, & Barlow, 1994), indicating acceptable sensitivity (75.4%) and specificity (78.7%). Ideally, greater use of brief screening measures such as the SAST will allow accurate identification of anxious older adults, particularly in nontraditional settings (e.g., primary care offices, senior citizen centers). Given the fact that anxiety disorders often may go unidentified in older adults (Smyer & Gatz, 1995), further development of this type of assessment appears to be of paramount importance.

Self-Report Questionnaires

A growing amount of research has begun to examine the psychometric attributes of self-report questionnaires that traditionally have been used to evaluate worry and related parameters of anxiety in younger adults. Because worry is a central construct in GAD, its measurement is particularly germane for older adults with this disorder. To date, two self-report worry scales have been examined in older adults. The Worry Scale (WS; Wisocki, Handen, & Morse, 1986) was developed specifically to evaluate the severity of worry about finances, health issues, and social concerns in older adults. Initially validated with community-dwelling and homebound older adults (Powers et al., 1992; Wisocki et al., 1986), the psychometric properties of this scale have subsequently been examined in well-defined samples of older patients with GAD (Stanley, Beck, & Zebb, 1996; Stanley, Novy, Bourland, Beck, & Averill, 2001). In the first report, data indicated strong internal consistency for both the total and subscale scores of the WS, and adequate test–retest reliability (with the exception of the Health subscale). Adequate convergent validity was noted, as the WS showed positive significant correlations with measures of trait anxiety and obsessionality. These findings subsequently were replicated in a separate sample of older patients with GAD (Stanley et al., 2001). Unfortunately, the WS also showed positive significant correlations with two measures of depression (Stanley et al., 2001), leaving open to question the specificity of this measure for the assessment of worry. It is possible that this reflects a genuine lack of specificity in the relationship of worry to GAD versus depression, although this hypothesis has not been examined within the psychopathology literature. Recently, the WS has been revised to assess more domains of worry (Wisocki, 2000); psychometric evaluation of the revised scale is underway.

The Penn State Worry Questionnaire (PSWQ; Meyer, Miller, Metzger, & Borkovec, 1990) has also been used for older patients with GAD. In contrast to the WS, which focuses on the content of worry, the PSWQ focuses more on the controllability of worry. In an initial report involving 47 older patients with GAD and 94 nonpsychiatric control participants, the PSWQ showed good internal consistency and adequate convergent validity (J. G. Beck, Stanley, & Zebb, 1995). A factor analysis indicated a two-factor solution, reflecting a tendency to worry and its opposite, the absence of worry. Similar findings have been reported by Watari and Brodbeck (1997), using a sample of older adults recruited from community-based nutritional programs and senior centers. These authors also note no differences in scores reported by older Japanese Americans versus European Americans on the PSWQ (Watari & Brodbeck, 2000). Recently, Stanley and colleagues (2001) have reported that the PSWQ may not be reliable over time—a finding that has not been noted in the literature on younger adults. Importantly, however, this measure appears to assess worry as a distinct construct from depression, based on obtained correlations with the GDS and the Beck Depression Inventory (A. T. Beck, Ward, Mendelson, Mock, & Erbaugh, 1961). Recently, Hopko and colleagues (2003) proposed that an abbreviated eight-item version of the PSWQ might be preferable for use with older adults, based on an improved single-factor model fit, slightly better test–retest reliability, high internal consistency, and comparable convergent and divergent validity with other self-report and clinician-rated scales. This shortened scale also has the advantage of greater ease of use, which may be helpful for older participants. Thus the PSWQ appears to be a useful measure for the evaluation of worry in older adults, although further study of its test–retest reliability is in order.

A number of other self-report questionnaires may be used in the evaluation of elderly patients with GAD. These include the State–Trait Anxiety Inventory (STAI; Spielberger, Gorsuch, & Lushene, 1970), the Beck Anxiety Inventory (BAI; A. T. Beck & Steer, 1991), the Anxiety Sensitivity Index (ASI; Reiss, Peterson, Gursky, & McNally, 1986), the Fear Survey Schedule–II (FSS-II; Geer, 1965), and the Fear Questionnaire (FQ; Marks & Mathews, 1979). To date, the STAI has been shown to be useful in the assessment of anxiety in elderly persons (e.g., Fuentes & Cox, 2000; Himmelfarb & Murrell, 1983; Kabakoff, Segal, Hersen, & VanHasselt, 1997; Stanley et al., 1996), although there is mixed support for the discriminant validity of the Trait Anxiety subscale. Investigations of the BAI suggest that this scale is useful in discriminating anxiety from depression in older adults (e.g., Kabakoff et al., 1997; Morin et al., 1999). Scores on the BAI have been shown to be unrelated to ethnicity, gender, and education (Wetherall & Arean, 1997), indicating that this measure has considerable promise for providing an unbiased assessment of anxiety. The ASI has been shown to have good internal consistency, although the data on convergent and divergent validity are mixed (Fuentes & Cox, 2000). Although psychometric data for the FSS-II are somewhat limited, this instrument has been used to document the prevalence and distribution of fears in older adults (Liddell, Locker, & Burman, 1991). More data are available for the FQ (Fuentes & Cox, 2000; Stanley, Beck, & Zebb, 1996; Stanley et al., 2001), but they suggest poor psychometric qualities (e.g., little evidence of internal consistency, mixed support for validity). As noted by Stanley and Beck (2000), the FQ does not appear viable for the assessment of specific fears in older adults.

Initial efforts are underway to examine brief questionnaire screening measures to identify anxiety problems in older adults. For example, Spinhoven and colleagues (1997) examined how the Hospital Anxiety and Depression Scale (HADS) would perform when utilized with older adults. The HADS was originally developed to indicate the presence of anxious and depressive symptoms in medical outpatients. Spinhoven and colleagues found that the dimensional structure of the HADS and its test–retest reliability were good, and (of particular importance) that scores were not correlated highly with age. Initial comparison with psychiatric diagnoses suggested that the total HADS score had adequate sensitivity and positive predictive value in identifying cases of psychiatric disorder. Unfortunately, these authors did not highlight anxiety disorders as a specific focus for this study. As such, future studies utilizing brief screening measures such as the HADS will be needed to examine their utility in identifying GAD in medical settings.

TREATMENT OF GAD IN OLDER ADULTS

In considering the developing literature on the treatment of GAD in elderly patients, it is important for us to place these efforts against the background of what we know about utilization of mental health services by older adults. In particular, only 38% of older adults in the community with diagnosed GAD reported use of mental health services during the year prior to evaluation (Blazer et al., 1991). Instead of seeking assistance from mental health professionals, many older adults with anxiety-based problems consult their primary care providers (e.g., Blazer et al., 1991) and typically receive medication. In fact, older adults are the primary consumers of anxiolytic medications in this country (Wetherell, 1998). Unfortunately, some of these medications can be dangerous to older adults—increasing their risk of falls or accidents, causing impairment to memory and other cognitive functions, and potentially interacting negatively with medication required for the management of medical conditions (Satlin & Wasserman, 1997). Although a thorough discussion of pharmacological treatment of GAD in older adults is beyond the scope of this chapter, a brief review of this literature is relevant.

Benzodiazepine medications probably are the most frequently prescribed agents used with anxious older adults (Salzman, 1991). Unfortunately, the empirical support for this medication is not strong, as the literature has numerous methodological problems (e.g., unsystematic diagnostic procedures, lack of appropriate control groups, etc.). Nevertheless, clinical recommendations are consistent with respect to the use of benzodiazepines in anxious older adults, based on clinical trials with younger adults with GAD. Clearly, this is an arena that deserves considerably greater research effort, particularly given the gulf between the available empirical studies and clinical practice. For further information on the pharmacological treatment of GAD, the interested reader is referred to Satlin and Wasserman (1997) and to Stanley and Beck (2000).

On the other hand, sound data are accumulating regarding psychosocial treatments of GAD in older adults. Early efforts to examine psychosocial treatments in this population focused on anxiety symptoms, rather than on anxiety disorders per se (e.g., DeBerry, 1982; Scogin, Rickard, Keith, Wilson, & McElreath, 1992). As reviewed by Wetherell (1998), evidence from these studies suggests that time-limited courses of relaxation training, cognitive-behavior therapy (CBT), psychodynamic treatment, supportive therapy, life review, and biofeedback may be useful in treating anxiety symptoms in elderly persons. Although these studies have laid important groundwork for research on the treatment of anxiety in older adults, it is important to recognize that their findings are limited by reliance on community-dwelling individuals without diagnosable disorders. In addition, some of these studies lacked the necessary methodological controls. As such, it is difficult to know whether one can generalize these findings to older adults with more severe forms of psychopathology.

At present, several investigative groups are studying treatments for older adults with GAD. Each of these groups is working with a CBT protocol that is similar to treatments developed for younger adults (e.g., Craske, Barlow, & O'Leary, 1992; Otto, Jones, Craske, & Barlow, 1996). In an initial effort, Stanley, Beck, and Glassco (1996) examined the efficacy of CBT relative to supportive psychotherapy for the treatment of GAD in adults aged 55–81. In this study, the treatment protocol mirrored the package developed initially by Craske and colleagues (1992); it contained education and training in self-monitoring of anxiety, muscle relaxation, cognitive therapy, and graduated exposure practice in worry-producing situations. Participants were treated in small groups over the course of 14 weeks. Results indicated significant reductions in self-reported and clinician-rated worry, anxiety, and depression for both the CBT and supportive psychotherapy conditions. Follow-up assessment 6 months later indicated maintenance or continued improvement on most measures. Unfortunately, this study is limited by the lack of a no-treatment control group. Stanley and colleagues have replicated and extended this work by contrasting CBT with a minimal-contact control condition. Participants included 85 individuals aged 60 and above with GAD who were withdrawn from psychotropic medication prior to beginning their research involvement. Results indicated significant improvement in worry, anxiety, depression, and quality of life following CBT, relative to the control condition. Forty-five percent of patients in CBT were classified as "responders," although these individuals did not return to normative levels on several self-report questionnaires (e.g., PSWQ, HARS). Most gains for patients in CBT were maintained or enhanced over 1-year follow-up.

A related effort was conducted by Wetherell, Gatz, and Craske (2003). In this study, the CBT protocol developed by Craske and colleagues (1992) was being compared with a structured discussion group and a wait-list control. Participants included 75 older adults with GAD.

Both CBT and the discussion group were more effective than the wait-list control condition. Although CBT participants improved on more assessment measures than patients enrolled in the discussion group, only one significant difference was noted between these two conditions immediately after treatment and no differences were noted at 6-month follow-up. The effect size for CBT was large (although smaller than noted in comparable studies with younger adults) while the effect size for the discussion group was medium sized. From this set of results, it would appear that interventions developed for the treatment of GAD in younger adults can be adapted successfully for older adults. Modifications include devoting greater emphasis to the education phase of treatment, increased reliance on visual and written aids, attending to practical issues (e.g., concerns about driving during times when the roads are crowded), and utilization of a small-group treatment format to facilitate social support. For greater information concerning the specific modifications of treatment, see Bortz and O'Brien (1997) or Stanley and Averill (1999).

Gorenstein and colleagues have recently developed a CBT protocol to reduce dependence on anxiolytic medication and to reduce anxiety symptoms in older adults with GAD (e.g., Gorenstein, Papp, & Kleber, 1999a). This treatment approach includes a blend of Craske and colleagues' (1992) treatment and the intervention package developed by Otto and colleagues (1996) to assist patients in managing withdrawal from benzodiazepines. Additional components of treatment include training in problem solving, providing guidelines for sleep hygiene, and daily activity scheduling. The CBT is administered in an individual format, spanning 13 sessions, and is contrasted with a medical-management-only condition. Preliminary data indicate that both groups reported approximately equivalent reduction in medication usage, with the CBT recipients reporting additional reductions in anxiety and depression that were not observed in the patients in the medical-management-alone condition (Gorenstein, Papp, & Kleber, 1999b). Continued attention to this study will allow us to determine whether this treatment approach receives empirical support and produces lasting changes in older adults with GAD.

CONCLUSIONS

As we have noted throughout this chapter, information on GAD in elderly persons is beginning to accumulate. Although prevalence data have been reported, questions remain about the presence of GAD with aging-related disorders (such as medical conditions and cognitive impairment). Because this work may be hampered by a lack of assessment instruments that do not rely on self-report, it will be important for future work to include the development of alternative methods for the assessment of worry and anxiety. Of equal importance will be work clarifying the interrelationship between anxiety and depression in older adults. Although some authors have suggested that these disorders "de-differentiate" as one ages (e.g., Krasucki, Howard, & Mann, 1998), a number of alternative hypotheses are equally plausible at this stage. Continued work on this topic has the potential to be most beneficial to our understanding of GAD in elderly individuals. Likewise, greater integration of current theories about the etiology and maintenance of GAD will be helpful as we continue to explore the origins of this disorder in older adults.

Examination of the available assessment and treatment literature suggests that we are making progress in these domains. At present, a growing amount of research supports the use of well-established clinician-administered and self-report assessment strategies for older patients with GAD. Clearly, there is a notable need to expand this focus to include behavioral and physiological assessment strategies. The availability of these assessment tools can advance research on the psychopathology of GAD in elderly persons as well. Finally, accumulating evidence indicates that treatments shown to be helpful for alleviating excessive worry and anxiety in younger adults are also useful for older adults. To date, the primary focus has been upon CBT, although it is likely that investigative efforts will branch out to include alternative treatment methods. Given the prevalence of GAD in the elderly, combined with the potential dangers that the use of anxiolytic medications poses for this population, this area is ripe for future development. Indeed, as our population grows older, the need for this knowledge will become more pressing and important.

REFERENCES

American Psychiatric Association. (1994). *Diagnostic and statistical manual of mental disorders* (4th ed). Washington, DC: Author.

Beck, A. T., Brown, G., Steer, R. Eidelson, J., & Riskind, J. (1987). Differentiating anxiety and depression: A test of the cognitive content-specificity hypothesis. *Journal of Abnormal Psychology, 96*, 179–183.

Beck, A. T., & Emery, G., with Greenberg, R. C. (1985). *Anxiety disorders and phobias: A cognitive perspective.* New York: Basic Books.

Beck, A. T., & Steer, R. (1991). Relationships between the Beck Anxiety Inventory and the Hamilton Anxiety Rating Scale with anxious outpatients. *Journal of Anxiety Disorders, 5*, 213–223.

Beck, A. T., Ward, C., Mendelson, M., Mock, J., & Erbaugh, J. (1961). An inventory for measuring depression. *Archives of General Psychiatry, 4*, 53–63.

Beck, J. G., Novy, D. M., Diefenbach, G. J., Stanley, M. A., Averill, P. M., & Swann, A. C. (2003). Differentiating anxiety and depression in older adults with generalized anxiety disorder. *Psychological Assessment, 15*, 184–192.

Beck, J. G., Stanley, M., & Zebb, B. (1995). Psychometric properties of the Penn State Worry Questionnaire in older adults. *Journal of Clinical Geropsychology, 1*, 33–42.

Beck, J. G., Stanley, M. A., & Zebb, B. J. (1996). Characteristics of generalized anxiety disorder in older adults: A descriptive study. *Behaviour Research and Therapy, 34,* 225–234.

Beck, J. G., Stanley, M., & Zebb, B. J. (1999). Effectiveness of the Hamilton Anxiety Rating Scale with older generalized anxiety disorder patients. *Journal of Clinical Geropsychology, 5,* 281–290.

Beekman, A. T., Bremmer, M. A., Deeg, D. J., van Balkom, A. J., Smit, J. H., de Beurs, E., van Dyck, R., & van Tilburg, W. (1998). Anxiety disorders in later life: A report from the Longitudinal Aging Study Amsterdam. *International Journal of Geriatric Psychiatry, 13,* 717–726.

Beekman, A. T., de Beurs, E., van Balkom, A. J., Deeg, D. J., van Dyck, R., & van Tilburg, W. (2000). Anxiety and depression in later life: Co-occurrence and communality of risk factors. *American Journal of Psychiatry, 157,* 89–95.

Beidel, D., & Turner, S. (1991). Anxiety disorders. In M. Hersen & S. Turner (Eds.), *Adult psychopathology and diagnosis* (pp. 226–278). New York: Wiley.

Blazer, D., George, L. K., & Hughes, D. (1991). The epidemiology of anxiety disorders: An age comparison. In C. Salzman & B. Lebowitz (Eds.), *Anxiety in the elderly: Treatment and research* (pp 17–30). New York: Springer.

Blazer, D., Hughes, D., & George, L. (1987). Stressful life events and the onset of generalized anxiety syndrome. *American Journal of Psychiatry, 144,* 1178–1183.

Borkovec, T., Roemer, L., & Kinyon, J. (1995). Disclosure and worry: Opposite sides of the emotional processing coin. In J. Pennebaker (Ed.), *Emotion, disclosure, and health* (pp. 47–70). Washington, DC: American Psychological Association.

Borkovec, T., Shadick, R., & Hopkins, M. (1991). The nature of normal and pathological worry. In R. M. Rapee & D. H. Barlow (Eds.), *Chronic anxiety: Generalized anxiety disorder and mixed anxiety–depression* (pp. 29–51). New York: Guilford Press.

Bortz, J., & O'Brien, K. (1997). Psychotherapy with older adults: Theoretical issues, empirical findings, and clinical applications. In P. Nussbaum (Ed.), *Handbook of neuropsychology and aging* (pp. 431–451). New York: Plenum Press.

Brown, T., DiNardo, P., & Barlow, D. (1994). *Anxiety Disorders Interview Schedule for DSM-IV (ADIS-IV).* Albany, NY: Graywind.

Christensen, H., Mackinnon, A., Korten, A., Jorm, A., Henderson, A., Jacomb, P., & Rodgers, B. (1999). An analysis of diversity in the cognitive performance of elderly community dwellers: Individual differences in change scores as a function of age. *Psychology and Aging, 14,* 365–379.

Clayton, A., Holroyd, S., & Sheldon-Keller, A. (1997). Geriatric Depression Scale vs. Hamilton Rating Scale for Depression in a sample of anxiety patients. *The Clinical Gerontologist, 17,* 3–13.

Craske, M., Barlow, D., & O'Leary, T. (1992). *Master of your anxiety and worry.* Albany, NY: Graywind.

Davey, G. (1994). Pathological worry as exacerbated problem solving. In G. C. L. Davey & F. Tallis (Eds.), *Worrying: Perspectives on theory, assessment, and treatment* (pp. 35–59). Chichester, UK: Wiley.

DeBerry, S. (1982). An evaluation of progressive muscle relaxation on stress related symptoms in a geriatric population. *International Journal of Aging and Human Development, 14,* 255–269.

Diefenbach, G. J., Stanley, M. A., & Beck, J. G. (2001). Worry content reported by older adults with and without generalized anxiety disorder. *Aging and Mental Health, 5,* 269–274.

Diefenbach, G. J., Stanley, M. A., Beck, J. G., Novy, D. M., Averill, P. M., & Swann, A. R.

(2001). Examination of the Hamilton scales in assessment with anxious older adults: A replication and extension. *Journal of Psychopathology and Behavioral Assessment, 23,* 117–124.

DiNardo, P., Moras, K., Barlow, D., Rapee, R., & Brown, T. (1993). Reliability of DSM-III-R anxiety disorder categories: Using the Anxiety Disorders Interview Schedule—Revised (ADIS-R). *Archives of General Psychiatry, 50,* 251–256.

Dugas, M. J., Freeston, M. H., & Ladouceur, R. (1997). Intolerance of uncertainty and problem orientation in worry. *Cognitive Therapy and Research, 21,* 593–606.

Dugas, M. J., Gagnon, F., Ladouceur, R., & Freeston, M. H. (1998). Generalized anxiety disorder: A preliminary test of a conceptual model. *Behaviour Research and Therapy, 36,* 215–226.

Fisher, J. E., & Noll, J. (1996). Anxiety disorders. In L. Carstensen, B. Edelstein, & L. Dornbrand (Eds.). *The practical handbook of clinical gerontology* (pp. 304–323). Thousand Oaks, CA: Sage.

Flint, A. (1994). Epidemiological and comorbidity of anxiety disorders in the elderly. *American Journal of Psychiatry, 151,* 640–649.

Fuentes, K., & Cox, B. (2000). Assessment of anxiety in older adults: A community-based survey and comparison with younger adults. *Behaviour Research and Therapy, 38,* 297–309.

Fulop, G., Strain, J., Fahs, M., Schmeidler, J., & Snyder, S. (1998). A prospective study of the impact of psychiatric comorbidity on length of hospital stays of elderly medical–surgical inpatients. *Psychosomatics, 39,* 273–280.

Ganzini, L., McFarland, B., & Culter, D. (1990). Prevalence of mental disorders after catastrophic financial loss. *Journal of Nervous and Mental Disease, 178,* 680–685.

Geer, J. (1965). The development of a scale to measure fear. *Behaviour Research and Therapy, 3,* 45–53.

Gorenstein, E., Papp, L., & Kleber, M. (1999a). Cognitive behavioral treatment of anxiety in later life. *Cognitive and Behavioral Practice, 6,* 305– 320.

Gorenstein, E., Papp, L., & Kleber, M. (1999b, November). *CBT for anxiety and anxiolytic drug dependence in later life: Interim report.* Paper presented at the 33rd annual meeting of the Association for Advancement of Behavior Therapy, Toronto.

Gurian, B., & Miner, J. (1991). Clinical presentation of anxiety in the elderly. In C. Salzman & B. Lebowitz (Eds.), *Anxiety in the elderly: Treatment and research* (pp. 31–44). New York: Springer.

Hamilton, M. (1959). The assessment of anxiety states by rating. *British Journal of Medical Psychology, 32,* 50–55.

Hamilton, M. (1960). A rating scale for depression. *Journal of Neurology, Neurosurgery and Psychiatry, 23,* 56–62.

Heun, R., & Muller, H. (1998). Inter-informant reliability of family history information on psychiatric disorders in relatives. *European Archives of Psychiatry and Clinical Neuroscience, 248,* 104–109.

Himmelfarb, S., & Murrell, S. (1983). Reliability and validity of five mental health scales in older persons. *Journal of Gerontology, 38,* 333–339.

Hopko, D. R., Stanley, M. A., Reas, D. L., Wetherell, J. L., Beck, J. G., Novy, D. M., & Averill, P. M. (2003). Assessing worry in older adults: Confirmatory factor analysis of the Penn State Worry Questionnaire and psychometric properties of an abbreviated model. *Psychological Assessment, 15,* 173–183.

Howell, T. (1996). Anxiety disorders. In W. Reichman & P. Katz (Eds.), *Psychiatric care in the nursing home* (pp. 94–108). New York: Oxford University Press.

Junginger, J., Phelan, E., Cherr, K., & Levy, J. (1993). Prevalence of psychopathology in elderly persons in nursing homes and the community. *Hospital and Community Psychiatry, 44,* 381–383.

Kabacoff, R., Segal, D., Hersen, M., & VanHasselt, V. (1997). Psychometric properties and diagnostic utility of the Beck Anxiety Inventory and the State–Trait Anxiety Inventory with older adult psychiatric outpatients. *Journal of Anxiety Disorders, 11,* 33–47.

Kant, G., D'Zurilla, T., & Maydeu-Olivares, A. (1997). Social problem solving as a mediator of stress-related depression and anxiety in middle-aged and elderly community residents. *Cognitive Therapy and Research, 21,* 73–96.

Katz, I. (1996). On the inseparability of mental and physical health in aged persons: Lessons from depression and medical comorbidity. *American Journal of Geriatric Psychiatry, 4,* 1–16.

Kinsella, K., & Taeuber, C. (1993). *An aging world II* (International Population Reports, Publication No. P95/92–3). Washington, DC: U. S. Department of Commerce.

Knauper, B., & Wittchen, H.-U. (1994). Diagnosing major depression in the elderly: Evidence for response bias in standardized diagnostic interviews? *Journal of Psychiatric Research, 28,* 147–164.

Krasucki, C., Howard, R., & Mann, A. (1998). The relationship between anxiety disorders and age. *International Journal of Geriatric Psychiatry, 13,* 79–99.

Lawton, M., Kleban, M., & Dean, J. (1993). Affect and age: Cross-sectional comparisons of structure and prevalence. *Psychology and Aging, 8,* 165–175.

Levenson, J., Hamer, R., & Rossiter, L. (1990). Relations of psychopathology in general medical inpatients to use and cost of services. *American Journal of Psychiatry, 147,* 1498–1503.

Liddell, A., Locker, D., & Burman, D. (1991). Self-reported fears (FSS-II) of subjects aged 50 years and older. *Behaviour Research and Therapy, 29,* 105–112.

Light, L. L. (1996). Memory and aging. In E. Bjork & R. Bjork (Eds.), *Memory* (pp. 443–490). San Diego, CA: Academic Press.

Lipton, M., & Schaffer, W. (1988). Physical symptoms related to post-traumatic stress disorder (PTSD) in an aging population. *Military Medicine, 153,* 316–318.

Lowe, P., & Reynolds, C. (2000). Exploratory analyses of the latent structure of anxiety among older adults. *Educational and Psychological Measurement, 60,* 100–116.

MacLeod, C. (1999). Anxiety and anxiety disorders. In T. Dalgleish & M. Power (Eds.), *Handbook of cognition and emotion* (pp. 447–477). Chichester, UK: Wiley.

Marks, I., & Mathews, A. (1979). Brief standardized self-rating for phobic patients. *Behaviour Research and Therapy, 17,* 263–267.

Meyer, T., Miller, M., Metzger, R., & Borkovec, T. (1990). Development and validation of the Penn State Worry Questionnaire. *Behaviour Research and Therapy, 28,* 487–495.

Morin, C., Landreville, P., Colecchi, C., McDonald, K., Stone, J., & Ling, W. (1999). The Beck Anxiety Inventory: Psychometric properties with older adults. *Journal of Clinical Geropsychology, 5,* 19–29.

National Center for Health Statistics. (1993). Advance report for health statistics, 1991. *Monthly Vital Statistics Report, 42.*

Novy, D., Stanley, M., Swann, A., Averill, P., Breckenridge, J., Akkerman, R., & Beck, J. G. (1997, November). *An observational approach to assess anxiety behaviors in elders.* Poster presented at the 31st annual meeting of the Association for Advancement of Behavior Therapy, Miami Beach, FL.

Otto, M., Jones, J., Craske, M., & Barlow, D. (1996). *Stopping anxiety medication: Panic control therapy for benzodiazepine discontinuation.* San Antonio, TX: Psychological Corporation.

Palmer, B. W., Jeste, D. V., & Sheikh, J. I. (1997). Anxiety disorders in the elderly: DSM-IV and other barriers to diagnosis and treatment. *Journal of Affective Disorders, 46,* 183–190.

Parmelee, P., Katz, I., & Lawton, H. (1993). Anxiety and its association with depression among institutionalized elderly. *American Journal of Geriatric Psychiatry, 1,* 46–58.

Pearson, J. (1998). Research in late-life anxiety: Summary of a National Institute of Mental Health workshop on late-life anxiety. *Psychopharmacology Bulletin, 34,* 127–138.

Person, D., & Borkovec, T. (1995, August). *Anxiety disorders among the elderly: Patterns and issues.* Paper presented at the 103rd annual meeting of the American Psychological Association, New York.

Powers, C., Wisocki, P., & Whitbourne, S. (1992). Age differences and correlates of worrying in young and elderly adults. *The Gerontologist, 32,* 82–88.

Regier, D., Boyd, J., Burke, J., Rae, D., Myers, J., Kramer, M., Robins, L., George, L., Karno, M., & Locke, B. (1988). One-month prevalence of mental disorders in the United States: Based on five Epidemiologic Catchment Area sites. *Archives of General Psychiatry, 45,* 977–986.

Reiss, S., Peterson, R., Gursky, D., & McNally, R. (1986). Anxiety sensitivity, anxiety frequency, and the prediction of fearfulness. *Behaviour Research and Therapy, 24,* 1–8.

Reynolds, C., & Richmond, B. (1978). What I think and feel: A revised measure of children's manifest anxiety. *Journal of Abnormal Child Psychology, 6,* 271–280.

Riskind, J., Beck, A. T., Brown, G., & Steer, R. (1987). Taking the measure of anxiety and depression: Validation of the reconstructed Hamilton scales. *Journal of Nervous and Mental Disease, 175,* 474–479.

Robins, L., Helzer, J., Croughan, J., & Ratcliff, K. (1981). National Institute of Mental Health Diagnostic Interview Schedule: Its history, characteristics, and validity. *Archives of General Psychiatry, 38,* 381–389.

Salzman, C. (1991). Pharmacological treatment of the anxious elderly patient. In C. Salzman & B. D. Lebowitz (Eds.), *Anxiety in the elderly: Treatment and research* (pp. 149–173). New York: Springer.

Sanderson, W., & Wetzler, S. (1991). Chronic anxiety and generalized anxiety disorder: Issues in comorbidity. In R. M. Rapee & D. H. Barlow (Eds.), *Chronic anxiety: Generalized anxiety disorder and mixed anxiety–depression* (pp. 119–135). New York: Guilford Press.

Satlin, A., & Wasserman, C. (1997). Overview of geriatric psychopharmacology. In L. Dickstein, M. Riba, & J. Oldman (Eds.), *American Psychiatric Press review of psychiatry* (Vol. 16, pp. IV-143–IV-172). Washington, DC: American Psychiatric Press.

Scogin, F. R. (1998). Anxiety in old age. In I. H. Norhus, G. R. VandenBos, S. Berg, & P. Fromholt (Eds.), *Clinical geropsychology* (pp. 205–209). Washington, DC: American Psychological Association.

Scogin, F. R., Rickard, H., Keith, S., Wilson, J., & McElreath, L. (1992). Progressive and imaginal relaxation training for elderly persons with subjective anxiety. *Psychology and Aging, 7,* 419–424.

Segal, D., Hersen, M., VanHasselt, V., Kabacoff, R., & Roth, L. (1993). Reliability of diagnosis in older psychiatric patients using the Structured Clinical Interview for DSM-III-R. *Journal of Psychopathology and Behavioral Assessment, 15,* 347–356.

Shapiro, A., Roberts, J., & Beck, J. G. (1999). Differentiating symptoms of anxiety and depression in older adults: Distinct cognitive and affective profiles? *Cognitive Therapy and Research, 23,* 53–74.

Sheikh, J. (1992). Anxiety disorders and their treatment. *Clinical Geriatric Medicine, 8,* 411–426.

Sinoff, G., Ore, L., Zlotogorsky, D., & Tamir, A. (1999). Short anxiety screening test: A brief instrument for detecting anxiety in the elderly. *International Journal of Geriatric Psychiatry, 14,* 1062–1071.

Smyer, M., & Gatz, M. (1995). The public policy context of mental health care for older adults. *The Clinical Psychologist, 48,* 31–36.

Spar, J., & LaRue, A. (1990). *Concise guide to geriatric psychiatry.* Washington, DC: American Psychiatric Press.

Spielberger, C., Gorsuch, R., & Lushene, R. (1970). *Manual for the State–Trait Anxiety Inventory.* Palo Alto, CA: Consulting Psychologists Press.

Spinhoven, P., Ormel, J., Sloekers, P., Kempen, G., Speckens, A., & VanHemert, A. (1997). A validation study of the Hospital Anxiety and Depression Scale (HADS) in different groups of Dutch subjects. *Psychological Medicine, 27,* 363–370.

Spitzer, R., Williams, J., Gibbon, M., & First, M. (1988). *Structured Clinical Interview for DSM-III-R–Patient Edition.* New York: Biomedical Research Department, New York State Psychiatric Institute.

Stanley, M. A., & Averill, P. (1999). Strategies for treating generalized anxiety in the elderly. In M. Duffy (Ed.), *Handbook of counseling and therapy with older adults* (pp. 511–525). Chichester, UK: Wiley.

Stanley, M. A., & Beck, J. G. (1998). Anxiety disorders. In B. Edelstein (Ed.), *Comprehensive clinical psychology* (pp. 171–191). Oxford: Elsevier Science.

Stanley, M. A., & Beck, J. G. (2000). Anxiety disorders. *Clinical Psychology Review, 20,* 731–754.

Stanley, M. A., Beck, J. G., & Glassco, J. (1996). Treatment of generalized anxiety in older adults: A preliminary comparison of cognitive-behavioral and supportive approaches. *Behavior Therapy, 27,* 565–581.

Stanley, M. A., Beck, J. G., Novy, D. M., Averill, P. A., Swann, A. C., Diefenbach, G. J., & Hopko, D. R. (2003). Cognitive-behavioral treatment of late-life generalized anxiety disorder. *Journal of Consulting and Clinical Psychology, 71,* 309–319.

Stanley, M. A., Beck, J. G., & Zebb, B. (1996). Psychometric properties of four anxiety measures in older adults. *Behaviour Research and Therapy, 34,* 827–838.

Stanley, M. A., Novy, D., Bourland, S., Beck, J. G., & Averill, P. (2001). Assessing older adults with generalized anxiety: A replication and extension. *Behaviour Research and Therapy, 39,* 221–235.

U.S. Bureau of the Census. (1992). *Sixty-five plus in America* (Current Population Reports, Special Studies, Series No. P23–178). Washington, DC: U.S. Government Printing Office.

van Balkom, A., Beekman, A., de Beurs, E., Deeg, D., van Dyck, R., & van Tilburg, W. (2000). Comorbidity of the anxiety disorders in a community-based older population in The Netherlands. *Acta Psychiatrica Scandinavica, 101,* 37–45.

Vrana, S., Cuthbert, B., & Lang, P. (1986). Fear imagery and text processing. *Psychophysiology, 23,* 247–253.

Wands, K., Mersky, H., Hachinski, V. C., Fishman, M., Fox, H., & Boniferro, M. (1990). A questionnaire investigation of anxiety and depression in early dementia. *Journal of the American Geriatrics Society, 38,* 535–538.

Watari, K., & Brodbeck, C. (1997, November). *The Penn State Worry Questionnaire in older adults: Internal consistency and cultural diversity issues.* Poster presented at the 31st annual meeting of the Association for Advancement of Behavior Therapy, Miami Beach, FL.

Watari, K., & Brodbeck, C. (2000). Culture, health, and financial appraisals: Comparison of worry in older Japanese Americans and European Americans. *Journal of Clinical Geropsychology, 6*, 25–39.

Wetherell, J. (1998). Treatment of anxiety in older adults. *Psychotherapy, 35*, 444–458.

Wetherell, J., & Arean, P. (1997). Psychometric evaluation of the Beck Anxiety Inventory with older medical patients. *Psychological Assessment, 9*, 136–144.

Wetherell, J., Gatz, M., & Craske, M. G. (2003). Treatment of generalized anxiety disorder in older adults. *Journal of Consulting and Clinical Psychology, 71*, 31–40.

Wetherell, J., Gatz, M., & Pedersen, N. (2001). A longitudinal analysis of anxiety and depressive symptoms. *Psychology and Aging, 16*, 187–195.

Wisocki, P. (2000). *Worry Scale–Revised.* Unpublished manuscript, University of Massachusetts.

Wisocki, P., Handen, B., & Morse, C. (1986). The Worry Scale as a measure of anxiety among homebound and community active elderly. *The Behavior Therapist, 5*, 91–95.

World Health Organization. (1990). *Composite International Diagnostic Interview.* Geneva: Author.

Yesavage, J., Brink, T., Rose, T., Lum, O., Huang, V., Adey, M., & Leirer, V. (1983). Development and validation of a geriatric depression screening scale: A preliminary report. *Journal of Psychiatric Research, 17*, 37–49.

Zarit, S., & Zarit, J. (1998). *Mental disorders in older adults.* New York: Guilford Press.

Index

Page numbers followed by an *f* indicate figure; *t*, table.

435